An
Introduction
to
Clinical Immunology

An Introduction to Clinical Immunology

FRANCES K. WIDMANN, M.D.
Associate Professor of Pathology
Duke University Medical Center
Durham, North Carolina

 F. A. DAVIS COMPANY • Philadelphia

Printed in the United States of America

Last digit indicates print number: 10 9 8 7 6 5 4 3 2 1

Library of Congress Cataloging-in-Publication Data

Widmann, Frances K., 1935–
   An introduction to clinical immunology.
   Includes bibliographies and index.
   1. Immunology.   2. Immunopathology.   I. Title.   [DNLM:
1. Immunity.   QW 504 W641i]
QR181.W65   1989   616.07′9   88-33562
ISBN-0-8036-9311-7

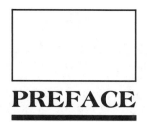

PREFACE

An Introduction to Clinical Immunology is exactly what the title promises: an explanation of immunology for those with little or no experience in immunology or clinical medicine. Written to meet the needs of students and practitioners in the allied health professions, this book should also prove useful to any reader seeking to understand the sometimes bewildering flood of recent advances in immunology. Moreover, student and practicing nurses will appreciate the close integration of basic-science concepts and practical clinical concerns. My primary goal is to help healthcare practitioners understand what the immune system does, how it protects the body, how it sometimes works to the apparent disadvantage of the body, and how immunologic principles are related to an increasingly sophisticated array of laboratory tests.

By the end of the first section, "Basic Principles," the reader will have a thorough grasp of classical immunologic concepts as well as sophisticated recent developments. This section explains the role immunity plays in overall bodily defenses; how immune processes arise in, expand upon, and differ from other physiologic processes; and how these uniquely specific and sensitive functions evolve. Presuming no more than a modest understanding of general biology and chemistry on the part of the reader, I explain every immunologic term and concept before incorporating them into progressively complex contexts.

The second section, "Clinical Applications," discusses the physiologic and pathologic consequences of immune activity, the ways in which these can be manipulated, and the highlights of transplantation immunology. Comprehensive summaries of immunodeficiency conditions, neoplasms of the immune system, and diseases of immune etiology provide a solid clinical foundation for allied health practitioners as well as a basis for understanding more complex material.

The third section, "Applications of Immunologic Principles to Laboratory Testing," is not merely a manual of laboratory techniques.

I believe that those who perform laboratory tests, those who order them, and those who interpret them need to understand how tests exploit different immunologic principles and the relative advantages and disadvantages they provide for laboratory analysis. This section unites the seemingly disparate realms of basic immunology and technical laboratory activities, fostering an appreciation of analytic procedures.

Because understanding the language of immunology facilitates understanding its concepts, I have devoted special attention to vocabulary. At their first use, potentially unfamiliar terms are highlighted in boldfaced print and followed by an explanation of the term in context. This approach is also used to explain some terms outside of the boundaries of immunology. A comprehensive glossary lists the immunologic terms that the reader needs in understanding not only this book but other immunology literature as well.

There are certain topics in immunology that students frequently find troublesome, and I have devoted particular attention to making these as lucid as possible. This book should be especially helpful in clarifying the following:

☐ CD terminology for leukocyte antigens, and how the new terms correlate with other descriptive systems
☐ The immunologic concepts underlying Western blot, ELISA, and other widely used test methods
☐ The increasing importance of soluble mediators and receptor-ligand events in initiation and evolution of immune events
☐ The physiologic relevance of the complement system, with descriptions and drawings that explain the cascade and the mechanisms that control these protein interactions
☐ The most recent specificities in the HLA system
☐ The practical and theoretical considerations on which strategies to induce protective immunity are based
☐ The ways in which immune-based disease conditions resemble one another, as well as their distinguishing features

It is a pleasure to acknowledge the support and assistance that others have unstintingly provided. I am especially grateful to Joan Jones, of the Medical Art service of Duke University Medical Center, who did the line drawings; and to the personnel of the Medical Media Production Service at the Durham VA Medical Center, for their advice and assistance in many aspects of illustration. Moreover, this text has been enriched by the cumulative expertise of several dedicated reviewers. My thanks to: Kathleen Becan-McBride, Ed.D., MT(ASCP), CLS, University of Texas, Health Science Center, Houston; Laurence R. Draper, Ph.D., The University of Kansas; Robert P. Ellis, Ph.D., Colorado State University; Denise Fountain, MT(ASCP), SBB, New England Blood Center; Cara R. Fries, Ph.D., University of Delaware; Nancy Johnson, MT(ASCP), SBB, Memorial Blood Center of Minneapolis; Sharon Kutt, MT, MHE, Medical College of Georgia; and Rene La Chapelle, Ph.D., MT(ASCP), CLS(NCA), University of Vermont. A number of people helped me with secretarial support, but Andrea Tillotson and Karen Bethea carried most of the load and did a fine job.

It has been a challenge to encompass the rapidly expanding and rewarding field of immunology in a book suitable for those new to the topic. Writing this book has taught me a great deal. I hope it will bring the same sense of excitement to readers that it did to me as the author.

F.K.W.

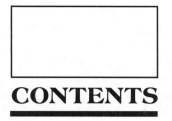

CONTENTS

xvi

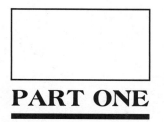

PART ONE

Principles of
Immune Function

CHAPTER 1

Introductory Concepts

INNATE AND ADAPTIVE
IMMUNITY
  Cells Involved
  Inflammation
  Immunity
BIOLOGICALLY SIGNIFICANT
MOLECULES

Classification and Terminology
Structure and Shape
CELLS AND CELL PROPERTIES
  Genes and Their Actions
  Membrane Markers
  Receptors and Ligands
  Cell Replication

The term **immunity** comes from a Latin word that means "exempt" or "free from." Immunity encompasses the body's mechanisms to protect itself from external agents, notably microorganisms and foreign materials; internal abnormalities, such as degenerative changes or tumors; and harmful environmental influences such as toxins, radiation, or extreme heat or cold. To maintain its equilibrium, the body must have ways (1) to exclude potentially harmful invaders or stimuli, (2) to neutralize or to eliminate such stimuli if they succeed in entering, and (3) to repair whatever damage has been inflicted. The first requirement, **exclusion,** depends largely on physical barriers between the body and the environment: intact surfaces, such as skin and mucous membranes, and the secretions that flow over these surfaces, such as saliva, respiratory secretions, urine, intestinal fluid, sweat, and the like. The requirement of **repair** embodies an infinite range of cell replication, adaptation, and modification. The remaining requirement, that of **neutralization** or **elimination** of injurious agents, can be considered immunity.

——— INNATE AND ADAPTIVE IMMUNITY ———

Even the most primitive organisms can defend themselves against injury. In organisms on all rungs of the evolutionary ladder, cells can surround and engulf molecules or particles, a process called **phagocytosis,** and can synthesize products that degrade, denature, or otherwise alter the materials they encounter. Phagocytosis and production of active substances are non-specific mechanisms; the same weapons are deployed against disturbing agents of all sorts. These ubiquitous non-specific activities constitute the innate physiologic process called **inflammation**. Discrimination, memory, and modification of physiologic response according to previous bodily experience constitute adaptive **immunity**, a capacity present only in vertebrates. Table 1–1 summarizes these processes.

CELLS INVOLVED

Cells that achieve defined effects are called **effector** cells for those activities. Cells that support performance of the activities are called **accessory** cells. Effector cells for inflammation and for adaptive immunity share a common precursor, and inflammatory cells often play crucial accessory roles in immune activities.

A cell capable of differentiation into many different cell types is called **pluripotential**. The primordial cell from which immune and inflammatory effectors descend originates in the embryonic yolk sac and later migrates to the bone marrow. The pluripotential cell whose

---

TABLE 1–1. Innate and Adaptive Immunity

	Innate Immunity (Inflammation)	Adaptive Immunity (Immune system)
Evolutionary distribution	All multi-celled organisms	Vertebrates only
Major effector cells	Neutrophils, macrophages, lymphocytes	Lymphocytes
Major accessory cells	Epithelium, through barrier function	Macrophages
Other accessory influences	Products of immune stimulation	Products of inflammation
Target specificity	Non-specific	Highly specific recognition
Effect of previous exposure	None	Markedly alters nature of response

descendents include both inflammatory and immune effectors is called the **hematopoietic stem cell**. Progeny of the hematopoietic stem cell differentiate into red blood cells; several different kinds of white blood cells; megakaryocytes, which generate coagulation-promoting cell fragments called platelets; and phagocytic cells resident in solid tissues (Fig. 1–1). We need not pursue, in this discussion, the evolution of red blood cells or platelets.

The hematopoietic stem cell differentiates into precursor cells that are themselves pluripotent: The **lymphoid** precursor cell gives rise to several populations of lymphocytes, the effector cells of specific, adaptive immunity; the **myeloid** precursor differentiates into the many cells that perform non-specific inflammatory activities. All descendents of the hematopoietic stem cell have enormous capacity for

DIFFERENTIATION OF CELLS IN BONE MARROW

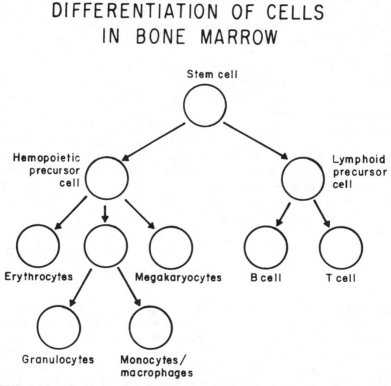

FIGURE 1–1. The totipotential stem cell differentiates first into the lymphoid precursor and the precursor for cell lines that remain and perpetuate themselves in the bone marrow. The lymphoid line differentiates into T and B lines. Precursors for the monocyte/macrophage population and cells of the circulating blood differentiate within the marrow. Granulocytes and the monocyte/macrophage line are closely related, through descent from a common pluripotent precursor.

cell division; the differentiated cell lines manifest continuous growth and multiplication throughout life, some within the bone marrow and some at other tissue sites.

Characteristics of Cells

Two main types of inflammatory cells evolve from the myeloid precursor: **granulocytes** and mononuclear phagocytic cells variously called **monocytes, macrophages,** and **histiocytes.** Granulocytes have cytoplasmic granules that contain enzymes and other products characteristic of various subtypes, which are described as **neutrophils, eosinophils,** or **basophils,** according to the staining characteristics of the granules. Eosinophils and basophils have highly specialized roles in inflammation that will be described in later sections. Neutrophils have an irregularly shaped multilobed nucleus; another name for the neutrophilic granulocyte is **polymorphonuclear leukocyte,** often shortened to "PMN" or "poly." Monocytes have a large nucleus and abundant cytoplasm that may have a granular appearance but lacks the specific granules that distinguish granulocytes. Both neutrophils and monocytes can move through tissues or across surfaces, a property described as **motility.** They engage in phagocytosis when their membranes are suitably stimulated; and they synthesize a wide variety of proteins, many of which are enzymes capable of cleaving a broad range of proteins.

Descending from the lymphoid precursor are lymphocytes, which characteristically have a round, dense nucleus and relatively scant cytoplasm. Lymphocytes present a relatively uniform appearance on light microscopic examination, but two major subpopulations and several less well-defined categories exist. The major populations are **T lymphocytes** and **B lymphocytes.** Lymphocytes do not exhibit phagocytosis or conspicuous motility; they do synthesize proteins, but few are proteolytic enzymes.

INFLAMMATION

Inflammation is described as non-specific because the same reactions follow stimulatory events of all sorts. Anything that damages cells or alters normal tissue elements elicits inflammation, involving various proportions of neutrophils and monocytes, as well as vascular changes and many fluid-phase proteins. Table 1–2 summarizes significant features of inflammation. **Acute inflammation** is a short-lived, clearly defined process in which the first visible events are changes in blood vessels induced by damaged cells or products derived from microorganisms or altered tissue. Capillaries and small veins dilate, bringing increased amounts of blood to the area; fluid and proteins leak out of altered vessels into the interstitial fluid. Neutrophils exit from the blood to accumulate at the site of damage and

TABLE 1–2. Acute vs. Chronic Inflammation

	Acute Inflammation	Chronic Inflammation
Time sequence	Short-term; clearly defined	Prolonged; difficult to determine onset and cessation
Predominant cells	Neutrophils; some macrophages	Lymphocytes; macrophages
Gross appearance of tissue	Reddened, swollen	Pale, retracted
Condition of interstitium	Edema; increased proteins in fluid	Increased collagen; scarring
Condition of tissue elements	Rapid destruction by enzymes from neutrophils	Gradual destruction by enzymes from macrophages

phagocytize damaged cells and foreign particles. Neutrophilic enzymes degrade phagocytized material and also exert proteolytic effects on material outside the cell, notably cells and proteins at the site of injury. Acute inflammation may affect the entire body, resulting in increased bone marrow production of neutrophils, elevated body temperature, and elevated blood levels of several proteins collectively described as **acute phase reactants**. The goal of acute inflammation is elimination of injurious stimuli and removal of damaged tissue elements.

Chronic inflammation lasts longer and has less sharply defined onset and disappearance than acute inflammation. The predominant effector cells are macrophages, which evolve from monocytes. Vascular dilatation and protein-rich interstitial fluid are not conspicuous; normal tissue constituents tend to suffer gradual destruction and replacement by fibrous scar tissue. Macrophages participating in chronic inflammation generate numerous proteins that influence blood coagulation and cell growth, as well as proteolytic enzymes that act less rapidly but more persistently than those of neutrophils.

IMMUNITY

Unique to adaptive immune reactions is **recognition** of identifying characteristics specific for the eliciting agent. Substances and materials derived from the host's own cells or extracellular substances constitute **self;** anything other than these constituents is **non-self,** or **foreign**. Encounter with non-self material initiates adaptive changes that result in an altered reactive state. On encountering the same non-self material again, the reactive host responds in a manner different from that of the non-exposed individual. The altered response is **specific,** conditioned by the identity (the specificity) of the stimulating agent.

The major features of adaptive immunity are **recognition, memory,** and **reactivity;** lymphocyte populations in various stages of differentiation and activation perform these functions. Effector lymphocytes are assisted by accessory actions of other lymphocytes and of several types of mononuclear cells.

Variations in Immune Response

It is customary to divide immune reactions into two principal categories: **humoral** and **cell-mediated** responses. The hallmark of humoral immunity is production of **antibodies,** proteins uniquely constructed to interact with the stimulating material. Cell-mediated immunity includes a range of actions unified by the requirement that **viable effector cells** be present. Material capable of eliciting immune activity is described as **immunogenic.** An **antigen,** or **immunogen,** is defined as material capable of eliciting an immune response when introduced into an immunocompetent host to whom it is foreign. Nearly infinite numbers of non-self materials exist to which hosts potentially can be exposed. Many variables affect the evolution of immune events. Some agents are more effective than others in provoking an immune response; some individuals are more responsive than others to certain immunogens; internal or environmental circumstances may influence the intensity of the immune response; and immune responses may alter the host's overall economy in ways that influence later reactivity.

─────── BIOLOGICALLY SIGNIFICANT ─────── MOLECULES

The constituent elements of cells and multicelled organisms are proteins, carbohydrates, and lipids; these molecules may be simple or complex. A single copy of an independent molecular structure is called a **monomer.** A molecule in which two or more identifiable units are joined is called a **polymer;** the prefix poly means "many." The individual units that combine as a polymer are sometimes called **residues.** Constituent monomeric units may be identical or different. When subunits of differing constitution join as a polymer, the description **hetero,** meaning "other" or "different," may be used; for example, a heterodimer consists of two unlike subunits; a heterotrimer has three constituents, all different.

CLASSIFICATION AND TERMINOLOGY

Proteins, which are chains of amino acids linked by peptide bonds, are often designated **polypeptides**. The building blocks for mammalian proteins are 20 different amino acids; like letters of the alphabet combined into words, these 20 units can be combined into an infinite array of large or small proteins. Small polypeptide molecules may contain 10 to 20 amino acids; larger examples include hundreds or thousands of amino acids. Proteins are the working molecules of cells; they confer structure, carry out reactions, control metabolic processes, transport and transform other materials, produce movement, and regulate genetic activity.

Carbohydrates have somewhat less structural and functional diversity. Carbon, hydrogen, and oxygen are the fundamental constituents of carbohydrates; the so-called simple sugars consist of 5 or 6 carbons and their associated hydrogen and oxygen atoms joined in characteristic linkages. The combining forms **glyco-** and **sacchar-** refer to sugars. Carbohydrates fuel animal metabolism and contribute structural elements for plant and animal cells. Combinations of carbohydrates and amino acids are called **glycoproteins;** carbohydrates with fatty elements are **glycolipids**. Simple sugars frequently polymerize; chains that contain a variety of simple sugars are called **polysaccharides**.

Lipids are hydrophobic, meaning they do not mix with water. The basic building blocks are **hydrocarbons,** carbon and hydrogen residues that combine into chains of various lengths, often with attached side chains of diverse composition. Lipids contribute the principal element of biological membranes, which surround and define cells and intracellular structures. Hydrocarbons combined with other substituent groups provide a wide range of biologically important materials such as phospholipids, sphingolipids, alcohols, and steroids.

STRUCTURE AND SHAPE

The molecules we have described are not just formulas on a page. Every combination of atoms displays behavior determined by physicochemical principles. Complex molecules assume a characteristic three-dimensional configuration that reflects the selection and sequence of constituent parts (Fig. 1–2). The shape and properties of a molecule may change as changing environmental conditions influence physicochemical behavior, but specific structural composition confers predictable configurations and interactions. The properties of self mentioned earlier reflect the shape and the activities of molecules characteristic of the individual's cells and cell products. Responses to injury and change depend upon interactions between inciting and re-

(a) Primary Structure

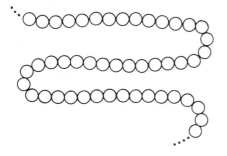

(b) 3-Dimensional Configuration

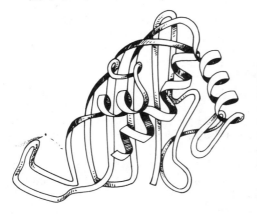

MOLECULAR SHAPE

FIGURE 1–2. The sequence in which constituent parts are assembled is the primary structure of any molecule, schematized in a. The attracting and repelling forces inherent in chemical groups impose a three-dimensional shape, as shown in b. Each molecule of a specific primary composition assumes the same three-dimensional configuration under consistent environmental conditions.

sponding molecules of complementary shapes. Such interactions are predictable and consistent, occurring whenever molecules of complementary configurations encounter each other.

Proteins exhibit enormous diversity of structure and activity, reflecting complex but consistent correspondence between structural formula and physical shape. The primary structure of a protein is its linear sequence of amino acids. Internal and external influences affect the shape that the protein finally displays; this final configuration determines the function of the molecule and the ways in which it interacts with surrounding materials. Alteration of a single amino acid in a complex protein can radically modify these dependent interactions and cause two molecules, differing only in a single detail, to have completely different functional properties. Variations in the number, selection, and sequence of constituent amino acids confer infinitely variable properties upon polypeptides.

―――――― **CELLS AND CELL PROPERTIES** ――――――

Mammalian cells are defined by a membrane that separates the cell from its environment. The nucleus, also defined by a membrane, contains the genetic material that controls the cell's structural and functional capacities. Numerous intracellular structures, called **organelles,** carry out cell functions. Fundamental to multicelled existence is the fact that cells can multiply, respond to external stimuli, and synthesize numerous products; all these properties depend upon the nature and the actions of genetic material present.

GENES AND THEIR ACTIONS

A structural **gene** is the deoxyribonucleic acid (DNA) sequence necessary for production of a single polypeptide. The sequence of amino acids in the protein is determined by the sequence of nucleotides in the DNA helix. Every cell of a single individual contains the same set of DNA sequences arranged in chromosomes, which transmit genes from cell to cell during cellular division. Ova and sperm have a single set of 23 chromosomes and are described as **haploid**. Somatic cells have 46 chromosomes and are described as **diploid,** meaning that they have two copies of each chromosome, including two copies of each of the 22 paired **autosomes;** females have two copies of the X sex chromosome, whereas males have one X and one Y. One chromosome of each pair derives from the individual's father and one from the mother. Every cell contains exactly the same genetic material as every other cell; an individual's total genetic endowment is called the **genome**. Cells that are genetically identical assume different appearances and functions through the process of **differentiation**.

How Cells Differ

All cells start with the same potential to produce all the proteins encoded in the genes present, but any one cell synthesizes only those few proteins characteristic of the particular cell type. As cells divide and the embryo develops, DNA undergoes rearrangement and redistribution. Some sequences permanently disappear; most sequences persist but exhibit activity only after activation by complex combinations of internal and external stimuli that are not fully understood. Protein synthesis seems to occur in response to discrete messages that may be present at some times and absent at others. In most cases, manufacture of structural or functional proteins changes the cell so that it expresses one set of properties but permanently loses the potential for other products or properties. Fully differentiated cells are capable only of a limited number of highly specialized actions. Other cells retain the potential to perform various actions; environmental events determine what course such a cell pursues. Different cell types possess different ranges of potential function; within cell types, differences in maturation determine what material each cell manufactures.

MEMBRANE MARKERS

Features that characterize cells have diverse origins: structural proteins that confer shape, motility, contractility, or other properties; metabolically active internal molecules; and molecules on the cell membrane through which environmental influences affect the cell's interior. Membrane molecules exhibit tremendous diversity. In a single individual, cells of different types display different membrane markers; even among cells of a single type, membrane markers vary with the level of cellular maturity. Increasingly sophisticated identification of membrane markers has expanded our understanding of cell populations and their dynamics.

Some marker molecules exist on all cells of all organs of a single individual; these help determine the self characteristics of that individual. Other molecules characterize all cells performing a certain function and serve as markers for that functional capacity. If the activity occurs in a broad range of cells, the marker will be found on many types of cells. Highly differentiated cells have membrane molecules that mediate their specialized functions. Such molecules will be present only on cells capable of performing that activity, but the same marker can be present on comparable cells from many different individuals and even from many different species. Cells express a changing selection of membrane molecules; molecules often disappear after performing their function and may or may not reappear with changes in internal and external circumstances. Table 1–3 summarizes categories of markers significant in immune processes.

RECEPTORS AND LIGANDS

A molecule so shaped that it interacts optimally with some other molecule is called a **receptor** for that material; the material complementary to the receptor is called a **ligand**. Receptor-ligand interactions allow cells to receive instruction or stimulation from outside. Intercellular communication occurs when one cell manufactures and

---

TABLE 1–3. Categories of Identifying Features

Self Determinants
    Present on all cells in a single individual
    Determined by genetic constitution
    Different in each individual, except monozygotic ("identical") twins
    May be immunogenic for other members of same species
Species Determinants
    Present on cells or proteins of all individuals of a given species
    Determined by genetic information common to the species
    May be immunogenic for individuals of other species
Functional Determinants, Inherent
    Reflect proteins that perform characteristic functions
    Examples: contractile proteins, enzymes, structural proteins
    Present in all cells, from any species, that perform that function
    Immunogenic only under pathologic or experimental circumstances
Functional Determinants, Variable
    Reflect phase of differentiation process or activation state
    Membrane receptors may disappear after interacting with ligand
    Stimulation of one receptor may initiate appearance or disappearance of others
    Immunogenicity may be part of physiologic network of immune regulation

---

releases a product that engages the receptor molecule of another cell. The receptor-ligand complex has physical and physiological properties different from those of the unbound receptor molecule; the changed state alters the membrane or affects other molecules on the interior of the cell. Sometimes the flexible membrane engulfs the receptor-ligand complex, which ends up inside the cell in a process called **interiorization**. Interiorization is one example of the phenomenon called **modulation,** in which cells exhibit altered structural features in response to external events (Fig. 1–3).

Receptor-Ligand Events

In multicelled organisms, a broad range of receptor-ligand events occurs continually. For example, most cells have receptors for insulin; when insulin molecules combine with intact insulin receptors, insulin-mediated metabolic events occur within the cell. For other hormones, only one or a few cell types may possess suitable receptors, and such hormones have rather restricted metabolic effects. In neural transmission, stimulation passes from cell to cell when neurotransmitter substances generated by the sending cell interact with complementary receptors on the receiving cell. Many types of cells produce various growth-promoting factors that stimulate multiplication of

RECEPTOR-LIGAND INTERACTION

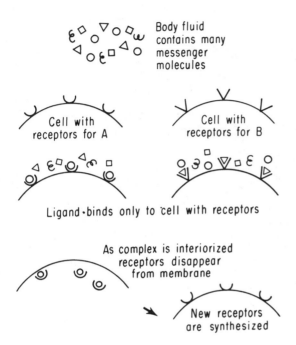

FIGURE 1-3. Receptors and ligands interact through reciprocal characteristics of their configurations. Mediator molecules convey messages only to cells possessing the complementary receptor molecule. If the receptor-ligand complex is incorporated into the interior, the membrane remains bare of receptors and unable to receive new messages until additional receptor molecules are expressed.

cells that have suitably configured receptors. Phagocytosis occurs when membrane receptors of inflammatory cells interact with molecular complexes of other cells or particles. Each cell has many different receptor molecules, enabling it to respond to various stimuli as they occur. A cell unable to manufacture a particular receptor will not respond to the presence of the complementary mediator substance, no matter how high its concentration.

Interiorization of the receptor-ligand complex leaves the cell without receptors and unable to respond to additional ligand, a condition described as being **refractory** to further stimulation. Reappearance of newly synthesized receptors reestablishes a responsive state. Many receptor-ligand interactions, however, provoke internal changes that cause the cell to synthesize different products or to express different capabilities. This may cause a different set of receptors to appear, initiating avenues for stimulation and function quite different from those originally present. The genetic composition of the cell is unchanged, but structure and function can change dramatically with changing external events.

CELL REPLICATION

Genetic material present in the diploid nucleus undergoes duplication during cell division, so that each of the two daughter cells contains identical sets of chromosomes. **Mitosis** is the asexual process whereby diploid cells generate chromosomal material to provide each daughter cell with 46 chromosomes. Occasional mishaps occur as chromosomes replicate and divide, but daughter cells are, for all practical purposes, identical to the cell of origin. Suitably stimulated, the daughter cells can divide and their offspring can divide in geometric expansion to produce a cell population genetically identical to the original cell. A **clone** is a cell population that evolves without sexual recombination; if all cells in a population derive from successive divisions of a single cell, the population is described as **monoclonal**. If many different cells divide, the accumulating cells embody the differing genetic properties of diverse progenitor cells. A cell population that reflects division of many different cells is called **polyclonal** (Fig. 1–4). Polyclonal cell multiplication occurs when an extensive growth stimulus affects several or many individual cells. Monoclonal expansion occurs if some stimulus activates the receptors only of a single cell, or if there is defective internal regulation so that an individual cell divides in the absence of any external growth stimulus.

Meiosis is the form of cell division whereby an original diploid cell evolves into 4 haploid cells, each containing a single copy of the 22 autosomes and a single sex chromosome, either X or Y. The **germ cells,** ova and sperm, are the only haploid cells in normal individuals. During meiosis, genetic material often exchanges between duplicated copies of individual chromosomes in a process called **crossing over;** or between segments of different chromosomes in a process called **translocation**. As the complex nucleic acid molecules undergo replication, the sequence of nucleotides may change, causing new genetic information to develop, a process called **mutation**.

Cellular Aggregates

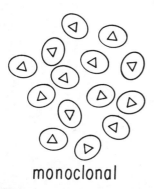

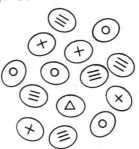

monoclonal   polyclonal

FIGURE 1–4. A group of cells is described as monoclonal if every member derives from a single progenitor; all cells have identical genetic constitution. In a polyclonal aggregate, many different cells of origin are represented and the genetic constitution of the accumulated cells manifest many differences, some of them subtle and some quite pronounced.

─────────── **SUGGESTIONS FOR** ───────────
FURTHER READING

Darnell J, Lodish H, Baltimore D: Molecular Cell Biology. New York: Scientific American Books, 1986:51–104 (Molecules in cells); 105–129 (Synthesis of proteins and nucleic acids); 131–186 (Principles of cellular organization and function)

Dexter TM, Spooncer E: Growth and differentiation in the hemopoietic system. Ann Rev Cell Biol 1987; 3:423–41

Guyton AC: Human Physiology and Mechanisms of Disease. 4th ed, Philadelphia: WB Saunders, 1987:1–31 (The cell and general physiology); 194–205 (Red blood cells, white blood cells and resistance of the body to infection)

Lehrer RI, moderator. Neutrophils and host defense. Ann Int Med 1988; 109:127–42

CHAPTER 2

The Immune System

A brief overview of immunity is necessary to provide a context for description of the cells, tissues, and organs that constitute the immune system. Later chapters will discuss at greater length the concepts that this account introduces.

NATURE OF IMMUNE REACTIONS

The essential features of immunity are **recognition** of specific stimuli and **adaptive response** to later encounters with the stimulating material. Under normal conditions, immune responses occur only to "foreign" materials, with configurations that differ from those of the host's cells and cell products.

ANTIGEN RECOGNITION

Lymphocytes are the cells that recognize foreign material as potentially antigenic and respond to its presence by the cellular and humoral changes that constitute the immune response. These responsive lymphocytes have receptor molecules configured so as to interact optimally with a single antigen; the lymphocyte is said to exhibit **specificity** for that material.

Interaction between antigen and receptor is a complex process. Antigenic material must enter the body through or across the physical barrier of surface epithelium. Before stimulating the receptive lymphocyte, antigen must undergo modification that enhances physical interaction with the receptor; this modification is called **antigen processing**. Cells that process antigen are called **accessory** or **antigen-presenting** cells and are frequently macrophages or related cells (Fig. 2–1). Macrophages also elaborate products that stimulate

ANTIGEN PROCESSING

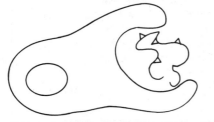

Macrophage phagocytizes antigenic material

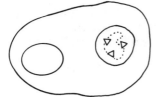

Macrophage processes native material, enhances antigenicity

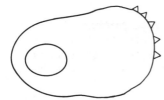

Macrophage presents antigen in accessible, effective form

FIGURE 2–1. The antigen-presenting cell incorporates potentially antigenic material, modifies its chemical and/or physical characteristics, and presents the altered material in a manner that facilitates interaction with the antigen-specific receptor of a lymphocyte. Macrophages and specialized epithelial cells perform most antigen processing and presentation.

and modify the effector cells that exhibit specific recognition. Cell products that influence the actions of other cells are called **cytokines**. Cytokines derived from macrophages and from lymphocytes have crucial regulatory roles in the immune process.

RESPONSE TO ANTIGENIC STIMULATION

Contact between antigen and cell-membrane receptor activates intracellular message systems that prepare the cell for replication. A lymphocyte that has never encountered its antigen is described as a **resting** cell; antigenic stimulation causes **transformation** into an **immunoblast,** the lymphocyte beginning to undergo multiplication. Multiplication involves replication of nuclear material and division into successive generations of daughter cells. A variety of cytokines, many of which come from accessory lymphocytes activated by the same antigen, influence these processes. A complex sequence of cytokine production, receptor interactions, and modulation of membrane receptors orchestrates generation of daughter cells cloned from the original stimulated cell. Daughter cells, responding to recent antigen contact and expressing receptors for various cytokines, exist in a state of **activation**.

As activated antigen-specific cells proliferate, individual members of the clone experience contact with any of several cytokines at various concentration levels; the result of these varied influences is that cells exhibit a range of different membrane and internal products. Many daughter cells evolve into effector forms that produce antibodies or initiate the cell-to-cell activities described as cell-mediated immu-

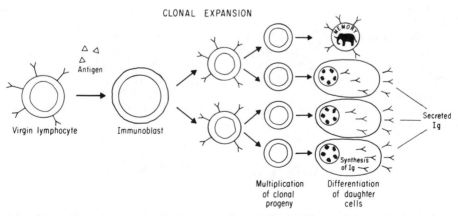

FIGURE 2–2. The virgin lymphocyte transforms into an immunoblast after stimulation of the idiotypically unique receptor molecule. Clonal expansion generates progeny that are genetically identical but evolve into different effector cells after contact with mediators of different sorts.

nity. Most of these highly differentiated effector cells survive only for hours or days, performing their functions and then disappearing. Some activated cells do not become effector cells; they cease active division and become quiescent, although maintaining intracellular changes that reflect prior activation. These become **memory** cells, retaining a state of heightened reactivity such that subsequent encounter with antigen provokes rapid proliferation. Figure 2–2 illustrates the changes that follow contact with antigen.

DIFFERENT CELL POPULATIONS

Many stimuli, including cytokines and externally derived materials, affect various cell characteristics, but predetermined cellular capabilities restrict the magnitude of change. For example, macrophages modify and present antigens and produce cytokines but never recognize specific antigenic configurations. In differentiating from the common hematopoietic precursor (see Fig. 1–1), macrophages lose the capacity to synthesize a receptor molecule, just as lymphocytes lose the capacity for phagocytosis. In differentiating from the common lymphoid precursor, T cells and B cells acquire differing properties.

Human and other mammalian B lymphocytes are exposed very early to the maturational effects of yolk-sac and liver elements. B cells undergo gene rearrangements that confer the ability to manufacture immunoglobulins, the proteins with antibody activity. Activation and subsequent differentiation cause antigen-stimulated B lymphocytes to evolve into **plasma cells,** which secrete the antibody into body fluids. After activation, B lymphocytes evolve either to short-lived antibody-producing plasma cells or to long-lived memory cells that are capable of rapid multiplication but are not actively synthesizing antibody.

By contrast, T lymphocytes perform numerous different functions, and several different populations of T cells can be seen to have various roles. Precursor forms experience the distinctive genetic event that marks them as T cells either just before or just after entering the thymus, where more complete evolution occurs. Different T-cell populations can be identified by antibodies against characteristic membrane markers.

THE LYMPHORETICULAR SYSTEM

The organ that executes immunity is a dispersed array of cells and tissues collectively termed the **lymphoreticular system;** other synonymous terms are the **lymphocyte-macrophage** system, the **reticuloendothelial** system, and, simply, the **immune** system. Lymphocytes and macrophages are free-living cellular constituents. Solid-tissue components of the lymphoreticular system are the bone marrow; the lymph nodes; the spleen; the liver; the thymus; and elements of the mucosal lining of alimentary, respiratory, and, to a lesser extent, genitourinary tracts. Many of these tissues perform additional functions besides immune reactivity.

CIRCULATORY PATTERNS

Lymphocytes and macrophages lead a nomadic existence, traveling continuously through tissues, blood, and lymphatic fluid. The body has several fluid compartments, all in dynamic equilibrium with one another. Sixty percent of body weight is water. Of this volume, approximately 60 percent is inside cells; the fluid part of blood constitutes 5 to 7 percent of total water in the body. Water that is neither inside cells nor inside blood vessels is called **interstitial fluid;** this surrounds and bathes cells in all organs and tissues and is the medium across which gases and metabolites pass as they enter and leave cells, blood, and the external environment. In performing their inflammatory and immune functions, lymphocytes, macrophages, and granulocytes move between blood and interstitial fluid.

Two Different Systems

It is convenient to consider the heart and blood vessels as a closed system, in which the plasma and cells of blood remain confined unless trauma or abnormal permeability allows elements to escape. This is not strictly true. Water and metabolites enter and leave the blood across capillary walls; lymphocytes enter and leave the blood at different sites; and certain proteins of blood origin accumulate to substantial concentrations in the interstitial fluid. By comparison with lymphatic circulation, however, the bloodstream is a closed circle.

The **lymphatic system** is open-ended. The watery low-protein fluid called **lymph** originates from interstitial fluid. The smallest lymphatic vessels are funnellike traps in the interstitium, into which fluid, particles of all sorts, and wandering macrophages and lymphocytes are pushed when tissue pressures rise. The flow of lymph fluid is **centripetal,** meaning from the periphery toward the center of the body. In their centripetal course, lymphatic vessels pass through **lymph nodes,** aggregates of tissue located at numerous regional intervals. As lymphatic vessels leave lymph nodes, they coalesce to form ever-larger vessels. The largest lymphatic vessel, the **thoracic duct,** receives lymph from the entire body and empties it into the bloodstream in one of the two veins that returns blood to the heart for repeated circulation. The fluid and cells present in lymph mingle with the blood and reenter the circulatory cycle.

Sinusoidal Flow

An important aspect of lymphatic flow is sinusoidal drainage through lymph nodes. **Sinusoids** are circulatory channels of relatively wide caliber, with irregular contours and thin walls. Fluid passing through these broad, meandering paths moves relatively slowly, so material carried in the fluid has prolonged and intimate contact with cells and membranes that line the sinusoids. Lymph fluid enters lymph nodes through **afferent** lymphatics at the periphery; it percolates through sinusoids toward the center of the node, where a slightly larger **efferent** vessel continues the centripetal route that leads eventually to the bloodstream. Macrophages, which line sinusoids or lie immediately beneath the walls, experience prolonged contact with material present in the lymph fluid. Particulate matter—such as microorganisms, bits of foreign material, or debris from the body's own cells—is cleared from the tissues by entering the lymphatics; it is cleared from lymph by sinusoidal macrophages. Macrophages either degrade the material permanently or process it for presentation to immune effector cells.

In several portions of the cardiovascular system, the bloodstream passes through sinusoids, allowing comparable contact of macrophages with the contents of flowing blood. In the spleen, the liver, and the bone marrow, flowing blood has intimate contact with macrophages associated with the walls of sinusoids. If the blood contains cellular, particulate, or molecular material with antigenic properties, macrophages can extract these elements and process them as needed. Sinusoidal macrophages also have repeated contact with circulating cells and act to remove aging or damaged blood cells from the circulation.

LYMPHORETICULAR ORGANS

The quintessential immune tissue is the **lymph node**. Lymph nodes are ovoid masses of tissue present in clusters along the routes that lymphatic vessels follow before joining the bloodstream. Sinusoidal architecture results from the arrangement of the delicate fibrillar protein called **reticulin;** a denser structural protein, **collagen,** surrounds lymph nodes and constitutes a capsule that confines the tissue into a compact, bean-shaped mass. Lymph nodes contain both T and B lymphocytes. In the outer portion of the node, called the **cortex,** B cells form circular aggregates, called **follicles**. T lympocytes cluster around the follicles and in deeper portions, the **paracortical** area. Deeper still, in the **medulla,** B cells and their differentiated plasma-cell progeny are the predominant cells, along with the macrophages that hug the walls of sinusoids. Figure 2–3 shows a schematized lymph node.

FIGURE 2–3. Lymph fluid enters the periphery of the lymph node through the afferent lymphatics and percolates through the sinusoids to emerge from the node through the centrally located efferent lymphatic vessel. Follicles, which consist largely of B cells, are conspicuous in the outer cortex. Around the follicles and in the slightly deeper paracortical portions of the node, T cells predominate. In the deepest portion, the medulla, there is a mixed population of lymphocytes, in which B cells and plasma cells are the most numerous.

ARCHITECTURE OF LYMPH NODE

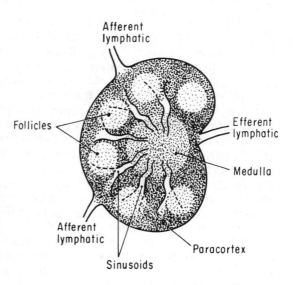

Functions of Marrow

Bone marrow occupies the central portion of nearly all the 206 bones in the body, but in adults, most marrow spaces contain largely fat, with little reticuloendothelial activity. Reticuloendothelial elements of bone marrow perform the function of **hematopoiesis,** the production of blood cells, as well as immune-related functions. Hematopoietic and lymphoreticular tissue occupies more marrow space in the fetus than in postuterine life, and more in young children than in adults. In normal adults, active bone marrow is almost entirely confined to the vertebral column, the breast bone, and the bones of the pelvis, although both physiologic and pathologic stimuli can reexpand adult bone marrow activity to the ribs, the long bones of the extremities, and the bones of the skull.

Bone marrow consists of sinusoids defined by reticulin fibers and surrounded by macrophages; between the sinusoids are masses of proliferating erythrocyte, granulocyte, monocyte, and platelet cell lines. Maturing cells enter the blood by slipping across the sinusoidal walls into the flowing blood. Macrophages resident in the bone marrow phagocytize particulate material and damaged cells and secrete cytokines that affect both hematopoietic and immune elements. Relatively few lymphocytes proliferate in the marrow after fetal maturation, unless there is neoplastic or other unusual stimulation.

Liver and Spleen

The **spleen** is a fist-sized organ in the upper left quadrant of the abdominal cavity. Blood circulating through the spleen pursues a tortuous course. The arterial tree branches into arterioles that run adjacent to follicles of lymphocytes: B cells occupy the centers; and T cells, the periphery of these follicles. Blood traversing the spleen leaves the arterial side and percolates slowly through venous sinusoids, allowing intimate contact with splenic macrophages. During this interaction, aging or damaged cells are removed from the circulation, and antigenic material is extracted for processing and presentation. The spleen contains numerous antigen-presenting cells, called **dendritic cells,** in close association with follicular B cells. The normal spleen is the major site for blood filtration, serving a function comparable to the cleansing effect that lymph nodes exert on lymphatic fluid. If the spleen is absent or circulation is impaired, liver and bone marrow take over these activities.

Like the bone marrow, the **liver** has substantial lymphoreticular elements in an organ that serves other functions. Between the macrophage-lined sinusoids of the liver lie **hepatocytes,** cuboidal cells of epithelial origin that constitute most of the approximately 1500 grams (about 3 pounds) that the liver weighs. Hepatocytes synthesize many blood proteins and perform metabolic conversions that manufacture and degrade most body constituents. Blood that traverses the hepatic sinusoids comes largely from the gastrointestinal tract and other abdominal organs, bringing with it antigenic material as well as the nutrients essential for continuing metabolism. Hepatic macrophages are called **Kuppfer cells;** the combined actions of hepatocytes and Kuppfer cells regulate antigenic exposure from the many substances entering the body as food and drink. The normal liver contains very few lymphocytes and appears to generate very little immune effector activity.

Non-sinusoidal Tissues

The **thymus,** a fleshy, lobulated organ in the anterior chest, is at its largest and most active during intrauterine life and early childhood. It virtually disappears in older children and adults, but its early presence and activity are crucial for immune development. The thymus is demarcated into a highly cellular outer portion called the **cortex** and a smaller central area called the **medulla**. Early in fetal life, lymphoid precursor cells enter the outermost portion of the cortex and acquire the markers characteristic of T cells. Progressive maturation and proliferation occur as the cells migrate through cortex and medulla to emerge as circulating T lymphocytes. These events are discussed more fully in chapter 5 and are illustrated in Figure 5–3. Lymphocytes within the thymus are called **thymocytes;** they become **peripheral** T cells after leaving the thymus. Differentiation and sub-

SITES OF LYMPHORETICULAR TISSUE

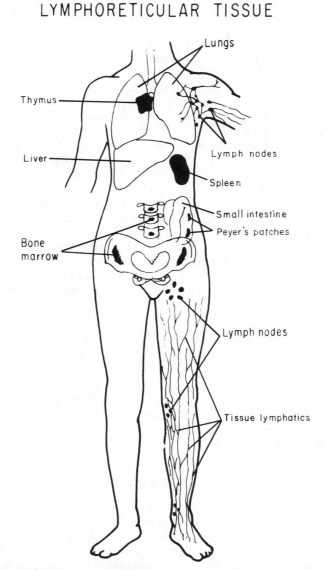

FIGURE 2–4. Elements of the lymphoreticular system are present throughout the body. Lymphatic vessels drain every organ and tissue; on its way to join the bloodstream, lymph fluid passes through lymph nodes at many sites. The spleen, liver, and bone marrow are important lymphoreticular organs at all stages of life, while the thymus is prominent only in fetal life, infancy, and early childhood. The respiratory and gastrointestinal tracts contain most of the mucosa-associated lymphoid tissue.

sequent maturation are mediated by hormones, including **thymosin** and **thymopoietin,** produced by thymic epithelial cells. A lifetime supply of dedicated T-cell precursors develops during the migration and proliferation that occur in the large, active thymus of early existence.

Approximately a third of the body's lymphocytes are found in superficial mucosal locations. Large numbers of lymphocytes and plasma cells lie beneath surface epithelial cells in the respiratory and alimentary tracts, close to the cells that metabolize incoming material and secrete the fluids that bathe these surfaces. The superficial portions of the genitourinary system have a smaller lymphoid component. Lymphocytes in these locations are collectively described as the **mucosa-associated lymphoid tissue,** abbreviated as MALT. Lymphocytes, mostly B cells, form follicles in the upper portions of the respiratory and alimentary tracts; these are most easily seen as the tonsils, the adenoids, and the Peyer's patches of the small intestine. A thick layer of lymphocytes is diffusely arranged among the epithelial elements in most segments of these mucosal surfaces. These lymphocytes express a very strong functional sense of place; lymphocytes travel continuously through the tissues, the lymphatics, and the bloodstream, but cells initially present in specific mucosal locations consistently return to these sites after their migrations.

Figure 2–4 depicts the major sites of lymphoreticular elements.

THE MONONUCLEAR-PHAGOCYTE SYSTEM

Macrophages, which are intimately involved in the processes of antigen recognition, immune stimulation, and the tissue consequences that follow immune stimulation, have different lineage and functional properties from those of lymphocytes.

BONE MARROW ORIGIN

Development and replenishment of mononuclear phagocytic cells occur continuously throughout life. Macrophages and granulocytes descend from a common bone marrow precursor; the two populations diverge into the precursor forms **monoblast** and **myeloblast,** respectively. In the physiologic steady state, unidentified mediator substances in the marrow stimulate monoblast proliferation and differentiation; in inflammatory conditions, factors have been identified that promote increased monocyte development and others that reduce this activity when the stimulus ceases.

Each monoblast divides to form two **promonocytes,** which in turn divide to generate four **monocytes** from the original blast. Within 24 hours of their generation, monocytes enter the circulating blood, where they constitute approximately 3 to 8 percent of peripheral-blood white cells. Circulating monocytes are cells that have not reached full differentiation; further evolution occurs at the various tissue sites to which the blood carries them.

LOCATIONS AND FUNCTIONS IN TISSUE

The mononuclear-phagocyte population occupies many tissue sites and exhibits a wide range of differentiated appearance. Features common to cells of this overall category include the presence of several cytoplasmic enzymes, notably **non-specific esterase** and **lysozyme**. Several membrane receptor molecules consistently occur on macrophages but are not lineage-specific, being present on other cell types as well. Particularly important in immune activity are the receptors for immunoglobulin molecules (the **Fc receptor**) and the **C3 receptor,** which binds one of the proteins in the complement system (see chapter 8). Mononuclear phagocytes have the capability to phagocytize particles (Fig. 2–5), especially those coated with antibody or complement proteins. Antigen-presenting cells exist that have features suggestive of monocyte origin but lack phagocytic capacity.

Differentiation into Macrophages

Upon leaving the bloodstream, monocytes migrate to tissue locations where they remain as **resident macrophages**. We have already mentioned macrophage elements in lymph nodes, spleen, and liver. Additional populations of resident macrophages include (1) **alveolar macrophages,** which live in the lungs; (2) macrophages that monitor and protect the **peritoneal** lining around abdominal organs and the **pleural** surfaces that surround the lungs; (3) **osteoclasts,** which perform degradative activities in bone; (4) macrophages in the central nervous system, sometimes called **microglia;** (5) **histiocytes,** the name given to macrophages that are free in connective tissue; and (6) macrophages present in joint linings and in the renal glomeruli. As compared with circulating monocytes, macrophages have a wider repertory of internal enzymes, greater phagocytic capacity, and the ability to synthesize a wide range of cytokines and other proteins. Macrophages in tissue retain some capacity to multiply, but this potential is exercised only after pronounced stimulation; under normal conditions, macrophage populations are replenished from the bone marrow.

Resident macrophages occupy predictable locations within each tissue. Following a stimulus to inflammation, the macrophages that

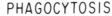

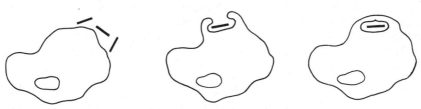

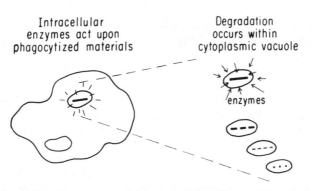

FIGURE 2–5. Phagocytosis begins with surface contact between the particle and the cell membrane, which invaginates to enfold the material and incorporate it into the cytoplasm. A complex system of enzymes and energy-requiring reactions causes degradation of the phagocytized material.

accumulate constitute a population described as **exudate macrophages**. Such macrophages elaborate cytokines that activate cells of the immune system and influence other aspects of inflammation. In turn, the lymphokines from antigen-specific lymphocytes cause macrophages to manifest heightened reactivity. Stimulated by immune cytokines, activated macrophages become larger, exhibit more numerous and more active organelles, and engage in more effective phagocytosis and enzyme production. Products of activated macrophages include proteolytic enzymes and numerous proteins that affect coagulation, complement activity, and multiplication of cells that generate new tissue and repair damaged tissue.

SUGGESTIONS FOR FURTHER READING

David J: Organs and cells of the immune system. In: Rubenstein E, Federman DD, eds. Scientific American Medicine. New York: Scientific American Books, 1987:6:I:1–14

Johnson RB, Jr: Monocytes and macrophages. NEJM 1988; 318:747–52

Nossal GJV: The basic components of the immune system. NEJM 1987; 316:1320–25

Ritter MA, Rozing J, Schuurman H-J: The true function of the thymus? Immunol Today 1988; 9:189–93

Unanue ER, Allen PM: The immunoregulatory role of the macrophage. Hosp Pract 1987; 22 (issue 4):87–104

CHAPTER 3

The HLA System

Crucially important in immune regulation are several classes of membrane antigens collectively designated the **HLA system**. Their physiologic role seems to be internal immunomodulation, but they were first studied on circulating leukocytes and were soon noted to be significant in survival of transplanted tissues. HLA is sometimes said to stand for "human leukocyte antigens"; other sources derive the term from "histocompatibility locus A." It is preferable to consider HLA a free-standing independent term, not an acronym for some other concept. A discussion of the origin, function, and significance of the HLA system requires preliminary consideration of several basic genetic and molecular concepts.

POLYMORPHISMS, INHERITANCE, AND THE MHC

HLA antigens are polypeptides, the structures of which are encoded by genetic material located on the short arm of chromosome 6.

This segment determines structures of HLA antigens and of several serum proteins and also exerts systemic immunoregulatory activities; the entire segment is called the **major histocompatibility complex,** or **MHC**.

ALLELES AND POLYMORPHISM

The amino acid sequence of a polypeptide is a direct reflection of the nucleotide sequence in chromosomal deoxyribonucleic acid (DNA). Deoxyribonucleic acid sequences may experience substitutions, transpositions, additions, or deletions; these changes—called **mutations**—cause predictable changes in amino acid sequence of the corresponding protein. For some proteins, any alteration in amino acid sequence destroys functional capacity; if the function of that protein is essential for survival, the affected cell or organism does not survive to transmit the altered DNA to offspring. Many mutations, however, induce protein alterations that do not affect reproductive capacity, and offspring of the original individual exhibit the same genetic trait. Different forms of a gene, occupying the same chromosomal location and determining variant forms of the same product, are called **alleles**. The structural differences that result are called **allotypic** variants. Figure 3–1 depicts the effects of allelic variation.

Some proteins have exactly the same structure in every individual; the gene for those products is presumably the same in everyone. For many proteins, however, slight structural variations exist; individuals expressing different forms of the polypeptide possess different alleles. The existence of many different alleles for a given characteristic in a population is described as **polymorphism,** from Greek words

FIGURE 3–1. Alleles are alternative genes for the production of a single protein. Differences in DNA sequence cause the resulting proteins to differ in amino acid sequence at localized sites. For the protein shown above, the products of three different alleles (designated *a, b,* and *c*) differ in structure at a single segment. The overall nature of the protein is the same, but the allelic characteristics may affect functional or antigenic properties of the molecule.

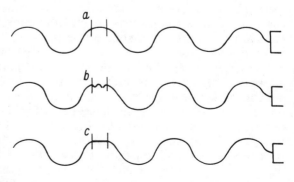

ALLELIC DIFFERENCES

Same protein
Different allelic characteristics

meaning "many forms." The HLA system is highly polymorphic, with numerous alleles that determine subtle differences among cells from different humans.

Significance of Polymorphism

Allelic variants may determine products that vary in functional efficiency. Certain variants of the hemoglobin molecule, for example, cause significant health problems; genetically aberrant enzymes cause diseases of many sorts. Other allelic differences have few or no apparent physiologic effects. HLA polymorphism falls into the latter category; there is no evidence that one or another polypeptide performs any better or any worse than comparable molecules of different sequence. HLA structures modify how immune effector cells interact with both accessory and target cells, but specific alleles confer no advantage or disadvantage.

HLA antigens differ sufficiently in structure that exposure to cells bearing foreign HLA molecules can provoke an immune response in a host exposed to cells from another human. Characterization of this highly polymorphic cell-surface system resulted from observations made in women exposed to the foreign HLA antigens of the fetus they carried, in patients exposed to transfused cells, and in experimental tissue-grafting systems.

CHROMOSOMAL ORGANIZATION AND HAPLOTYPES

Genes performing a given function occupy the same position on the same chromosome in all individuals of a species; that position is called the **locus** (plural: **loci**) for that gene. Loci for many human genes have been identified; for example, genes for manufacture of immunoglobulin chains reside on chromosomes 14, 2, and 22; those for ABO red cell antigens are on chromosome 9. Genes controlling the HLA antigens are on chromosome 6.

Diploid cells possess two copies of every chromosome except the sex chromosomes, hence they have two copies of every gene. If that locus on both chromosomes is occupied by the same allele, the cell is said to be **homozygous** for that gene; if each chromosome has a different allele, the cell is **heterozygous** for the gene. Numerous factors determine whether one or both alleles will produce a detectable product, but these need not concern us here. Each HLA gene in a cell produces a detectable product, regardless of what allele occupies the other chromosome. Heterozygotes express two different sets of antigen-bearing molecules. Homozygotes, who have the same allele on both chromosomes, do not produce twice as much of that material; their cells simply display molecules of a single antigenic structure.

Manner of Transmission

When chromosomal material is apportioned to germ cells during meiosis, genes located very close to one another tend to remain together. Genes some distance apart on a chromosome may become entangled with strands of condensed chromosomal material and **crossover** from one chromosome to the opposite member of the pair; the alignment of genes on the resulting chromosomes is different from that in the original cell. Genes so close together that crossing-over rarely occurs are transmitted as a consistent unit of genetic material, called a **haplotype**. Genes constituting the MHC pass from one generation to the next in predictable haplotypes, although crossing-over occurs occasionally.

HLA molecules on cell surfaces display at least six different categories of activity, designated **series,** which are identified by letters. Each series is determined by alleles at a specific site within the MHC. The combined sequence of genes within that segment of chromosome 6 comprises the MHC haplotype on that chromosome. Each individual possesses two haplotypes, one from each parent; when the individual reproduces, each offspring will receive one—and only one—of those haplotypes. No matter how many different alleles exist in a population, and how many ways these alleles can align into haplotypes, the offspring of a single mating can express only those haplotypes present in the original couple. Starting with two maternal haplotypes and two paternal haplotypes, each offspring will express one of only four possible combinations.

In characterizing the HLA constitution of siblings, it is customary to describe those siblings who have received the same haplotypes from the mother and the father as **HLA-identical;** if they received the same haplotype from one parent but different haplotypes from the other, they are considered **haploidentical**.

CLASSES OF MHC PRODUCTS

The six series of HLA molecules can be divided into two categories, called **classes,** according to their size and molecular structure. **Class I** products of the MHC genes include the A, B, and C series. Class I molecules have two chains, one of which is a large glycoprotein that penetrates the membrane; the other is a much smaller chain attached only to the larger chain and not to the membrane at all. **Class II** products, designated the DP, DQ, and DR series, also consist of two chains, but these are nearly equal in size, and both penetrate the cell membrane. Certain non-HLA products of genes within the MHC are sometimes called **class III** products; these include serum proteins involved in the **complement system,** which is discussed in chapter 8. Figure 3–2 shows the location of these gene sites within the MHC. There are thought to be genes in the MHC that influence how individ-

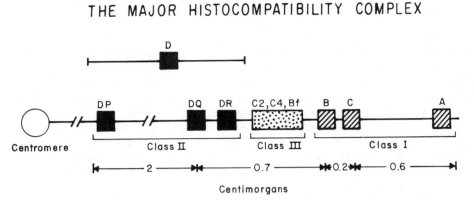

FIGURE 3–2. The major histocompatibility complex (MHC) on chromosome 6 has been mapped in detail. Discrete portions encode the class I products (HLA series A, B, and C), the class II products (HLA-D and DP, DQ, and DR series) and the class III products, largely proteins that participate in the complement system.

uals respond to different antigenic stimuli, but no products have been identified that perform these functions.

STRUCTURE AND NOMENCLATURE OF HLA ANTIGENS

The HLA antigens were discovered through deliberate efforts to find antigens on white blood cells comparable to those on red cells; as reagents, investigators used sera from persons previously exposed to cells from other individuals. Patterns of positive and negative reactions demonstrated antigenic features compatible with allelically determined traits. The first white-cell polymorphism was demonstrated in 1958, and others soon followed. Since then, discoveries of numerous antigens and complex relationships have required a systematic approach to nomenclature. International workshops in 1967 and 1970 generated a system of terminology that continues to be workable and is reexamined and expanded at successive workshops now held approximately every 4 years.

BIOCHEMISTRY OF HLA ANTIGENS

Class I MHC products, comprising the HLA-A, -B, and -C antigens, express a large glycoprotein chain, called alpha, the structure of which is determined by genes within the MHC. For the smaller chain, called **beta-2-microglobulin,** the determining gene is on chromosome 15. The polymorphic sites that embody antigenic specificity are on the alpha chain. The beta-2-microglobulin component is unvarying; all class I molecules possess the same chain structure: a looped configuration of molecular weight 12 kD. The beta-2-microglobulin polypeptide also exists as an independent fluid-phase molecule in serum and urine, but its function is unknown. The larger, alpha, chain has 338 amino acid residues and a molecular weight of 44 kD. Its configuration includes three looped segments, called **domains;** the variations in amino acid sequence that produce antigenic differences exist on the two distally located domains.

The class II MHC products that have been clearly characterized are the DP, DQ, and DR series of HLA antigens. For both chains of class II products, the determining genes lie within the MHC. Both chains are glycoproteins that penetrate the cell membrane; the alpha chain is slightly larger than the beta, MW 34 kD and 29 kD, respectively. Both chains are configured into domains. For the DR series, antigenic specificity resides in domains only on the beta chain. The other two series are less well characterized. Figure 3–3 shows the structures of the class I and class II molecules.

STRUCTURE OF MHC PRODUCTS

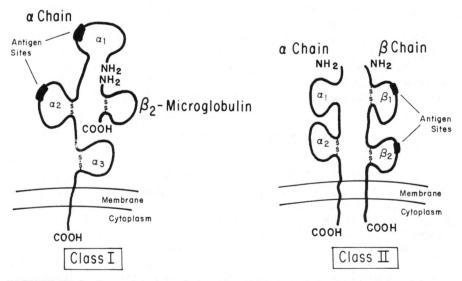

FIGURE 3–3. In molecules of class I, structure of the large alpha chain is determined by genes of the MHC. The beta-2-microglobulin chain is the same in all class I molecules; its manufacture is directed by a gene on chromosome 15. In class II molecules, both chains are products of genes in the MHC. The chains are similar in size and general configuration, but sites that determine allotypic antigens are not uniformly distributed. For the DR series, antigenic activity resides in sequences on the beta chain only.

ALLOGENEIC SERIES

Early workers assigned idiosyncratic names and numbers to the antigens they discovered; it was difficult to discern genetic relationships or even to determine that a single antigen had been assigned several different names. Terms adopted at the 1970 workshop embodied the concept that HLA antigens derived from two separate genetic loci. Antigens of the series designated A reflected alleles at one locus, those of the B series, another. Numbers were assigned to those antigens with clearly defined serologic characteristics. Antigens about which uncertainty existed received a number prefixed by "w," standing for "workshop." Succeeding workshops have incorporated newly discovered antigens into this scheme, removing the "w" as ambiguous findings were clarified.

Since establishment of the A and B series in 1970, additional genetic loci have been discovered and new antigenic series established. The first workshop worked with many antigens already established in the vocabulary, and it seemed undesirable to assign numbers arbitrarily to each series as parallel sequences. Instead, the numbers 1, 2, and 3 went to A antigens; 4, 5, 6, 7, and 8 to B; 9 and 10 to A antigens, and so on. The A and B series continue to share a single numerical sequence as new observations are incorporated; for example, numbers 41 and 42 are B-series antigens, whereas 43 is an A antigen. As new antigenic series emerged, however, later workshops assigned new letters and a sequence starting with 1, continuing the "w" designation until full characterization of each antigen was achieved. All antigens of the C series, no matter how well characterized, are prefixed by "w" because the letter C followed by numbers from 1 to 9 has been preempted by proteins of the complement system (see chapter 8). Table 3–1 lists the letters and numbers that constitute the HLA system as of the 1987 workshop.

SIGNIFICANCE OF TEST METHODS

White-cell antigens were first discovered through agglutination reactions induced by serum antibodies. In **agglutination,** interaction between antibody and surface antigen causes cells that express the antigen to clump together. Agglutination was used to test white cells because it was so satisfactory for studying red-cell antigens, but it proved less well suited to leukocytes. Other techniques were developed that used different end points for the specific interaction between antibody and antigen, but all employed serum antibody as the indicator. The term **serologically defined** was applied to leukocyte antigens identified by reactions in a serum system.

With increasing understanding of cellular immune events, new test methods were adopted that exploited cell-mediated immunity. In test systems that employed cultured lymphocytes, new patterns of membrane reactivity emerged. Antigens could be observed that provoked predictable cellular changes but for which no identifying antibodies existed. This series of antigens, assigned the letter D, was described as **lymphocyte defined**. The HLA-D antigens have been characterized from the behavior of carefully standardized reagent lymphocytes, but antigenically distinctive molecules have not been isolated for biochemical characterization.

Changing Concepts of D

Discovery of new membrane activities, especially the class II MHC products, enlarged and complicated understanding of the HLA system. DR and DQ antigens are identified through reactions with antibodies; they are serologically defined. Reactivity of DP antigens is apparent only in cell-culture procedures. The relationship between the class II antigens and those properties classified as the D series of antigens is not clear. The DR series acquired its name because reaction patterns seemed closely **D related;** these serologically defined antigens seemed promising surrogates for D antigens, which required laborious cellular testing for demonstration. DR reactions do not correspond perfectly to D reactivity. Many workers believe that the cellular reactions described as D antigens actually reflect the combined effects of all the class II molecules on the cell surface. Although DR exerts the preponderant effect, it does not exclusively control the behavior defined as the HLA-D series. At present, most workers are studying DP, DQ, and DR antigens individually, and much less attention is given to D.

GENETIC AND CELLULAR SIGNIFICANCE

The combination of three class I and three class II alleles present on a chromosome constitutes the HLA haplotype, of which there are two in all somatic cells. Inasmuch as HLA genes produce detectable products when present in either homozygous or heterozygous expression, an individual's cells can express up to 12 different HLA molecules. The combination of detectable traits that an individual expresses is called the **phenotype;** the composite of genetic material present in the nucleus is the **genotype**. "HLA typing" means testing with available reagents to generate information necessary for some clinical or investigational indication. Complete phenotyping is seldom performed. The antigens for which reagents are most widely available and from which the most useful clinical and investigational information is derived are those of the A, B, and DR series. From the antigens detected, it is usually possible to infer which alleles are present, but

---

TABLE 3–1. HLA Nomenclature: November 1987 (WHO Report 10th Workshop)

HLA-A	HLA-B	HLA-B	HLA-C
A1	Bw4*	Bw48	Cw1
A2	B5	B49 (21)	Cw2
A3	Bw6*	Bw50 (21)	Cw3
A9	B7	B51 (5)	Cw4
A10	B8	Bw52 (5)	Cw5
A11	B12	Bw53	Cw6
Aw19	B13	Bw54 (w22)	Cw7
A23 (9)	B14	Bw55 (w22)	Cw8
A24 (9)	B15	Bw56 (w22)	Cw9 (w3)
A25 (10)	B16	Bw57 (17)	Cw10 (w3)
A26 (10)	B17	Bw58 (17)	Cw11
A28	B18	Bw59	
A29 (w19)	B21	Bw60 (40)	
A30 (w19)	Bw22	Bw61 (40)	
A31 (w19)	B27	Bw62 (15)	
A32 (w19)	B35	Bw63 (15)	
Aw33 (w19)	B37	Bw64 (14)	
Aw34 (10)	B38 (16)	Bw65 (14)	
Aw36	B39 (16)	Bw67	
Aw43	B40	Bw70	
Aw66 (10)	Bw41	Bw71 (w70)	
Aw68 (28)	Bw42	Bw72 (w70)	
Aw69 (28)	B44 (12)	Bw73	
Aw74 (w19)	B45 (12)	Bw75 (15)	
	Bw46	Bw76 (15)	
	Bw47	Bw77 (15)	

The numbers in parentheses indicate the original specificity from which the listed antigen was split.

*Bw4 and Bw6 are broadly specific antigens whose expression is associated with many other specificities.

phenotyping cannot illuminate how the alleles are distributed in haplotypes. That information can come only from family studies, which show groups of alleles transmitted as consistent units. Figure 3–4 depicts the arrangement of alleles into haplotypes and the way in which these traits are transmitted to progeny.

CELLULAR EXPRESSION
OF ANTIGENS

All cells possess all HLA genes, but expression varies among cells. Class I antigens have far wider distribution than class II. Virtually all

TABLE 3–1. HLA Nomenclature: November 1987 (WHO Report 10th Workshop) *Continued*

HLA-D	HLA-DR	HLA-DQ	HLA-DP
Dw1	DR1	DQw1	DPw1
Dw2	DR2	DQw2	DPw2
Dw3	DR3	DQw3	DPw3
Dw4	DR4	DQw4	DPw4
Dw5	DR5	DQw5 (w1)	DPw5
Dw6	DRw6	DQw6 (w1)	DPw6
Dw7	DR7	DQw7 (w3)	
Dw8	DRw8	DQw8 (w3)	
Dw9	DR9	DQw9 (w3)	
Dw10	DRw10		
Dw11 (w7)	DRw11 (5)		
Dw12	DRw12 (5)		
Dw13	DRw13 (w6)		
Dw14	DRw14 (w6)		
Dw15	DRw15 (2)		
Dw16	DRw16 (2)		
Dw17 (w7)	DRw17 (3)		
Dw18 (w6)	DRw18 (3)		
Dw19 (w6)	DRw52†		
Dw20	DRw53†		
Dw21			
Dw22			
Dw23			
Dw24			
Dw25			
Dw26			

†DRw52 and DRw53 are broadly specific antigens whose expression is associated with many other specificities.

Adapted from: HLA Nomenclature Committee. Nomenclature for factors of the HLA system, 1987. Immunogenetics 1988; 28:391–398.

nucleated cells express HLA-A, -B, and -C antigens, with the probable exception of ova and sperm. Mature red blood cells have no nucleus and do not have consistent HLA reactivity. Free molecules of HLA-active material exist in blood plasma, and unpredictable amounts of fluid-phase material adsorb to red cells and to platelets, which also lack a nucleus. HLA expression on circulating red cells and platelets is clinically significant because transfusion of these components may immunize the recipient to the donor's HLA antigens. When organs are transplanted, the HLA antigens on solid tissue and bone marrow cells cause continuing antigenic stimulation.

Class II antigens are expressed primarily on immunologically reactive cells. Mature B lymphocytes and monocyte/macrophages manifest class II molecules at all stages of maturity; cytokines that enhance

TRANSMISSION OF HLA HAPLOTYPES

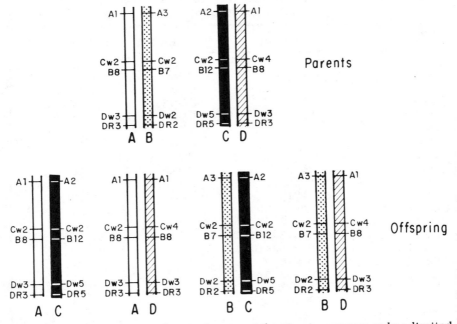

FIGURE 3—4. Offspring of a single parental pair can express only a limited number of HLA haplotypes. In the mating shown above, one parent will transmit *either* the A or the B haplotype; the other will transmit *either* C or D. Combination occurs at random, but only four different combinations are possible.

overall reactivity cause MHC-II expression to increase. Resting T lymphocytes express weak or non-detectable activity, but activated T cells have fairly strong class II expression. Functional cells of most other tissues and organs have little class II antigenic activity but, because solid tissues include variable numbers of monocyte/macrophages, most organs express appreciable class II activity.

Selection of Target Cells

HLA molecules are identification markers for cellular specificity, serving as a target to focus T-cell reactivity. In order to recognize any membrane antigen, T cells with helper functions require that the antigen-presenting cell express class II antigens on its surface. T cells with suppressor or cytotoxic actions recognize antigens only if presented simultaneously with class I antigens. Helper cells interact primarily with antigen-presenting macrophages and antigen-stimulated B lymphocytes, cells that strongly and consistently express class II activity. Class II expression may additionally occur, during states of altered immune reactivity, on tissue cells normally devoid of these molecules; class I molecules, which engage cytotoxic T cells, are a consistent membrane component on cells of all types.

EXPRESSION IN POPULATIONS

Genes for the HLA antigens exhibit striking differences in geographic distribution, but there is no convincing evidence that these genetically determined differences influence immunologic competence, susceptibility to disease, or capacity to defend against injuries. The antigens do, however, provide markers useful for determining parentage and, on a larger scale, for evaluating migrations of population groups. There are marked differences among populations in frequency of different alleles; such differences increase the power of these markers in evaluating parentage. If an allele rare in a given population proves to be present in a child and in the man alleged to be the father, the probability of paternity becomes quite high; if the allele that child and man share is widespread in the population, the common finding could be a chance occurrence.

HLA genes often manifest **linkage disequilibrium,** a phenomenon in which alleles at different loci occur in the same haplotype either more often or less often than the absolute frequency of each allele would predict. The most notable example is the combination of A1 with B8; the independent occurrence of each allele in the white population would predict a frequency of association of 0.0124 (present in 124 persons out of 10,000); the observed frequency is nearly five times that—0.0609. Less striking but still significant associations have been observed between A3 and B7, Aw30 and B13, and A26 and Bw38.

─────────── **CLINICAL SIGNIFICANCE** ───────────

TRANSPLANTATION

A major impetus for studying the HLA system has been tissue transplantation. Animal experiments and, later, human transplantation made obvious the fact that genetic constitutions of donor and host affect the survival of transplanted tissue. Early work with leukocytes made it clear that antigens present on white blood cells reflect genetic properties significant for successful transplantation. Two decades of experience with human kidney grafts demonstrated that congruence for HLA types improves graft survival; this is especially striking when donor and recipient are closely related. Among siblings or parent-child pairs, shared HLA antigens indicate that the same MHC haplotype is present. Unrelated individuals whose two A and two B antigens are the same could not be expected to share all the remaining material of the MHC; "matching" A and B antigens of unrelated individuals leaves much genetic disparity at other loci that affect histocompatibility. As techniques for HLA testing change and posttransplant immunosuppressive regimens improve, the significance of HLA matching for tissue transplantation seems to exert a less striking effect.

TRANSFUSION

Red blood cells express HLA antigens weakly and inconsistently. Although repeated red-cell transfusions can elicit HLA immunization, the resulting antibodies do not affect survival of red cells transfused later. Platelets consistently display HLA material and are far more immunogenic for these antigens than red cells. Recipients of platelet transfusions often develop antibodies against several or many HLA antigens, and transfused platelets expressing these antigens survive poorly. It is more difficult to type donors and patients for HLA groups than for red-cell antigens, and pretransfusion procedures to establish compatibility have been less successful for platelet transfusions than for red cells. Methods to select optimum platelet donors and to achieve the best possible posttransfusion survival continue as subjects of intense investigation.

ASSOCIATION WITH DISEASE

Experiments with mice have suggested that mouse genes analogous to the human MHC affect certain forms of immune responsiveness; these are called **Ir genes** in the mouse. There is no clear evidence for Ir genes in the human MHC, but individuals exhibit obvious differences in immune manifestations. In this context, it is significant that occurrence of many diseases of immune etiology correlate with presence of certain HLA antigens. This need not mean that HLA molecules influence the occurrence, magnitude, or direction of immune responses; more likely the HLA genes are markers for disease-producing genes the presence and nature of which remain to be determined. These disease associations are far from absolute. Persons possessing the antigen will not inexorably manifest the disease, nor does every person with the disease express the antigen. Degrees of association vary, some being quite striking and others merely suggestive or modestly greater than chance would predict.

B27 and Skeletal Inflammation

The firmest association of specific antigen and specific disease is B27 and the inflammatory condition of the vertebral column called

ankylosing spondylitis. In patients of all races with this disease, 70 to 95 percent possess the B27 antigen; the prevalence of B27 in the white population is only 8 to 9 percent, and for blacks and Asians it is even lower. The relative risk, which is the degree to which possessing the trait predicts present or future disease, is extremely high in Asians, among whom the B27 antigen is very uncommon; it is somewhat lower in blacks. In whites, the relative risk is considered moderate, inasmuch as the antigen is present in many healthy individuals who never acquire the disease. There is no plausible explanation for this association; the B27 antigen is associated, but less impressively, with several other immune-mediated diseases that involve the skeletal system.

Other Associations

The form of diabetes termed **insulin-dependent diabetes mellitus** (IDDM), or type I diabetes, is strongly associated with DR3 and DR4. Both genetic and environmental factors affect development of IDDM, and the association with the HLA system is far from straightforward. One interpretation is that the gene promoting development of IDDM is either the same as, or closely linked to, the genes that produce DR3 and DR4. Oddly enough, the likelihood of developing IDDM is greater in heterozygotes carrying both DR3 and DR4 than in homozygotes who have two expressions of either DR3 or DR4 alleles. Several other DR antigens have apparent association with immune-related diseases, among them DR2 with a particularly aggressive form of leprosy; DR4 with rheumatoid arthritis; DR3 with the intestinal condition called coeliac disease; and DR2 with an antibody-mediated disease of lung and kidney called Goodpasture's syndrome. The combination of A3 and B14 carries a high relative risk for idiopathic hemochromatosis, a disorder of iron metabolism.

SUGGESTIONS FOR FURTHER READING

Schwartz BD: The major histocompatibility complex and disease susceptibility. In: Wyngaarden JB, Smith LH, Jr, eds: Cecil Textbook of Medicine, 18th ed. Philadelphia: WB Saunders, 1988:1962–68

Simpson E: Function of the MHC. Immunol 1988; Suppl 1:27–30

Strominger JL: Biology of the human histocompatibility leukocyte antigen (HLA) system and a hypothesis regarding the generation of autoimmune diseases. J Clin Invest 1986; 77:1411–15

Trowsdale J: Molecular genetics of the MHC. Immunol 1988; Suppl 1:21–23

Yunis EJ: MHC haplotypes in biology and medicine. AJCP 1988; 89:268–80

CHAPTER 4

Principles of Immune Activation

DETERMINANTS OF IMMUNITY
  Nature of Antigen
  Route of Administration
  Recognition as Foreign
THE NATURE OF RECOGNITION
  The Cell-Surface Receptor
  Exposure to Self Determinants
PRIMARY EXPOSURE TO
ANTIGEN

The Antigen-Presenting Cell
Events in Activation
Differentiation of Daughter Cells
T-Independent Antigens
Time Sequence
SUBSEQUENT EXPOSURE TO
ANTIGEN
  Timing in Secondary Response
  Nature of the Response

An antigen is any material that elicits an immune response in an immunocompetent individual; between exposure to antigen and detectable presence of the immune response lie many variables. This chapter considers primarily the events that influence antibody production. This arm of the immune response has been more fully characterized than the cellular and molecular events of cell-mediated reactions. The principles underlying the two arms of the immune response are similar, but cell populations and mediator substances differ.

DETERMINANTS OF IMMUNITY

NATURE OF ANTIGEN

The general term for material that elicits immunity is **immunogen**. The smallest biochemical unit capable of eliciting an immune response is called an **epitope**. Some epitopes are very small, for example, polypeptides with just a few amino acids or certain simple sugars. Molecular weight of discrete epitopes may be less than 1 kD, but, under most circumstances, very small molecules do not elicit immunity without assistance. Epitopes are characteristically part of a larger molecule with substantial total mass (Fig. 4–1). A small epitope that cannot, as a free-standing molecule, stimulate immune reactivity may become immunogenic if joined to a larger molecule, called a **carrier**. The carrier molecule may or may not have immunogenic properties, but the complex of epitope plus carrier has the mass and configuration sufficient to initiate immune recognition.

Material that stimulates immunity only when complexed with a carrier is called a **hapten;** once antibody has been generated, independent molecules of hapten can combine with immunoglobulin without the need for a carrier. Hapten-carrier models are useful in experimental immunology and also occur in nature. Many small molecules in the environment elicit a primary immune response only if complexed to some protein molecule of the host's body; the small foreign molecule can later provoke immune reactions by itself. Poison ivy reactions are a familiar example of this phenomenon, which is depicted schematically in Figure 12–11.

FIGURE 4–1. In a complex molecule, different portions of the three-dimensional structure may have different antigenic attributes. In the molecule shown, configurations at each of the several lettered locations may interact with individual cells with receptors of the corresponding idiotypes. An epitope frequently exists at several locations in the same molecule, as shown above for B.

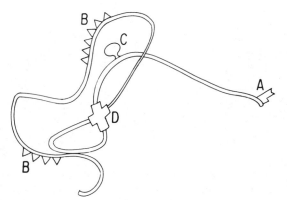

One molecule, several epitopes

Shape and Immunogenicity

Immune events reflect contact between three-dimensional receptors on effector cells and the ligand with an optimally complementary configuration. The three-dimensional shape of a molecule reflects its primary chemical structure and also the intramolecular attractions and repulsions that occur among individual constituents. Altering ionic composition or pH of the medium can alter these intramolecular events and change the shape of a molecule without disrupting its primary structure. Such configurational changes may enhance immunogenicity or, conversely, may abolish effective interaction with immune receptors. Molecules of consistent configuration are more immunogenic than those with shapes easily modified by changing ambient conditions. Proteins and complex polysaccharides are consistently effective immunogens. Most lipids have little or no independent immune activity.

ENHANCING ANTIGENICITY

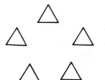

Unmodified antigen

Aggregated

Attached
to particle

Introduced
with adjuvant

FIGURE 4–2. Soluble material elicits an immune response less effectively than particulate material. Immunogenicity of an antigen can be increased by aggregating it into a macromolecular complex; by attaching it to the surface of an inert carrier; or by introducing it with an adjuvant substance that alters local tissue conditions.

ROUTE OF ADMINISTRATION

Material from the antigen-laden environment can enter the host in many ways. Most foreign elements enter the body across intact mucosal surfaces of lungs or alimentary tract, or across epithelium damaged by trauma, infection, or chemical abnormalities. Antigens can be introduced into blood or interstitial fluid by intravenous, intramuscular, or subcutaneous injection.

Within limits, the larger the dose of antigen, the greater the likelihood of initiating an immune response. Because antigen must be presented by accessory cells, and because most cells interact more effectively with particles than with soluble molecules, particulate or cellular antigens are more immunogenic than soluble antigens. Aggregating individual molecules into a complex or attaching them to a particle often makes them more antigenic (Fig. 4–2). Contact with antigen-presenting cells occurs in lymph nodes or in tissues with large populations of resident macrophages or accessory immune cells. Immunization tends to occur more rapidly when antigens enter tissues directly than when they enter the bloodstream.

Immunization can often by enhanced by introducing, along with the antigen, substances that heighten immune responsiveness, called **adjuvants**. Adjuvants act primarily by promoting an inflammatory response, attracting macrophages and lymphocytes to the area, and accelerating the interaction between effector and accessory cells.

RECOGNITION AS FOREIGN

The whole point of immunity is protection against the outside world. Constituents of the mammalian body embody many physical and chemical configurations that are also present in the outside world, in many different combinations and permutations. An example is the presence of identical combinations of simple sugars in certain bacterial cell walls and in the A and B antigens of human red blood cells. Some configurations of plants, animals, or microorganisms are similar or identical to host configurations, but others are very different. In general, the more completely an agent differs from materials in the host, the more likely it is to elicit an immune reaction. To provoke an immune response, materials that differ only modestly from host elements may require a larger dose, more frequent exposure, or a more effective route of administration than the immunizing conditions for massively dissimilar material.

Origin of Antigens

It is useful to classify the relationships between antigenic material and host constituents. Immune responses may develop against antigens arising within the host's own body; this is an abnormal pro-

TABLE 4–1. Types of Immunogens

Source	Descriptive Term for Antigen	Descriptive Term for Immune Response	Example
Material from host	Autoantigen	Autoimmune Autologous	Antibodies to hormones Cellular attack on liver cells
Material from some other human	Alloantigen	Alloimmune Homologous Allogeneic	Antibodies to transfused blood cells Cellular attack on transplanted organ
Material from plants, microorganisms, chemicals, other animals	Heteroantigen	Heterologous Xenogeneic	Antibodies to bovine or porcine insulin Cellular response to poison ivy

cess, called **autoimmunity** or **autologous** response, and the responsible antigen is described as an **autoantigen**. Immunity against material from other members of the host's species is called **alloimmunity** or **homologous** response; the immunity is directed against features that derive from allelic differences, and antigens are considered **alloantigens**. Antigenic material coming from outside the host species can be considered completely foreign; descriptive terms are **heterologous** or **xenogeneic** response, from Greek combining forms meaning "different" and "foreign," respectively. These terms are summarized in Table 4–1.

Mammalian hosts ordinarily mount less intense immune responses against allogeneic material than against the comparable substance from other species. Most antibodies used as laboratory reagents are raised by injecting antigen from one species into host individuals of other species. This can occur spontaneously as well as under laboratory conditions. An example is development of anti-insulin antibodies in humans repeatedly exposed to insulin from pigs or cows, whereas insulin derived from humans is far less immunogenic.

――――――――― **THE NATURE OF RECOGNITION** ―――――――――

Ligand-receptor interactions determine immune recognition, but comparable reactivity of membrane receptors underlies many other physiologic events. The difference between immune events and all others is that the immune receptor of each individual lymphocyte has a configuration optimally reactive with a different external agent; in most physiologic processes, entire populations of cells express the same receptor for a single ligand.

THE CELL-SURFACE RECEPTOR

Both T lymphocytes and B lymphocytes express receptor molecules of unique configuration; the receptors on T and B cells have different structures, but their function is the same. The differences in configuration restrict optimal binding of any one receptor to one specific molecular ligand. Differences in amino acid sequence at defined portions of the receptor polypeptides produce these differences in configuration. The unique amino acid sequence of the receptor is called the **idiotype** of the molecule or, by extension, of the cell that expresses it. The technical meaning of idiotype reflects the antigenic potential of the receptor molecule, but in practical terms, the idiotype can be considered the receptor structure that confers specificity for recognizing a unique antigen.

Differences Between T and B Receptors

B lymphocytes—cells destined for antibody secretion—have molecules of antibody on the exterior of the membrane where they recognize and react with antigen. Antibodies are proteins with a common structure described as **immunoglobulin** (Ig). This structure has four chains arranged as two pairs of identical chains in a longitudinally symmetrical pattern. The larger chains are called **heavy** chains, the smaller ones, **light** chains (Fig. 4–3). The decisive event whereby B-cell precursors differentiate from the pluripotent lymphoid stem cell is rearrangement of chromosomal deoxyribonucleic acid (DNA) in a way that commits each cell to manufacturing Ig of a single idiotype. As the cell matures, it synthesizes the two kinds of polypeptide chains, links them into the four-chain Ig molecule, and then positions Ig molecules on the exterior of the cell membrane. Membrane immunoglobulin (**mIg**) serves as receptor for antigenic activation; it is a sample of the product that will later be secreted.

The T-cell receptor is a molecule with no known site or role apart from the cell membrane. It consists of two idiotypically unique polypeptide chains synthesized after rearrangement of chromosomal

Immunoglobulin Monomer

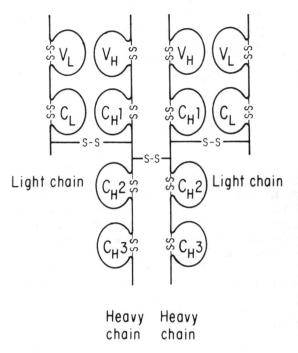

FIGURE 4–3. All immunoglobulins consist of two identical heavy chains and two identical light chains. Each heavy chain is linked, through a disulfide bond, to one light chain; the two heavy chains are linked by one or several disulfide bonds through the hinge region, which gives the molecule longitudinal symmetry.

DNA. Interaction between receptor and antigen is more complicated for T cells than for B cells because T cells have another aspect of the receptor additional to the heterodimer that expresses the idiotype. Common to all T cells in each individual is a recognition molecule that interacts with products of the major histocompatibility complex (MHC). It recognizes only the MHC products of that individual's HLA phenotype, so T cells respond to antigen only if the antigen-presenting cell is of the host's HLA type. Antigen recognition by T cells is said to be **MHC restricted;** antigens presented without MHC products or in combination with the wrong MHC products will not initiate immune activity. (See chapter 3 for more detailed discussion of MHC products and HLA phenotype.)

EXPOSURE TO SELF DETERMINANTS

T and B cells acquire their idiotypes early in fetal life, and subsequent continuous circulation throughout the body brings them into prolonged, intense contact with all antigenic configurations present in the individual. There is every reason to believe that circulating immunocompetent cells exist with idiotypes specific for autologous antigens. During maturation and early circulation, cells that recognize autoantigens experience intense exposure to their target antigens; this exposure suppresses, rather than stimulates, the response they are programmed to make. Failure to display a response for which innate capability exists is called **tolerance**. Early exposure to self constituents produces tolerance to self.

The mechanisms of self tolerance are not fully understood. One possibility is that early exposure to its target material inactivates the cell expressing that idiotype. This theory does not explain how pathologic autoimmune reactivity can later develop, nor does it explain persistence of tolerance in cells produced late in life by the mature individual. A more satisfactory theory is that contact with self determinants stimulates suppressor cells with idiotypes that recognize autoantigens. In this view of tolerance, self-specific suppressor cells respond to continuing antigenic contact by exerting continuous suppressive action against self-specific effector cells that could produce antibodies or autoaggressive cellular activities. These two concepts are not mutually exclusive. Deletion or inactivation of self-responding cells could occur before, or in addition to, ongoing immunosuppression. The consequence of self tolerance is that the normally functioning immune system does not exhibit actions against autologous cells or cell products. Everything else is a potential target for immune activity.

PRIMARY EXPOSURE TO ANTIGEN

Antigens enter the body after eating, drinking, breathing, or touching. Digestive enzymes and enzymes from inflammatory cells degrade complex entities into smaller fragments suitable for metabolic conversions, but further changes are necessary before immune reactions occur. The potential antigen becomes immunogenic only after **processing** and **presentation**.

THE ANTIGEN-PRESENTING CELL

The molecular changes characterized as "antigen processing" are not clearly understood. Most antigens undergo some degree of denaturation or enzymic cleavage, which seems to fragment or to reshape the native molecule for optimum exposure of specific epitopes. (See Fig. 2–1 for a schematic depiction.) Antigen-presenting cells must possess the enzymes necessary to perform these alterations; although macrophages are not the only cells with suitable enzymes, their pro-

ANTIGEN PRESENTATION

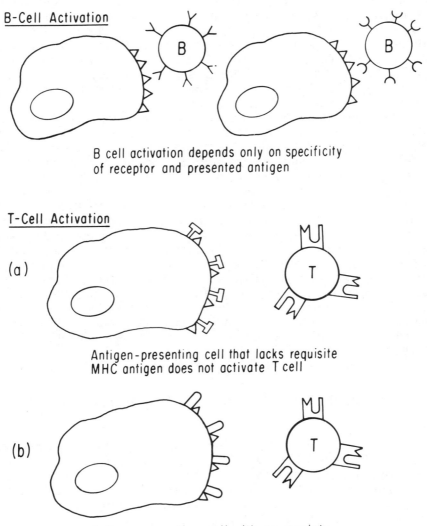

B-Cell Activation

B cell activation depends only on specificity of receptor and presented antigen

T-Cell Activation

(a)

Antigen-presenting cell that lacks requisite MHC antigen does not activate T cell

(b)

Antigen-presenting cell with appropriate MHC antigen does activate T cell

FIGURE 4—4. Activation of a B lymphocyte requires only that the antigen-presenting cell express antigen of the correct epitopic configuration, as shown in the top panel. The cell on the left will recognize and respond to the antigen but the one on the right will not. Activation of T cells requires that the antigen be presented in the context of the appropriate MHC product. In *panel a*, activation will not occur despite complementary epitope and receptor, because the presenting cell expresses the wrong MHC antigen. In *panel B*, the same antigen is presented by a cell with the MHC antigen corresponding to the receptor on the T cell.

pensity to encounter and to engulf foreign material makes cells of this lineage the most numerous antigen-presenting cells. Specialized cells in lymph nodes and skin, respectively called **dendritic** and **Langerhans** cells, present antigens encountered in these tissues. Cells with enzymes that have been inactivated cannot process antigens, although they retain the capacity to present antigen that is processed elsewhere. Some macromolecules are immunogenic without processing; presumably their epitopes are sufficiently accessible and concentrated that molecular reorganization or fragmentation is unnecessary.

Interactions with Receptors

Whether processed or effective in an unprocessed state, antigen stimulates effector cells only when presented on a cell surface. For stimulating B lymphocytes, the only requirement is arraying the antigenic epitopes on the surface of the antigen-presenting cell; T lymphocytes require the presenting cell to contribute MHC products as well. The T-cell receptor has two aspects. The idiotypic constituent recognizes the epitope, whereas the part of the receptor complex present on all T cells is what interacts with MHC material. Helper T cells—those positive for the CD4 antigen—require the antigen-presenting cell to express class II MHC products (Fig. 4–4). Macrophages, along with dendritic and Langerhans cells, are the major antigen-presenting cells and consistently express MHC class II products. B cells also express class II products. B lymphocytes are thought to assist in presenting antigen to some populations of helper cells; they probably perform some processing activity as well, but under standard immunizing conditions, B cells more often respond to antigen than present it.

Individual T and B lymphocytes have many copies of the receptor molecule on their exteriors. Effective antigen exposure requires numerous copies of epitope to engage simultaneously with numerous copies of receptor. When a binding substance reacts simultaneously with contiguous molecules, the receptor is said to be **crosslinked.** The stimulus to immune activation is crosslinking of receptor molecules (Fig. 4–5).

EVENTS IN ACTIVATION

Cells that have not yet encountered their antigen are called **virgin** or **resting** lymphocytes. Both T cells and B cells recirculate continuously. Constant circulation brings idiotypically specific cells into contact with antigen-presenting cells at many different sites. Idiotypic specificity develops as a random, independent genetic event in individual cells, and both T cells and B cells develop idiotypes of the same

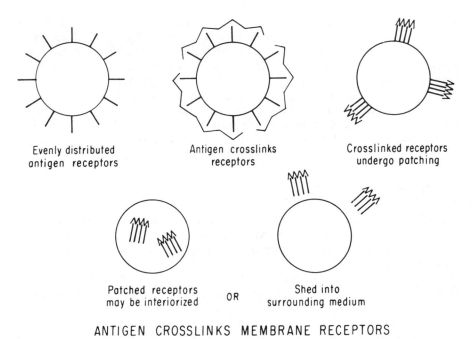

Evenly distributed
antigen receptors

Antigen crosslinks
receptors

Crosslinked receptors
undergo patching

Patched receptors
may be interiorized

OR

Shed into
surrounding medium

ANTIGEN CROSSLINKS MEMBRANE RECEPTORS

FIGURE 4–5. On a resting cell, receptors are distributed throughout the membrane. Cross-linking brings them together into aggregates, a process called patching. The patched antigen-receptor complexes are often incorporated into the cell cytoplasm, but may sometimes be shed into the surrounding medium as non-reactive macromolecular complexes.

specificities. Activation of most B cells requires simultaneous activation of helper T cells specific for the same epitope. T-cell responses do not require activation of B cells.

Stimulation of membrane receptors **activates** the virgin lymphocyte; the most conspicuous evidence of activation is a change in appearance called **lymphoblast transformation**. Lymphoblasts are larger than resting lymphocytes, owing primarily to enlargement of the nucleus where new DNA is synthesized preparatory to division into daughter cells. Lymphoblasts are recognized morphologically by their size and nuclear appearance and functionally by the metabolic activity that incorporates the bases necessary to construct new DNA. Contact with antigen is the physiologic stimulus to lymphoblast transformation, but other events can induce the same functional change.

Other Receptors

In addition to antigen-specific receptors, both T and B cells have membrane receptors for molecules that induce mitosis, the process of

WAYS TO CROSSLINK RECEPTORS

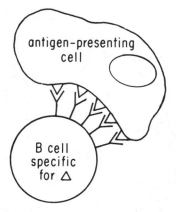

Receptors are crosslinked
by presented antigen

Receptors are crosslinked
by antibody to receptor
idiotype

FIGURE 4–6. Crosslinking of the idiotypically specific receptors on a cell membrane can occur through combination with suitably presented antigen, or through interaction with antibody reactive against the receptor molecules. The antibody may be directed against the idiotypic part of the molecule (anti-idiotype antibody) or against structural features of the receptor.

cell division. Non-antigens that combine with receptors to induce mitosis are called **mitogens**. Mitogens induce lymphoblast transformation and cellular division but do not promote production of antibodies or cytokines. Cells also can be activated by antibody directed against the antigen-specific receptor molecules. Antibodies that recognize the unique aspects of receptor molecules are called **anti-idiotype** antibodies. Other antibodies may react with structural elements common to receptor molecules of various specificities. Crosslinking by anti-idiotype or antistructural antibodies is a useful laboratory tool to induce transformation and cellular respones (Fig. 4–6). It is thought that anti-idiotype antibodies develop under physiologic conditions and play an important role in regulating immune activity.

After stimulation, the activated cell may express a different set of receptor molecules on the membrane from those present in the resting state. These receptors do not affect idiotype specificity; their function is to recognize various mediator molecules. Expression of new receptors enables the cell to respond to changing environmental conditions (Fig. 4–7). The presence of antigen provokes changes in the environment through effects on antigen-presenting cells and inflammatory cells as well as on immune cells. Environmental conditions change, the nature and number of mediator substances change, and the responsive capacities of the stimulated cell change.

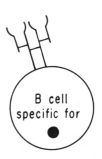
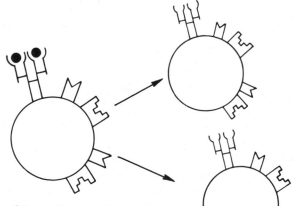

Unstimulated

Stimulation produces
daughter cells with
receptors on membrane

ANTIGEN-STIMULATED B CELLS
EXPRESS RECEPTORS FOR VARIOUS MEDIATORS

FIGURE 4—7. Activation causes the clonal progeny to synthesize molecules not produced by the resting cell. Membrane receptors appear that enable the activated cells to interact with mediators that would have no effect on unstimulated cells.

DIFFERENTIATION OF
DAUGHTER CELLS

Lymphoblast transformation is the first in a series of steps leading to **clonal expansion**. Successive mitotic divisions produce a population of genetically identical activated cells specific for the same initiating antigen. A variety of growth and differentiation factors modulate these steps; the presence of antigen induces macrophages and other lymphocytes to release these mediators. Macrophages produce the broadly reactive mediator, IL-1 (see page 107); T cells of the CD4 phenotype elaborate products that enhance growth, multiplication, and differentiation of B cells and of other T cells (see pages 109—111). IL-1 production occurs without regard to antigenic specificity, but helper T cells become active only after recognizing specific antigen.

The antigen-stimulated B cell evolves into antibody-producing plasma cells under the influence of growth-promoting factors generated by helper T cells that have recognized the same antigen that activates the B cell. Except for those antigens described as **T-indepen-**

dent (see later section in this chapter), antibody production occurs only if activated B cells receive help from comparably stimulated T cells. Lymphokines from the T cell bind to receptors newly expressed on the activated B cell. These provoke further changes that induce cell division, followed by differentiation into cells capable of synthesizing and secreting huge numbers of antibody molecules.

Types of Response

All members of a clone are genetically identical, but they may encounter different concentrations of mediators that influence separate aspects of multiplication and differentiation. This is shown schematically in Figure 4–8. Cells that become plasma cells lose the capacity to multiply. They survive for only a few days, generating many thousands of specific antibody molecules and secreting them into the body

HOW MEMBERS OF A CLONE DIFFERENTIATE

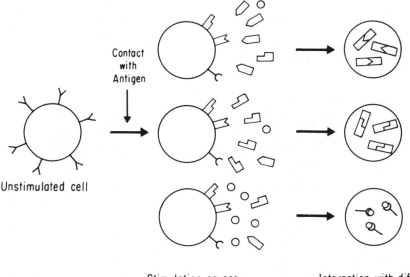

Contact
with
Antigen

Unstimulated cell

Stimulation causes
daughter cells to
express new receptors

Interaction with different
mediators stimulates
different events in
initially identical cells

FIGURE 4–8. Following activation, genetically identical clonal progeny may experience contact with numerous different mediators. As individual daughter cells encounter unique environmental conditions, they may differentiate along disparate functional lines. The genetic constitution is common to all members of the clone, but the way each cell expresses its genetic potential is influenced by materials in the environment.

fluids. Multiplying cells that do not evolve into plasma cells may cease dividing and resume the appearance of the unstimulated cell, but they do not return to the virgin state. They retain the activated state induced by antigen contact and are called **memory** cells. Memory cells survive and circulate for months or years in a state of suspended animation; exposure to only small amounts of antigen stimulates them to resume activity.

Helper T cells secrete mediator products that influence not only B cells but also the T lymphocytes active in several cell-mediated immune events, notably cytotoxicity and delayed hypersensitivity (see pages 114–119). T-cell activities are thus essential for production of most antibodies and for most manifestations of cell-mediated immu-

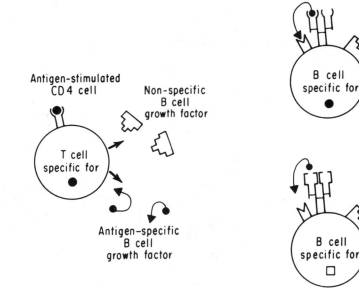

NON-SPECIFIC GROWTH FACTORS
VS.
ANTIGEN-SPECIFIC GROWTH FACTORS

FIGURE 4–9. Antigen-stimulated T cells secrete many different lymphokines. Some of these are capable of interacting only with cells that recognize the same antigen; others are broadly effective for any cell that has a receptor for the lymphokine molecule. Both the target B cells shown above have receptors for the non-specific growth factor, but only the upper cell can respond to the growth factor that requires antigenic identity with the stimulated T cell.

nity. Some of the growth- and differentiation-promoting mediators that antigenically specific T cells produce will act only on effector cells specific for the same antigen; others are not antigen-restricted and react with any cell possessing receptors for that mediator molecule (Fig. 4–9). By inducing formation of these non-restricted mediators, stimulation by one antigen or organism can affect the reactivity of cells specific for other antigens. In addition, many T-cell products enhance the functions of macrophages, which never express antigenic selectivity.

T-INDEPENDENT ANTIGENS

Certain antigens elicit antibody formation without conspicuous participation of T cells. Antigens characterized by a well-defined epitope in multiple, closely repeated copies can stimulate target B cells through crosslinking alone, inducing transformation, multiplication, and plasma-cell differentiation without the usually identified T-cell mediators. Such antigens are called **T independent**. Polysaccharide antigens of bacterial cell walls are the most notable examples and are thought to affect B lymphocytes through specialized antigen-presenting cells that are particularly numerous in the spleen. T-independent antigens never provoke cell-mediated immunity, and they elicit antibodies only of restricted Ig characteristics. T-cell factors appear to be necessary for production of other antibody classes and for evolution of memory cells.

TIME SEQUENCE

Between the first encounter with antigen and the appearance of detectable antibody or cell-mediated activity, days or weeks may elapse. The nature and dose of the antigen, the route of administration, and the host's overall metabolic state influence the rate of immunization, but a minimum of several days is necessary.

The earliest antibody class to appear is immunoglobulin M (IgM, see chapter 6), followed in days or weeks by IgG antibody, which has the same idiotype but different structural features. IgM production tapers off promptly if the antigen disappears, but IgG production persists somewhat longer. The antibody sequence in primary immunization is: early appearance of IgM, later appearance of IgG, subsequent disappearance of IgM, and fairly prolonged manufacture of IgG (Fig. 4–10). All protein molecules are subject to enzymic degradation. Individual antibody molecules survive only for several weeks. Unless plasma cells continue to produce new molecules, antibody of a particular specificity will disappear from body fluids after all the molecules with that idiotype have been degraded.

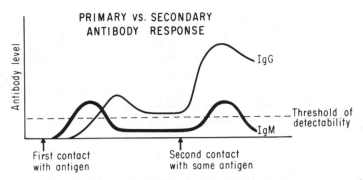

FIGURE 4–10. Production of IgM follows the same time sequence after primary immunization and after all subsequent contacts with the antigen. Establishment of IgG-producing cells engenders memory. In the primary response, substantial time elapses between antigenic contact and appearance of IgG, but subsequent contact with the same antigen elicits rapid increase in antibodies of this class.

SUBSEQUENT EXPOSURE TO ANTIGEN

Immune events that follow the host's first exposure to an antigen are the **primary immune response,** which usually generates memory cells in addition to the measurable immune products. Later contact between memory cells and additional examples of antigen produces a **secondary** or **anamnestic** immune response. "Anamnestic" reflects the same linguistic origin as "amnesia"; it means that there has not been forgetting.

TIMING IN SECONDARY RESPONSE

The anamnestic response becomes apparent more rapidly than the primary response. Whereas days, weeks, or even months may pass before measurable antibody develops in a primary response, second and subsequent exposures boost antibody levels in a matter of hours. Several factors contribute to this acceleration. Because memory cells have already undergone some of the intracellular events necessary for immune activity, fewer differentiating events are needed after repeated antigen contact. In addition, previous clonal expansion has generated a larger number of cells capable of recognizing the antigen; following activation of memory cells, geometric expansion of each available cell rapidly generates effective numbers of plasma cells. Figure 4–10 contrasts antibody levels in the primary and the anamnestic immune responses.

Obvious benefits accrue from the rapidity of anamnestic reactions. Once the host has immune memory for a pathogenic organism, later exposures can provoke anamnestic protection that attacks the organism before it can cause full-blown disease. Often, the initial encounter with an organism causes clinical disease, from which the host recovers after mobilizing inflammatory defense and an effective primary immune response. With elimination of the organism, immune activity becomes quiescent, but if the organism is prevalent in the environment, the host will encounter it again and again. These later exposures do not cause disease; they promote anamnestic responses that prevent the organism from establishing itself. For many organisms, artificial immunization is possible, so that the primary encounter need not be clinical illness (see chapter 9).

NATURE OF THE RESPONSE

Antibody molecules can belong to any of five classes of immunoglobulin. These will be discussed in detail in chapter 6, but the distinction between IgG and IgM must be mentioned briefly here. IgM is the first antibody class that a newly stimulated B cell produces. In most T-dependent reactions, lymphokines induce some daughter cells to switch to IgG production, and some of these become memory cells. Memory cells that direct IgM production seem not to develop. Secondary contact with antigen can stimulate memory cells to prompt IgG production, but there is no memory mechanism for IgM. In second and subsequent exposures, the time between antigen contact and the detectable presence of IgM is as long as it was for the primary event. Whereas IgM precedes IgG by days or weeks in the primary immune response, anamnestic responses can be identified through the appearance, in 12 to 24 hours, of rising IgG levels. T-independent antigens cannot evoke anamnestic responses because they elicit the production only of IgM.

Accelerated immune events occur for at least some cell-mediated reactions (see discussion of the tuberculin reaction, pages 116–117), but the mechanisms are less clearly understood. Effector cells responsible for the "delayed hypersensitivity" type of cell-mediated immunity (see pages 114–116) exhibit accelerated activity after previous antigenic exposure, but memory-associated changes in these cells have not been precisely characterized.

SUGGESTIONS FOR FURTHER READING

Abbas AK: A reassessment of the mechanisms of antigen-specific T-cell dependent B-cell activation. Immunol Today 1988; 9:89–94

Butcher EC: The regulation of lymphocyte traffic. Curr Topics Microbiol Immunol 1986; 128:85–122

Fauci AS, moderator: Immunomodulators in clinical medicine. Ann Int Med 1987; 106:421–33

Feldman M: Lymphocyte interactions and their mediators. In: Marchalonis JJ, ed: The Lymphocyte: Structure and Function, 2nd ed. New York: Marcel Dekker, 1988: 121–42

Manger B, Imboden J, Weiss A: Role of the T3/T-cell antigen receptor complex in T-cell activation. In: Mak TW, ed: The T-Cell Receptors. Plenum, New York, 1988:133–149

Novotny J, Handschumacher M, Bruccoleri RE: Protein antigenicity: A static surface property. Immunol Today 1987; 8:26–31

Vitetta ES, Bossie A, Fernandez-Botran R, et al: Interaction and activation of antigen-specific T and B cells. Immunol Rev 1987; 99:193–239

CHAPTER 5

Lymphocyte Populations

The rich diversity of lymphocyte populations is a relatively new concept in cell biology. Neutrophils and macrophages have been studied since the introduction of the microscope, but lymphocytes remained an enigma long after inflammatory cells were clearly characterized. Until the 1950s, little more was known about these small, round cells than their association with immune events and with chronic inflammation. The past 30 years have disclosed a diversity of lymphocyte functions and populations far greater than those of inflammatory cells.

WAYS TO IDENTIFY CELLS

To understand what cells are doing, it is essential to identify them. Increasingly discriminating methods of examination can un-

63

WAYS TO IDENTIFY CELLS

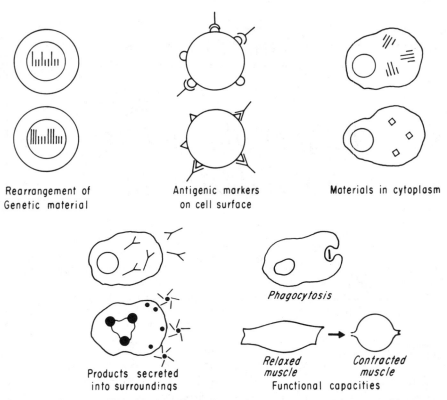

Rearrangement of
Genetic material

Antigenic markers
on cell surface

Materials in cytoplasm

Products secreted
into surroundings

Phagocytosis

*Relaxed
muscle*

*Contracted
muscle*

Functional capacities

FIGURE 5–1. Different identification techniques are useful in different circumstances. Genetic probes illuminate differences in DNA sequence, the most fundamental difference between cells. Consequences of genetic constitution include: antigenically distinctive molecules on the cell surface, nature and location of cytoplasmic constituents, composition and volume of secreted products, and functional activities that can be observed and measured.

cover distinguishing features in seemingly similar tissues, cells, or molecules. Some of these are illustrated in Figure 5–1.

STRUCTURE AND FUNCTION

The morphology, or appearance, of a cell or tissue is the simplest means of identification. With light microscopic examination, the location and number of lymphocytes can be determined in blood and tissue. Lymphocytes differ sufficiently from plasma cells in size, shape, and staining characteristics that these populations can be identified easily. Resting lymphocytes can be differentiated from lymphoblasts by their light microscopic appearance. Other microscopic techniques include transmission electron microscopy, which reveals details of intracellular structures, and scanning electron microscopy, which casts surface characteristics into sharp relief.

Important for studying function is the ability to isolate individual cells or purified cell populations and to propagate them in cell culture. Activity can be determined by examining which materials the cells remove from the culture medium and what substances they secrete. Mitotic activity in transformed immunoblasts, for example, is identified by uptake of radiolabeled DNA precursors; production of lymphokine or antibody is documented by harvesting these proteins from the supernatant fluid. Introducing agents that selectively inhibit or enhance metabolic steps allows identification of cells with differing intracellular processes. Study of viable cells permits delineation of dynamic events like growth, shape changes, motility, and responses to environmental agents.

IMMUNOLOGIC MARKERS

Antigen-antibody reactions reveal much about the nature and location of cell constituents. The critical problem is to develop antibodies that react specifically and exclusively with the desired target. Information derived from immune reactions is only as good as the identification and specificity of the antibody involved. Early experimenters introduced whole serum or other complex materials into a rabbit, guinea pig, or other immunologically responsive host and then attempted to purify the polyspecific serum by manipulation to remove unwanted reactivities. Current immunization protocols exploit highly purified antigens and sophisticated techniques to separate and to concentrate the resulting antibodies.

Monoclonal antibodies have expanded the scope of immunologic study. Monoclonal antibodies derive from individual immunoglobulin-producing cells stimulated to multiply indefinitely in cell culture. The multiplying cell is a hybrid of two very different initial cells: a B lymphocyte activated to produce a specific antibody, and a neoplastic cell capable of multiplying indefinitely in culture conditions. The tedious aspect of developing monoclonal antibodies is testing vast numbers of individual cell cultures to determine antibody specificity. Because a single-cell clone produces immunoglobulin of a single idiotype, any harvested antibody will be exquisitely specific. Once the specificity has been shown to recognize a desired antigen, it is relatively easy to prepare large quantities of antibody with consistent behavioral properties. Much of our current knowledge about surface antigens has come from studies with monoclonal antibodies. Antibodies also can be used to identify and to localize materials within the cell.

CLUSTERS OF DIFFERENTIATION

Innovative manipulation of antigen-antibody reactions has allowed detailed characterization of cell surfaces at different phases of maturation. As each group of workers developed its own system of letters and numbers to report newly discovered antigens, there arose enormous potential for terminologic chaos. In 1980, international collaboration through workshops on human leukocyte differentiation antigens began to organize mountains of data and rationalize seemingly unrelated observations. The dedication of imaginative scientists has combined with computerized analyses to generate a nomenclature for cell-surface antigens of all white-cell lines.

The cell-surface attributes identified primarily by monoclonal antibodies are called **clusters of differentiation** or **cluster determinants,** abbreviated **CD.** Well-characterized CDs receive numbers; as with the HLA nomenclature, the letter "w" precedes a number until the specificity is fully characterized. Cluster determinant antigens are molecules of many different structures and cell origins, and classification into unifying categories has been impossible. Instead of assigning dedicated alphanumerics to different cell lines or receptor functions, the workshops have assigned sequential numbers to characteristics as they are identified. Antigens receive a noncommittal designation like CD1 or CD10 or CDw26; correlation of antigens with different cell lines or different developmental phases cannot be inferred from the number. Many characteristics that received CD numbers were already current in scientific parlance by one or more other names. Usage continues non-standardized, but CD terminology is assuming increasing prominence. Table 5–1 summarizes CD antigens and their correlation with other cellular features.

MOLECULAR TECHNIQUES

Most molecules subjected to immunologic investigation are proteins or related complex structures, such as nucleoproteins. Proteins consist of amino acids joined through peptide bonds. It is possible to exploit the known behavioral characteristics of certain polypeptide sequences or associated chemical groups or side-chain linkages to characterize the molecules in which they appear. Chemical reactions and physical events like precipitation, migration through electrical fields, or crystallization have been useful for generations. An increasingly useful analytic tool is selective action of enzymes, which cleave only specific peptide bonds between specific amino acids. Certain enzymes act only on peptide bonds that include some single amino acid. If that amino acid appears many times in a polypeptide, the enzyme will divide the molecule into that number of fragments; if the amino acid is present only once or twice, treating the protein with enzyme

TABLE 5-1. Assignment of CD Numbers*

CD No.	Other Names	Distribution	Function, If Known
1	T6, Thy	Thymocytes; Langerhans cells	
2	T11	Thymocytes; T cells	Sheep RBC receptor
3	T3, TiT3 complex	Late thymocytes; T cells	Antigen receptor for T cells
4	T4	Helper subset of T cells	Assists in MHC-II recognition
5	T1	T cells; follicular B cells	
6	T12	T cells; some B cells	
7		Thymocytes; subset of T cells	Receptor for Fc-mu
8	T8	Suppressor subset of T cells	Assists in MHC-I recognition
9	p24	Monocytes; non-T, non-B ALL; platelets	
10	CALLA	1% of normal marrow cells; earliest T and B precursors; kidney cells	
11a	LFA-1	All leukocytes	Alpha chain of LFA-1 Participates in cellular adhesion
11b	Mac-1, CR3	Granulocytes; monocytes; NK cells	Receptor for C3bi
12–17		Granulocytes and/or monocytes; 16 is on NK cells	CD16 is low-affinity receptor for Fc-gamma
18	LFA-1	All leukocytes	Beta chain of LFA-1
19–24	21 is CR 2	B cells; 20, 21 and 24 on dendritic cells	21 is receptor for C3d, EBV
25	Tac	Activated T cells; ? activated B cells	Receptor for IL-2
w32		Granulocytes; monocytes; B cells; platelets	Receptor for Fc-gamma
35	CR 1	B cells; granulocytes; monocytes, dendritic cells	Receptor for C3b
45	LCA, T200	All leukocytes	Product of a structural gene common to leukocytes, absent from non-hematopoietic cells
45 R	Restricted T200	B cells; subsets of T cells; granulocytes; monocytes	High MW forms of gene product

*Adapted from McMichael, AJ, ed: *Leucocyte Typing III: White Cell Differentiation Antigens.* Oxford University Press, Oxford, 1987 (Proceedings of 3rd International Workshop and Conference on Human Leucocyte Differentiation Antigens).

generates only a few, fairly large fragments; if that amino acid is not present, enzyme treatment will not affect the protein. With well-characterized enzymes and suitable techniques to analyze the resulting fragments, the precise structure of individual proteins can be determined. Each constituent amino acid need not be identified; generating fragments of predictable behavior often provides adequate analytic information.

Significance of Paired Nucleotides

Enzymes with predictable activity against deoxyribonucleic acid (DNA) are also available; with techniques to isolate and to manipulate DNA, it has become possible to examine the DNA sequences that constitute individual genes. The enzymes, called **restriction endonucleases** or just **restriction enzymes,** target specific sequences within nuclear DNA; the resulting fragments, called **restriction fragments,** can be analyzed in several ways. The most ingenious exploit the fact that nucleic acids are double-stranded molecules that reproduce themselves by pairing restricted, predictable combinations of purines and pyrimidines in rigidly prescribed complementary relationships. Reagent sequences of known nucleotide composition can be exposed to restriction fragments; because the constituent elements pair only with complementary structures, the structure of the restriction fragments can be inferred from the structure of the known sequences with which they combine. The known sequences are called **gene probes**.

Differences of one or a few nucleotides in a gene can produce differences in protein structure that may exert profound physiologic effects. Even if the full nucleotide sequence in a gene is not identified, the existence of variant sequences can be demonstrated by observing which gene probes match with which restriction fragments. Sequence differences in genetic material at a single locus are called **restriction fragment length polymorphisms (RFLP)**. Gene probe examination has demonstrated substantial rearrangements in sequence when chromosomal segments that direct manufacturing processes switch from potential to activated function. Cells destined to synthesize different protein products display differences in DNA sequence at the relevant loci.

─────── DEVELOPMENT OF LYMPHOCYTES ───────

THE HEMATOPOIETIC STEM CELL

All cells of marrow origin are thought to derive from a single progenitor; irreversible developmental changes in progeny of this multipotential cell direct evolution into erythrocyte, platelet, granulo-

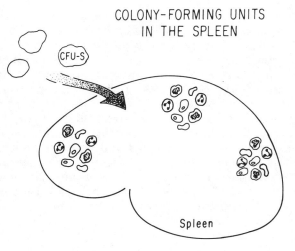

COLONY-FORMING UNITS
IN THE SPLEEN

FIGURE 5-2. The multi-potential capacity of individual stem cells (see Fig. 1-1) is shown when single cells introduced into the spleen of an irradiated experimental animal develop into colonies that contain many different cell types. Cells capable of establishing these multicellular splenic colonies are called CFU-S, which stands for *colony-forming units (spleen)*.

cyte/macrophage, and lymphocyte lines. Multipotential capacity of single cells has been demonstrated by injecting cells from a normal rat into a genetically identical rat whose bone marrow has been destroyed by irradiation. After a brief period, injected cells die off, but a few cells lodge in the spleen and begin producing hematopoietic colonies. After a period of cell division, the splenic colonies restore not only the circulating blood cells but also the immune system. Stem cells capable of differentiation into all cell lines are called colony-forming units (spleen), abbreviated **CFU-S** (Fig. 5-2). Human hematopoietic stem cells can be harvested from marrow or circulating blood for reconstitution of blood and immune systems in patients treated for malignant diseases. The differentiated daughter cells acquire properties unique for each hematopoietic cell line. Erythroid precursors grow in bursts rather than colonies and are called erythroid burst-forming units **(BFU-E);** megakaryocyte precursors are called **CFU-M;** the partially differentiated cell with granulocyte and monocyte potential is the **CFU-GM.** No single lymphoid cell has been cultured that has simultaneous T- and B-cell offspring, but it is clear that all lymphocytes derive from a common precursor.

EARLY LYMPHOID FEATURES

The idiotypically unique receptor molecules that typify lymphocytes are synthesized through the action of genes at known locations. Cells that have undergone DNA rearrangement at these sites are the earliest differentiated forms in each cell line. Rearrangement of chromosome 14 characterizes B-cell precursors; of chromosome 7 or 14,

T-cell precursors. Some cells with lymphocyte morphology and function lack identifiable membrane receptors for specific antigens. Cells called **NK cells** (see later section) and described as **large granular lymphocytes** do not have idiotypic specificity; nonetheless, they display some of the genetic rearrangements characteristic of T cells and are thought to be descended from the common lymphoid precursor.

Another feature of very early lymphoid differentiation is presence of the nuclear enzyme **terminal deoxynucleotidyl transferase (TdT),** which facilitates genetic rearrangements associated with synthesis of surface receptors. Terminal deoxynucleotidyl transferase disappears as cells become more mature, but it persists longer in developing T cells than in B cells. By the time cells display distinctive B-cell features, TdT has usually disappeared. By contrast, early T cells retain TdT until the last stages of full functional capability.

Ia Antigens

Very early in differentiation, class II major histocompatibility complex (MHC) products are present on the lymphocyte membrane. Confusing terminology applies to these surface properties, which were detected and studied long before the concept of class II MHC products was developed. The original observations were on mice. In mice, the region analogous to the MHC contains what is called the I region, which influences immune responsiveness; products of the I-region genes are called **Ia antigens**. The mouse I region is analogous to the human D region. The D-active antigens observed on human macrophages and B cells but not on mature T cells were called Ia antigens. B cells and macrophages are positive for Ia antigens. Mature T cells lack Ia, but undifferentiated lymphoid cells that lack T-cell characteristics do express Ia. Other hematopoietic lines are Ia negative. In current terminology, Ia activity correlates with expression of DR antigens.

——— DEVELOPMENT OF T LYMPHOCYTES ———

THE THYMUS

The thymus is a lobulated mass of lymphoid tissue in the upper anterior portion of the chest. At birth it weighs 12 to 15 grams, proportionately very large in the small body of the newborn; its largest absolute weight, 30 to 40 grams, is achieved just before puberty. The thymus is most active during fetal and early childhood development, when immunologic activity is expanding. Developing lymphocytes assume the properties of T cells as they pass through the thymus; this generates enough committed precursor cells that T-cell levels can be maintained for life, long after the organ disappears.

The outer portion of the thymus, the **cortex,** contains densely packed lymphocytes undergoing continuous cell division and proliferation. Most cortical lymphocytes survive only a short time and disintegrate before attaining maturity. Uncommitted cells enter the thymus at the outermost layer of cortex; cells of increasing maturity are seen toward the interior. In the inner part of the thymus, the **medulla,** lymphocytes are not proliferating; the cells are less densely packed and they experience intimate contact with epithelial cells. These epithelial cells secrete substances, collectively designated **thymosins,** that promote cellular differentiation. Cells traverse the thymus only once, spending 2 to 3 days in the thymus before emerging as immunocompetent cells. Cells within the thymus are called **thymocytes** and are, by definition, not fully mature. Fully instructed cells that have left the thymus are described as **peripheral T cells.** Figure 5–3 summarizes these relationships.

T CELLS IN THE THYMUS

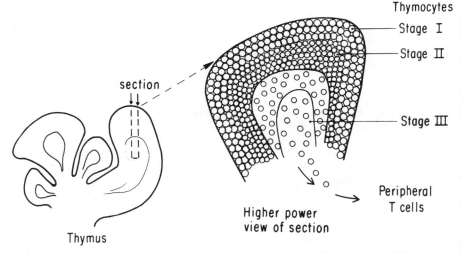

FIGURE 5–3. Each lobule of the thymus consists of a highly cellular outer *cortex* and an inner *medulla* in which cells are less densely concentrated. Cells enter the thymus at the periphery, and immediately acquire T-cell properties. Differentiation increases as the cells move toward the center. Stage II thymocytes, in the middle and inner cortex, exhibit tremendous proliferation and subsequent destruction. Cells that enter the medulla as Stage III thymocytes undergo full differentiation and emerge as immunocompetent peripheral T lymphocytes.

TABLE 5–2. Antigens of T Lymphocytes

All these surface molecules are glycoproteins, identifiable by native polyclonal antibodies or monoclonal antibodies or both

Antigen	T-cell Population	Non-T Cells Sharing Antigen	Comments
T1 (CD5)	All T cells, beginning at late cortical thymocyte	A B-cell subset	A pan-T marker; undergoes modulation after antigen binding
T3 (CD3)	Maturing thymocytes, as reciprocal T4/T8 subsets differentiate. Stronger on peripheral than thymic cells	None	A non-polymorphic part of the antigen receptor Approximately 30–40,000 on cell surface
Ti (CD3)	Same as T3	None	Contains variable region of antigen receptor A 90 kD MW heterodimer non-covalently linked to T3 Approximately 30–40,000 on cell surface
T4 (CD4)	Stage II and III thymocytes and 55–70% of peripheral T cells (those with helper-inducer function)	Some monocytes	Early medullary thymocytes have both T4 and T8; immunocompetent stage III and peripheral T cells have one or the other
T6 (CD1)	Stage II thymocytes, those with both T4 and T8	Langerhans cell of epidermis	Molecule is associated with β2-microglobulin Disappears with evolving immunocompetence
T8 (CD8)	Stage II and III thymocytes and 25–40% of peripheral T cells	None	As for T4

TABLE 5—2. Antigens of T Lymphocytes—*Continued*

All these surface molecules are glycoproteins, identifiable by native polyclonal antibodies or monoclonal antibodies or both

Antigen	T-cell Population	Non-T Cells Sharing Antigen	Comments
T9*	Stage I thymocytes; activated mature T4 and T8 cells	Bone marrow stem cells; many actively multiplying cells of various types	This is the transferrin receptor
T10 (CD38)	Stage I,II,III thymocytes but not peripheral cells	Bone marrow cells, immature B cells, plasma cells, most large granular lymphocytes	
T11 (CD2)	Earliest T-specific antigen, identifies stage I thymocytes and persists through full maturation.	None	Receptor for rosetting with sheep red cells
Tac (CD25)	Activated T4 or T8 cells	Activated B cells respond to IL-2, probably through Tac or very similar molecule	This is the receptor for IL-2. As CD3 expression modulates, IL-2 receptor expression increases reciprocally.

*No CD number assigned. Molecule is present on activated and proliferating cells of many different lineages.

ACQUISITION OF SURFACE ANTIGENS

As cells progress through the thymus, they acquire membrane antigens, some of which persist while others disappear. It is not clear what influences immature cells to express these changing characteristics; epithelial cells and resident macrophages are thought to exert these developmental influences. Some of these surface molecules participate in later immunologic interactions, but some have no discernible function.

The first membrane feature to develop identifies immature thymocytes in the outermost cortex and remains as a thymus-associated feature through every maturational stage, including circulating peripheral cells. This molecule—variously called the T11 antigen, the E-rosette receptor, or CD2—was the first cytologic feature found to distinguish T cells from B cells. The original observation was that cells possessing this antigen form rosettes of adherent cells when they are incubated with sheep red blood cells. Until more sophisticated tests became available, the only way to identify T cells in a blood sample was to induce rosettes by incubating the lymphocytes with sheep cells. The CD2 (T11) molecule is now seen as a receptor for intercellular communication of several kinds (see pages 112–113).

Developmental Features

Cells become more mature as they move centripetally through the thymus. The outer cortex contains about 10 to 20 percent of all thymocytes, considered to be at stage I. About 70 percent of the thymocytes are stage II, in the inner cortex. This is where seemingly inefficient multiplication and destruction are most prominent. Stage III cells, located in the medulla, constitute 10 to 20 percent of thymocytes; here they achieve complete differentiation and immune maturation. The peripheral T cell emerges from the thymus capable of recognizing antigen and performing programmed responses to antigen contact.

Various numbers have been assigned to the antigens of thymocytes and T lymphocytes. The numbers from 1 to 11 shown in Table 5–2 are one terminology that has enjoyed widespread but not universal acceptance. Table 5–2 describes the antigens, and Table 5–3 correlates the appearance and disappearance of these membrane features with the developmental stage of the T cell.

THE T-CELL RECEPTOR

T lymphocytes recognize their specific antigens through the complex membrane protein called the **T-cell receptor,** which has two parts. One part, Ti, is idiotypically unique for the specific antigen. The other, T3, is present on all T cells and probably conveys to the cell interior the message that Ti has combined with antigen. This receptor complex is depicted in Figure 5–4. Ti consists of two dissimilar chains, designated alpha and beta. The gene for alpha-chain manufacture resides on chromosome 14, at a site unrelated to that for the immunoglobulin heavy chain; the beta-chain site is on chro-

TABLE 5–3. Stages of T-Lymphocyte Maturation and Differentiation

	Location	% of Total	Antigens Present	Antigens Lost
Thymocytes				
Stage I	Outer cortex	10–20% of thymocytes	11, 10, 9	
Stage II	Inner cortex	Approximately 70% of thymocytes	11, 10, 6, 1 (weak), both 4 _and_ 8	9
Stage III	Medulla	10–20% of thymocytes	11, 10, 1 (strong), either 4 _or_ 8, T3-Ti (weak)	6
Peripheral T-Cells				
Unstimulated	Blood, lymph tissues	Approximately 70% of blood lymphocytes	11, 1, 4 _or_ 8 T3-Ti (strong)	10
Activated	Mostly tissues, some in fluids	Not applicable	4 _or_ 8 (enhanced), 11, Tac, Ia; 9 reappears	T3-Ti, 1

mosome 7. The idiotypically specific amino acid sequence results from rearrangement, in each individual cell, of the gene sequences on chromosomes 7 and 14 (see pages 98–101). The idiotypically specific configuration can, under experimental and physiologic conditions, elicit antibodies specific for the individual molecules that characterize individual T cells.

Two Parts of Receptor

T cells recognize antigen only when the presenting cell offers class I or Class II MHC products in association with the antigen. Recognition of the MHC products depends upon a receptor molecule closely associated with the Ti heterodimer. This portion of the receptor complex consists of three polypeptide chains synthesized independently of the Ti polypeptides. All T cells in an individual have the same molecular configuration in this part of the receptor complex. Stage III

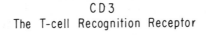

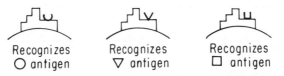

FIGURE 5–4. Immuno-competent T cells are identified by the presence of CD3, the membrane molecule that recognizes antigen. CD3 consists of 5 chains, of which 3 are common to all T cells of an individual. This portion, sometimes called T3, interacts with the MHC products of the antigen-presenting cell. The other two chains, which express the idiotype of each T lymphocyte, are sometimes called the Ti portion of the receptor.

thymocytes, in the medulla, are the earliest cells to express Ti and the MHC-recognition structure, which has been designated the T3 maturation marker. In CD terminology, the entire complex is designated CD3, comprising the Ti heterodimer unique to each cell and the three-chain structure that directly interacts with MHC products.

MAJOR T-CELL SUBPOPULATIONS

Stage III thymocytes and circulating T cells embody two antigenically distinct populations. One possesses the CD4 (T4) antigen, the other has CD8 (T8). The molecules that confer these identities are present in very low concentration on the cell membrane. They appear to stabilize or otherwise to influence the contact necessary for interaction between CD3 and the presentation of antigen and MHC product. Cells with CD8 recognize antigen only in the context of MHC I products; those with CD4 react only to antigen presented with MHC II products (Fig. 5–5). In broad functional terms, CD4-positive cells enhance and promote actions of other immune cells and are called **helper T** cells; CD8-positive cells have generally suppressive or cytotoxic effects and have been called **suppressor T** cells. This division clearly oversimplifies the situation. Some CD4-positive cells exert suppressive effects, and subpopulations of both CD4- and CD8-positive cells perform direct effector functions. These activities are discussed more fully in chapter 7. The CD4 molecule is also the receptor for attachment and cellular invasion by the virus that causes the acquired immune deficiency syndrome (AIDS), the retrovirus called **HIV-1**.

POSTACTIVATION T CELLS

After activation, T cells express receptors different from those of resting T cells. When the CD3 complex interacts with antigen, the receptor-ligand complex is interiorized, leaving few or no antigen re-

MHC RESTRICTION OF CD4 AND CD8 CELLS

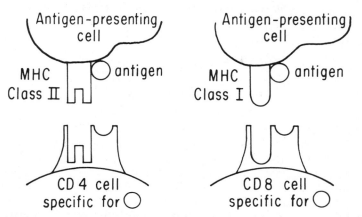

FIGURE 5–5. The CD4 molecule restricts interaction of the T cell to those cells that express MHC class II products along with antigen. The CD8 molecule requires that antigen be presented in the context of MHC class 1 products. Cells with intrinsic expression of class II products are less numerous than those with class I, but after immune activation, many cells that lack MHC II products in their resting state begin to express these antigens.

ceptors accessible. Instead, a new molecule appears, called **Tac** or CD25. This receptor is a marker for activation and is a receptor for IL-2, a lymphokine elaborated by activated T cells. This is **autocrine** stimulation, in which products of a cell stimulate the cell to further activity. CD25 and CD3 expressions are reciprocal. When CD25 is strongly expressed, CD3 is minimal, and vice versa.

Activation of the T cell has two aspects: one is the binding of antigen by CD3; the other is stimulation by IL-1, a cytokine derived from the macrophages that process and present the antigen. Under the influence of IL-1, the antigen-stimulated T cell begins producing IL-2 and expresses CD25. See pages 107 and 109–110 for a more detailed discussion of IL-1 and IL-2.

The activated T cell expresses another antigen absent from the resting cell. Ia activity—the expression of MHC class II products that characterizes lymphoid precursor cells, B lymphocytes, and antigen-presenting cells—becomes apparent on T cells after exposure to antigen and IL-1. Recrudescence of Ia on activated T cells suggests that cell-to-cell contact is involved in regulating immune reactivity.

——— **DEVELOPMENT OF B LYMPHOCYTES** ———

B lymphocytes undergo instruction and differentiation in the bone marrow, and possibly also in the fetal liver. Birds possess a distinct organ, called the **Bursa of Fabricius,** that provides instruction to B cells comparable to that of the thymus for T cells. Mammals have no single organ comparable to the avian Bursa, but their cells obviously experience effective instruction. The "B" in B lymphocytes originally meant "bursa equivalent"; it now seems reasonable to consider B to mean "bone marrow."

THE EARLIEST B CELL

Several features identify lymphoid cells committed to B-cell maturation. The irrevocable earliest event is rearrangement of the genetic sequences responsible for immunoglobulin manufacture. Genes for heavy-chain synthesis are on chromosome 14; those for light chains are on 2 and 22. Rearrangement of chromosome 14 signifies commitment to B-cell differentiation, inasmuch as heavy-chain genes rearrange before those for light chains. Actual protein manufacture occurs later in cell development.

Lymphoid precursors express MHC class II products, and these remain apparent on B cells through every stage up to the plasma cell. The membrane of fully developed plasma cells, however, lacks class II glycoprotein chains. MHC class II products, which were originally designated the Ia characteristic, are also present on macrophages, on certain accessory immune cells, and on mature T cells that have experienced antigenic activation.

Markers that Disappear

Very early B cells, like early T cells, have the enzyme TdT in the nucleus. This enzyme appears to be necessary for rearrangement of heavy-chain genes, but rearrangement of the light-chain genes occurs without it. Terminal deoxynucleotidyl transferase is no longer present in cells of the B lineage later than the pre-pre-B stage.

Another transient marker for early B cells is the membrane glycoprotein formerly called **CALLA,** now designated CD10. This protein was first identified as a leukemia marker. It was found on cells of nearly all acute lymphoblastic leukemias (ALL), most of which could not be assigned to either T or B origin (see page 201). The antigen, present in these undifferentiated leukemias, came to be called the **common-ALL-antigen,** or CALLA. Increasingly sensitive cell-typing techniques reveal that most CD10-positive leukemias have rearrangement of chromosome 14 in the leukemic cells, which are thus of B-cell lineage. Presence of CALLA does not connote leukemic cell proliferation; its presence indicates rapid multiplication of highly immature cells. Perfectly normal B-cell precursors are CD10 positive, and CD10 can be found on certain nonlymphoid cells as well.

CHANGES WITH MATURATION

The B-cell population is functionally more homogeneous than that of the T cell; virtually all cells mature toward immunoglobulin manufacture and potential activation into plasma cells. After rearrangement of chromosome 14, there is a brief phase in which heavy chains are synthesized in the cytoplasm without corresponding light chains. Once the genes for light chains have rearranged, light-chain synthesis begins, and the complete immunoglobulin molecule is assembled. For a short time, immunoglobulin molecules can be found in the cytoplasm but not on the membrane; the immunoglobulin molecules soon migrate to the membrane, rendering the cell capable of interaction with antigen.

Receptors for Proteins

Several additional receptors appear as B cells acquire functional maturity. One of these interacts with a structural element of the immunoglobulin molecule, the **Fc** segment (see chapter 6). Unstimulated B cells have relatively few Fc receptors. Contact with antigen generates strong Fc-combining capacity, allowing the activated B cell to interact with antibody molecules in the surrounding medium. Fully differentiated plasma cells engaged in antibody production do not have Fc receptors. Fc receptors are thought to mediate up and down regulation of antibody responses through mechanisms that are unclear. Some T-cell populations also have Fc receptors, suggesting an additional aspect of mutual regulatory effects between T cells and B cells.

B cells, but not T cells, have membrane receptors for several proteins of the complement system (see chapter 8). The complex interactions of the complement cascade generate a changing array of proteins and fragments. B cells express receptors for specific intermediate products, designated C3b and C3d. Complement receptors with various specificities are also present on macrophages and other accessory immune cells, on certain granulocytes, and on red blood cells. The receptor for C3d, designated CD21, is the target molecule whereby the Epstein-Barr virus (EBV) infects B lymphocytes. Although CD21 exists on certain antigen-presenting cells, B lymphocytes seem to be the only cells to experience EBV infection.

Evolution to Plasma Cell

The fully differentiated plasma cell loses most membrane markers characteristic of B cells and assumes appearance and function very different from the parent lymphocyte. Plasma cells are specialized to manufacture and to secrete immunoglobulin; they need no further environmental stimulation or regulation. Membrane immunoglobulin is no longer expressed; the class II MHC products disappear, as do receptors for immunoglobulin heavy chains and for complement proteins. After several days of manufacturing and releasing immunoglobulin molecules, the individual plasma cell dies without reproducing itself.

Figure 5–6 and Table 5–4 summarize aspects of B-cell maturation.

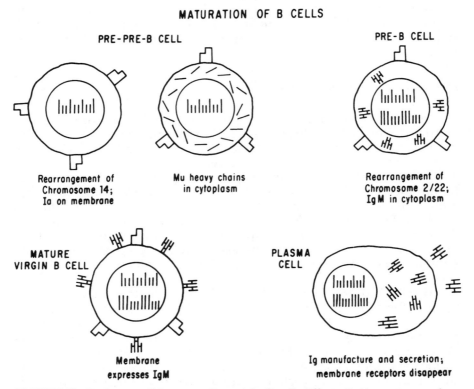

FIGURE 5–6. Irreversible commitment to B-cell differentiation occurs when the site for heavy-chain manufacture, on chromosome 14, undergoes rearrangement. Pre-pre-B cells are identified by rearrangement of the heavy-chain site and synthesis of heavy chains without corresponding events involving light chains. The Ia antigen, present on B cells at the earliest stages, persists through all B-cell phases but disappears from plasma cells. The pre-B cell has rearranged the light-chain gene and has immunoglobulin monomers in the cytoplasm but not on the membrane. Presence of membrane IgM marks the cell as a mature, immunocompetent B cell. After activation, proliferation and differentiation to a plasma cell, immunoglobulin production increases; immunoglobulin is secreted to the exterior; and membrane characteristics necessary for communication with the environment disappear.

TABLE 5—4. Markers for Cells of B-Lymphocyte Lineage

	1. Gene Rearr	2. cIg	3. mIg	4. Ia	5. Fc recept	6. CD 35	7. CD 21
Pre-pre-B	+	0	0	+	0	0	0
Pre-B	+	+	0	+	0	±	0
Mature B	+	0	+	+	+	+	+
Activated B	+	0	+	+	+ +	+ +	+
Plasma cell	+	+ +	0	0	0	0	0

1. DNA sequence of heavy-chain genes on chromosome 14 is rearranged
2. Immunoglobulin molecules are present in cytoplasm
3. Immunoglobulin molecules (IgM and IgD) are present on membrane surface
4. Class II MHC antigens (Ia antigen) are expressed on membrane
5. Membrane has receptor for Fc portion of IgG molecule
6. Membrane has receptor for C3b fragment of complement
7. Membrane has surface peptide that binds C3d and is receptor for EBV

NATURAL KILLER CELLS

Approximately 5 percent of blood lymphocytes have neither the membrane immunoglobulin characteristic of B cells nor the sheep-cell rosetting capacity characteristic of T cells. Originally called "third population" or "null" cells, these cells have acquired the more lurid appellation "natural killer" cells **(NK cells)**. Natural killer activity is the capacity to lyse target cells regardless of antigenic specificity, MHC expression, or previous exposure. NK activity resides in the population of cells described as **large granular lymphocytes** (LGL), which have abundant cytoplasm that contains numerous enzyme-containing granules.

IDENTIFYING FEATURES

Natural killer cells react with at least one "monocyte-specific" monoclonal antibody, but they seem to be most closely related to T lymphocytes; their development probably represents a differentiation event that occurs shortly after division into T and B lines. Natural killer cells have partial rearrangement of the site determining one chain of the Ti receptor; immature cells of this line found in bone marrow sometimes have weak expression of CD3. Although NK cells do not rosette when incubated with sheep cells, they do react with monoclonal antibodies specific for CD2. They also react with antibody to CD38 (T10), an antigen present not only on thymocytes but also on B cells at certain stages of differentiation and activation. Monoclonal antibodies have identified an antigen apparently unique to NK cells, designated HNK-1.

Natural killer cells have on their membranes a high-affinity receptor for the Fc portion of the IgG immunoglobulin class. Ig molecules are more strongly bound by Fc receptors on NK cells than on other lymphocytes; the binding capacity resembles that of the Fc receptor of neutrophilic granulocytes. Natural killer cells sometimes give positive results in tests for surface immunoglobulin, because their Fc receptor so strongly attracts and holds antibody molecules.

EFFECTOR FUNCTIONS

Natural killer cells attack target cells with which they have had no previous experience, and this cell-to-cell contact does not engender heightened activation or later memory. Natural killer activity does, however, increase under conditions of heightened immune activity; immune reactions generate cytokines that enhance NK activity, especially gamma interferon, a product of antigenically stimulated T cells, and IL-2, produced by T cells exposed to IL-1.

Intimate contact with the cell membrane is essential for NK-mediated cytolysis. The effect resembles a lethal injection, perhaps of proteolytic enzymes stored in the cytoplasmic granules. Natural killer cells can inflict a lethal "hit" on a target cell, disengage, and then repeat the process with the next target.

Laboratory Findings

Although NK cells act against a wide range of target cells, they display more discrimination than do macrophages and neutrophils, the totally non-specific inflammatory cells. The surface properties with which NK cells react include HLA antigens of all allotypes, viral products, and membrane markers present on immature cells of various lines. The less mature the cell, the more susceptible it is to NK-mediated cytolysis. Thus NK cells react strongly, *in vitro*, against such normally present cells as hematopoietic precursors, fetal cells, and the connective tissue cells that produce collagen. Their most conspicuous action in the laboratory is against abnormal populations such as tumor cells and virus-infected cells. Observations in patients with defective NK activity, in patients with various tumors and infections, and in experimental cell pairings invite the conclusion that NK cells defend against inappropriate cell proliferation. There is not yet, however, clear evidence for a defined physiologic or protective role for NK cells.

SUGGESTIONS FOR FURTHER READING

Boyd AW: Human leukocyte antigens: an update on structure, function and nomenclature. Pathology 1987; 19:329–37

Hersey P, Bolhuis R: "Nonspecific" MHC-unrestricted killer cells and their receptors. Immunol Today 1987; 8:233–38

Jalkanen S, Wu N, Bargatze RF, Butcher EC: Human lymphocyte and lymphoma homing receptors. Ann Rev Med 1987; 38:467–76

Janeway CA, Jr., Carding S, Jones B, et al: CD4+ T cells: specificity and function. Immunol Rev 1988; 101:39–80

Kay NE: Natural killer cells. CRC Crit Rev Lab Sci 1986; 22:343–359

Ling NR, Maclennan ICM, Mason DY: B-cell and plasma cell antigens: new and previously defined clusters. In: McMichael AJ, ed: Leucocyte Typing III. Oxford: Oxford University Press, 1987:302–335 (Proceedings of the Third International Workshop and Conference on Human Leucocyte Differentiation Antigens)

McMichael AJ, Gotch FM: T-cell antigens: new and previously defined clusters. In: McMichael AJ, ed: Leucocyte Typing III. Oxford: Oxford University Press, 1987:31–62 (Procedings of the Third International Workshop and Conference on Human Leucocyte Differentiation Antigens)

Meuer SC, Hercend T: Functional significance of human T-lymphocyte-associated antigens. In: Miyasaka M, Trnka Z, eds: Differentiation Antigens in Lymphopoietic Tissues. New York: Marcel Dekker, 1988:1–12

Shaw S: Characterization of human leukocyte differentiation antigens. Immunol Today 1987; 8:1–3

CHAPTER 6

Immunoglobulins

Immunoglobulins are proteins synthesized by B lymphocytes and their differentiated progeny, plasma cells. Immunoglobulin (Ig) molecules have a characteristic four-chain structure; those for which a corresponding antigen can be identified are called antibodies, but millions of molecules have not been matched with specific antigen. All antibodies are immunoglobulins, but not all immunoglobulins can be considered functional antibodies. Immunoglobulin molecules on the B-cell membrane serve as the receptor through which B lymphocytes interact with antigen; after secretion from the plasma cell, they function as antibodies.

THE GENERALIZED IMMUNOGLOBULIN

The basic Ig molecule has two pairs of identical polypeptide chains, one longer set and one shorter. The longer chains, called **heavy chains** (H chains), contain approximately 440 amino acids; the **light chains** (L chains) have approximately 220 amino acids. Only one half of the light chain and one quarter of the heavy chain participate in binding antigen; the remainder of the molecule contributes essential structural features. The four-chain unit is called the Ig **monomer** (Fig. 6–1). Molecules consisting of two or more monomers are called **polymers;** some immunoglobulins comprise 2, 3, or 5 monomers and are described as **dimers, trimers** or **pentamers,** respectively.

ISOTYPES AND Ig CLASSES

The antigen-recognition portion of the Ig monomer has a unique amino acid sequence for each specificity; this is the **idiotype** of the molecule. The remaining one half of the L chain and three quarters

FIGURE 6–1. The generalized immunoglobulin monomer has two identical heavy chains, composed of one variable domain and 3 or 4 constant domains; and two identical light chains, with one variable and one constant domain. Idiotypic specificity resides in the variable domains and requires simultaneous presence of both heavy and light chains. Treatment with papain cleaves the heavy chains just above the hinge region, yielding two identical fragments (called Fab, shown above) that contain the antigen-binding sites; and one fragment (Fc, shown above) that contains the carboxy-terminal ends of both heavy chains, joined by the disulfide bonds of the hinge region.

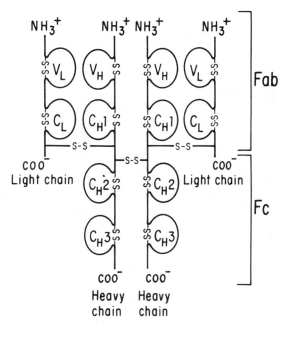

Immunoglobulin Monomer

of the H chain are common to large numbers of Ig molecules. Two different L-chain sequences exist, designated **kappa** and **lambda;** and five H-chain sequences, designated **alpha** (α), **delta** (δ), **epsilon** (ε), **gamma** (γ), and **mu** (μ). Immunoglobulins are categorized into **classes,** according to the H chain expressed. The Ig classes are **IgA, IgD, IgE, IgG,** and **IgM**. In all classes, approximately two thirds of the molecules have two kappa L chains, and one third have lambda; hybrids with one kappa and one lambda do not occur.

The individualized portion of H and L chains that determines the idiotype is called the **variable region** of the chain. The remaining amino acids, approximately 110 in the light chain and 330 in the H chain, constitute the **constant region**. Regardless of the antigen they recognize, all IgM molecules have the same amino acid sequence in their μ-chain constant region, and this is quite different from the constant-region sequence in immunoglobulins of other classes. When characteristic features are present in all members of a molecular category and that category is distinguishable from groups with other characteristics, the category is called an **isotype** (Fig. 6–2). There are two L-chain and five H-chain isotypes. Within a single isotype there may be consistent structural differences that confer subgroup identity within the larger isotype category. Differences within the H-chain isotypes allow subdivision of Ig classes into **subclasses**. There are four IgG subclasses, designated IgG1, IgG2, IgG3, and IgG4; IgA and IgM each have two subclasses; IgD and IgE molecules seem to be uniform within their class.

DOMAINS AND INTRAMOLECULAR BONDS

Amino acids are joined by peptide bonds, which link the amino group of one acid with the carboxy group of the next in a head-to-toe fashion. No matter how long the polypeptide chain, there is always an amino group at one end and a carboxy group at the other. The H and L chains of the Ig monomer join so that all amino terminals are at one end and all carboxy groups are at the other. The variable portion occupies the half of the L chain and the quarter of the H chain that are at the amino-terminal end.

Each L chain is joined by a **disulfide bond** (S–S bond) to one H chain. One or more disulfide bonds link the two H chains at approximately their midportions, in an area of considerable flexibility called the **hinge region**. Flexibility at this site allows the molecule to change shape while interacting with antigen epitopes located at irregular intervals or in awkwardly accessible sites. Disulfide bonds also join Ig monomers into polymers; but the S–S bonds that join monomers into a polymer are more easily broken than the S–S bonds in the hinge region or those joining L to H chains. IgM pentamers are easily dispersed into five monomers by treatment with reducing agents

ISOTYPE vs. SPECIFICITY

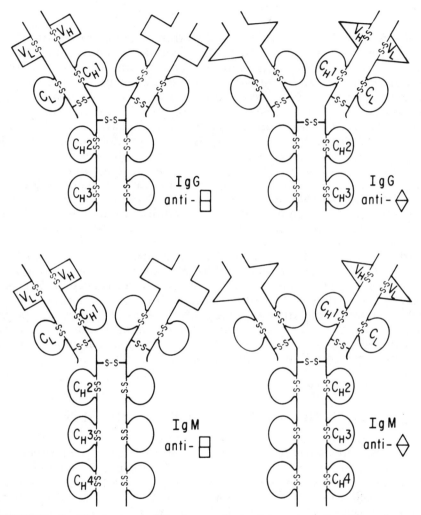

FIGURE 6–2. The isotype of the heavy chain determines the class of an antibody molecule; amino acid sequence of the variable domains determines the idiotype, which gives the molecule specificity. The amino acid sequence for a single idiotype can be attached to different heavy chains, causing a single specificity to be present in different immunoglobulin classes. In the drawing above, both antibodies on the left identify a square-shaped antigen; on the right, both recognize a triangle. The individual molecules are of different classes, however; the two molecules on the top have gamma heavy chains and those on the bottom have mu heavy chains.

like dithiothreitol or 6-mercaptopurine, whereas breaking the S–S bonds that link chains within the monomer requires intense reducing techniques not used in routine immunologic testing.

Characteristics of Domains

Protein molecules are not a two-dimensional string of amino acids. They have a complex three-dimensional configuration imposed by forces of attraction and repulsion among amino acids and their attached side chains. Disulfide bonds form within chains, linking strategically placed sulfur-containing groups and imposing a ballooned-out loop shape at several sites of both H and L chains; these looped areas are called **domains**. Light chains have two domains; H chains have either four or five. Antigen recognition involves the domains of H and L chains that are nearest the amino-terminal end. Inasmuch as variation in sequence of amino acids confers individual recognition capacity upon the molecule, the amino-terminal domains are called the **variable domains;** the other domains are the **constant domains**. Variable domains of H and L chains are denoted as V_H and V_L respectively. Light chains have only one constant domain, C_L. Alpha, delta, and gamma H chains have three constant domains, numbered C_H1, C_H2, and C_H3; epsilon and mu chains have an additional domain, C_H4. The physiologic and functional differences among antibody classes reflect properties of the constant domains characteristic of each class. The subclass differences within alpha, gamma, and mu isotypes result from differences in amino acid sequence in specific constant domains. Despite conspicuous differences among constant-domain sequences of isotypes and subclasses, many long amino acid sequences are common to segments of all Ig chains.

WHERE ANTIBODY JOINS ANTIGEN

Antibody does not recognize and combine with antigen unless the molecule includes both H and L chains. The three-dimensional configuration that interacts with the epitope gets half its shape from the variable domain of each chain. Only certain segments of the variable domain actually do vary; many sequences are exactly the same in molecules with different specificities. Invariant sequences within the variable domains provide the structural framework for the idiotypically unique amino acid sequences that recognize antigens. The portions of the variable domain that are unique for each idiotype are called the **hypervariable** or **complementarity-determining regions;** three such segments occur in both H-chain and L-chain variable domains. The intervening amino acid sequences that are common to molecules of all specificities are called the **framework regions**. In order to have distinctive amino acid sequences in the hypervariable regions, each Ig-producing cell must have a unique DNA sequence at the loci that determine manufacture of H and L chains. The genetic events that produce these unique sequences are detailed in the later section about protein diversity.

Enzymic Cleavage

Use of proteolytic enzymes to divide the molecules into constituent parts allows greater understanding of antibody structure and behavior. A useful technique is to separate the antigen-combining sites from the constant portions of the molecule. This must be done without breaking the disulfide bond that joins H and L chains, because antigen recognition requires simultaneous presence of both chains. The enzyme **papain** breaks the H chain at a point just above the hinge, generating three separate fragments: two identical fragments consisting of L chain linked to the amino-terminal half of the H chain, and one fragment that contains the hinge region and the remaining H-chain constant domains. The two fragments that carry the antibody activity are called **Fab** fragments (for **f**ragment with **a**ntigen-**b**inding capacity). The linked H-chain fragment is called **Fc,** denoting that it can be crystallized; it contains the constant domains that determine the biologic and serologic characteristics of the Ig class or subclass.

Another enzyme sometimes used to cleave immunoglobulins is **pepsin,** which cleaves the H chain below the hinge to yield a large fragment that includes both combining sites. This fragment, which has two recognition sites, is called **F(ab)'$_2$** and is capable of uniting with two epitopes simultaneously. The remainder of the H chains is degraded into small fragments with no immunologic activity.

THE J CHAIN

Immunoglobulin monomers comprise only H and L chains. Immunoglobulin polymers characteristically include an additional chain, called the **J** (for joining) **chain**. This is a short polypeptide manufactured by the plasma cell and added to the polymerized Ig just before it leaves the cell. IgM molecules that serve as antigen receptor on the B-cell membrane are monomers and do not express a J chain. Only secreted polymers include a J chain, and there is only one to a molecule, regardless of the number of monomers present.

IMMUNOGLOBULIN SYNTHESIS

Plasma cells have far more capacity to synthesize and to secrete Ig than their parent lymphocyte. All proteins are assembled in tiny spheres, **ribosomes,** which adhere to a web of internal membranes called the **endoplasmic reticulum**. Polypeptides destined to leave the cell of origin enter the space enclosed by these membranes and travel to a specialized intracellular site, called the **Golgi apparatus,** where proteins are processed for external secretion. The heavy concentration of ribosomes and endoplasmic reticulum necessary for intense protein synthesis and secretion gives the plasma cell its abundant cytoplasm and dark-blue color seen in most stained preparations.

Heavy and light chains are synthesized independently, in different ribosomes. It takes about 30 seconds to assemble an L chain and 60 seconds for an H chain. Constituent chains are linked through disulfide bonds while traveling through the endoplasmic reticulum. In the Golgi apparatus, Ig monomers are packaged into membrane-bound units that traverse the cytoplasm, merge with the cell membrane, and have their contents discharged to the exterior—a process called **reverse pinocytosis**. Polymerization of IgA and IgM occurs late in the process, shortly before the protein leaves the cell. Immunoglobulin polymers are not secreted until the J chain is attached. Plasma cells that secrete only monomeric IgG, IgD, or IgE manufacture J chains, but the chain goes unused and is subsequently degraded. The mechanisms and regulation of polymerization are not fully understood.

TECHNIQUES FOR STUDY

There are several ways to characterize Ig classes. Detailed amino acid sequences can be determined, but most investigations observe the behavioral characteristics of the molecules. Immunoglobulins migrate in an electrical field with other globulins, but this covers a range of rates. Gamma migration is the slowest (Fig. 6–3); antibodies are sometimes described collectively as **gamma globulins,** because IgG molecules are the most abundant antibody class and they migrate in the gamma range. The term is somewhat misleading because some Ig classes migrate more rapidly, in the beta part of the electrophoretic tracing.

When subjected to analytic ultracentrifugation, immunoglobulins sediment at characteristic rates that reflect molecular size and shape. The unit of measurement is the **Svedberg unit** (abbreviated S), and molecules are described by their **sedimentation constant**. IgM molecules are sometimes called 19S antibodies and IgG are 7S, properties that describe the entire class without regard to antigenic specificity.

Some Definitions

The different Ig classes express a variety of physiologic functions, which will be discussed in chapters 9 through 13. These activities

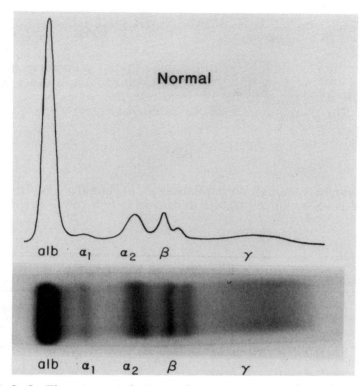

FIGURE 6–3. The strip at bottom shows migration of serum proteins through a gel. Molecules move at rates determined by their individual characteristics; concentration is reflected in the density of stain, which is graphically rendered in the tracing above the strip. At pH 8.6, large numbers of homogeneous albumin molecules move rapidly toward the anode, at left. The remaining bands are less sharply defined because molecules within these groups show greater diversity. Globulins designated gamma move toward the cathode (at right) at this pH. The gamma category includes so many different proteins that the migration band is indistinct. The aggregate concentration of gamma globulins, in this specimen, is virtually the same as that of the less heterogeneous beta and alpha-2 globulin categories.

have been evaluated through experimental manipulation and by observations of normal individuals and patients with various abnormalities. The H-chain constant domains carry the configurations that determine these activities. The study of antibodies in serum or other body fluids is called **serology;** observations demonstrate the **serologic** properties of immunoglobulins. The earliest serologic activities to be characterized were clumping of particles, called **agglutination,** and dissolution of red blood cells, called **hemolysis**. These and other ways to demonstrate Ig activities are described in chapters 14 through 18.

SPECIFIC IMMUNOGLOBULINS

Immunoglobulins constitute approximately 20 percent of plasma proteins and are present at varying concentrations in other body fluids. Wide differences in distribution and properties exist among Ig classes. These are summarized in Table 6–1.

IgM

It is logical, though not alphabetical, to consider IgM first. This is the first class produced by the maturing B cell, the first class to ap-

TABLE 6–1. Characteristics of Immunoglobulins

	IgM	IgG	IgA	IgE	IgD
Heavy-chain class	μ	γ	α	ξ	δ
Heavy-chain sub-classes	μ1,μ2	γ1,γ2, γ3,γ4	α1,α2	None	None
Constant domains on H chain	4	3	3	4	3
Approximate molecular weight (in kD)	900	150	160	190	180
Polymerization	Pentamer	No	Mostly dimers in secretions; Monomers in serum	No	No
Serum concentration (mg/dl)	120–150	1000–1500	100–300	1–3	0.003–0.005
% of serum Ig	8–12%	70–75%	10–20%	<1%	Trace
Serum half-life (days)	5	23–25	6	1–5	2–8
Complement fixation (classical pathway)	4+	1–3+	No	No	No
Crosses placenta	No	Yes	No	No	No
Skin sensitization	No	?Minimal	No	Yes	No
Transported across epithelium	Occasionally	No	Yes	No	No

pear in the serum of maturing infants, and the first class of antibody detected in primary immune responses.

In body fluids, IgM is a pentamer, but on the B-cell membrane, the antigen receptor is monomeric IgM. This section will consider only the pentameric secreted form, which is the largest of the Ig molecules. It has a molecular weight of 900 kD and a diameter of approximately 1000 Ångstrom units. The five monomers form a star-shaped molecule (Fig. 6–4) that can combine simultaneously with antigenic determinants widely separated from one another. Although the five monomers include 10 combining sites, only five are available for combination with most antigens. Only with very small, soluble haptens can all 10 sites react.

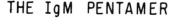

THE IgM PENTAMER

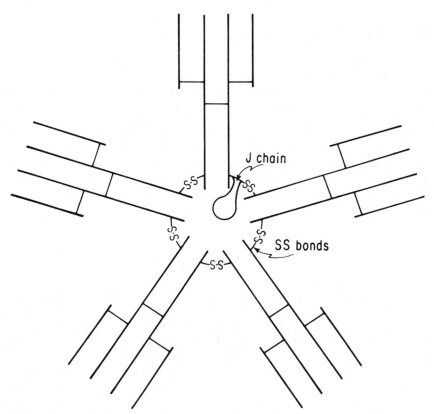

FIGURE 6–4. The Fc portions of 5 IgM monomers are joined by disulfide bonds into a pentamer, which contains, in addition, a small polypeptide called the J chain. The S–S bonds linking the monomers are more easily cleaved by reduction than the S–S bonds holding chains together within the monomer.

IgM as Agglutinin

Large molecular size has several consequences. Nearly all secreted IgM is found in the bloodstream. Very little is in tissue or other body fluids unless vessels become abnormally permeable or there is actual rupture of capillaries or other vessels. Because of their large diameter, IgM antibodies readily combine with antigens on the surface of dispersed particles, agglutinating them into easily observed clumps. IgM antibodies are effective agglutinins because of their size and their multiple combining sites. Although many laboratory tests use agglutination as an end point, agglutination is relatively insignificant in physiologic events. More important in the living host is the ability of IgM antibodies to initiate the classical pathway of complement activity (see chapters 8 and 9). A consequence of *in vivo* IgM antibody reactions is enhancement of macrophage activity.

Appearance and Disappearance

IgM antibodies appear earlier than IgG in the primary immune response, but synthesis continues only while antigen remains in the system. As antigen molecules are degraded or eliminated, IgM production declines and no memory cells develop for IgM secretion. Upon subsequent exposure to the same antigen, the interval before IgM antibodies become detectable is just as long as in the primary response (See Fig. 4–10). Like all proteins, IgM molecules are metabolized at a predictable rate. The disappearance of molecules from the circulation is often expressed as the **half-life,** the time required for half the molecules originally present to be degraded. IgM antibodies in the bloodstream have a half-life of 5 days.

IgG

The preponderant serum Ig is IgG, contributing 70 to 80 percent of circulating immunoglobulins and 20 to 25 percent of total serum proteins. Quantities of IgG accumulate for two reasons: individual molecules have a long half-life—23 to 25 days—and there is continuous high-level stimulation for IgG production. Once an individual develops immunity to antigens in the environment, there is frequent opportunity for repeated contact and anamnestic stimulation; anamnestic antibodies are IgG. As shown in Table 6–2, the four IgG subclasses differ substantially in biologic behavior and half-life; most generalized statements about IgG refer to IgG1, which constitutes 60 to 70 percent of serum IgG. IgG is found in tissue fluids as well as blood but is absent from external epithelial secretions. IgG is always a monomer, with a molecular weight of approximately 150 kD and a diameter of 250 Ångstrom units.

TABLE 6–2. Characteristics of IgG Subclasses

	IgG1	IgG2	IgG3	IgG4
Percent of total IgG	60–70	15–25	4–8	2–5
Serum half-life (days)	23	23	8	23
Fixes complement	2+	1+	3+	0
Crosses placenta	Yes	Yes	Yes	Yes
Macrophages have receptors for this Fc	Yes	No	Yes	No
Neutrophils have receptors for this Fc	Yes	Yes	Yes	±
Molecular weight of H chain (in kD)	51	51	60	51
Allotypic variation (Gm groups) present	Modest	Modest	Marked	Absent

Effects on Cells and Proteins

IgG antibodies unite with antigens on particle surfaces but seldom cause agglutination. Attachment of IgG antibodies to antigenically reactive cells or organisms has two major consequences. The most important is that the Fc portion of the gamma chain remains accessible on the particle surface; antigen-antibody recognition involves the Fab portions, leaving the Fc portions extending outward. Macrophages and neutrophils have high-affinity receptors for gamma-chain Fc, so particles coated with IgG antibody are far more susceptible to cellular attack than cells or organisms in their native state. Enhancement of phagocytic activity by alteration of a surface is called **opsonization;** IgG antibodies are potent **opsonins,** as are some of the protein fragments generated by the complement sequence. All IgG subclasses except IgG4 activate complement by the classical pathway; another consequence of IgG antibody reactions is complement activation, although this occurs less consistently and less intensely than with IgM antibody reactions.

Effects on Fetus

IgG is the only class of antibody that crosses the placenta from mother to fetus. The normal fetus occupies a sealed, sterile environment and experiences no stimulus to immune activity. If they did not have maternal antibodies, normal newborns would have little or no immune protection against the world. Infants born with the mother's antibodies rarely suffer infections with common environmental bacteria and viruses. Protein degradation, however, occurs more rapidly than immune maturation, so antibody levels fall dramatically after 6 to 8 weeks of age. In rare cases, transmission of maternal antibodies has harmful effects. Transfusion or other stimuli may have caused a woman to produce antibodies against antigens absent from her own cells but present on fetal cells. If these antibodies enter the fetus in high concentration, cell damage may ensue. The most conspicuous example of this is the condition called **hemolytic disease of the newborn,** which affects fetal red blood cells.

IgA

The body contains large quantities of IgA, but serum concentration is relatively low. Most IgA is in secreted fluids present on the epithelial surfaces of the alimentary, respiratory, and reproductive tracts, and in urine, saliva, and milk. Serum IgA circulates as a monomer, but the secreted forms are largely dimers. Secreted IgA has, in addition to the J chain present in polymerized immunoglobulins, a glycoprotein chain called the **S** (for secretory) **component**. The S component derives from epithelial cells, not from the plasma cells that synthesize Ig. IgA is generated largely by plasma cells in the mucosa-associated lymphoid tissue; to enter secreted fluid, it must enter and pass through epithelial cells. The S component originates from the receptor molecule through which epithelial cells bind and incorporate the IgA dimers. The Ig enters the cell, traverses the cytoplasm, and exits into the epithelial secretions, carrying a portion of the receptor molecule with it. The presence of the S component appears to protect the Ig polymer in secreted fluids from digestion by surface enzymes.

Antimicrobial Effects

IgA antibodies in secreted fluids deter microorganisms from penetrating epithelial cells. The mechanisms for this are far from clear, because IgA antibodies neither agglutinate particles nor activate the classical complement pathway nor remain affixed to the surface of cells or organisms. Aggregates of IgA molecules or of IgA complexed with protein can activate complement through the alternative pathway (see chapter 8), but this seems to play no direct role in epithelial protection. IgA provides variably effective protection against infection by various species of bacteria and viruses. Individuals with congenital failure of IgA synthesis do not exhibit any consistent pattern of increased respiratory-tract or other infections. Physiologic protection probably occurs by a substitute pathway, because the secretions of IgA-deficient individuals contain IgM antibodies that have used the S-component pathway to traverse epithelial cells (see page 166).

IgE

Serum and body fluids contain very little IgE. Nearly all of the body's IgE is attached to the membrane of highly specialized tissue granulocytes called **mast cells;** some is present on basophilic granulocytes in the blood. Basophils and mast cells have membrane receptors specific for the Fc of IgE; attachment occurs through the fourth constant domain of the epsilon heavy chain. Fab sites are not involved in this interaction, and cell-bound IgE antibodies remain capable of combining with antigen (Fig. 6–5). When the Fab sites unite with antigen, the change in molecular configuration signals the underlying cell to release substances stored in its granules.

Mast cells are heavily concentrated in the skin and the lining of the respiratory and alimentary tracts. Their densely basophilic cytoplasmic granules contain histamine, heparin, and other substances that affect smooth muscle contraction, vascular permeability, and inflammatory events. The physiologic consequence of IgE-mediated reactions is accumulation of substances that produce the events perceived as **immediate hypersensitivity reactions** (see chapter 12).

IgE antibodies have several names that reflect their biologic characteristics. The term **cytophilic antibody** denotes their propensity to bind firmly to cells, and **skin-sensitizing antibody** reflects the effects of IgE in the skin, where mast cells are abundant. A potentially confusing term sometimes applied to IgE antibodies is **reagin**. The same name is also used for the anticardiolipin antibody that develops in conditions of immune dysfunction, especially syphilis; the two anti-

IgE ON BASOPHILS

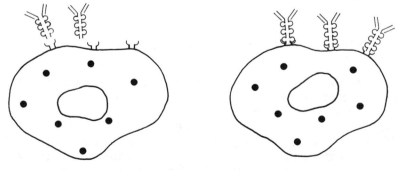

Basophil Receptors Link C_H4 of IgE

FIGURE 6–5. Basophils in blood and in tissue (where they are called mast cells) have membrane receptors that bind the fourth constant domain of the epsilon heavy chain. IgE molecules bound to the cell remain free to combine, through their Fab sites, with available antigen.

bodies designated "reagin" are completely different in structure, function, and clinical significance.

IgD

IgD remains the least understood of the immunoglobulins. Serum contains very small amounts of monomeric IgD molecules with a 2- or 3-day half-life. Most IgD is found on the surface of immunocompetent B lymphocytes that have not experienced primary stimulation. Although all mature B lymphocytes express membrane IgM, not all have IgD. It is thought that IgD participates in the feedback mechanisms that regulate levels of immune activity, but specific actions have not been described.

PROTEIN DIVERSITY FROM GENETIC HOMOGENEITY

All cells in an individual possess identical genetic information encoded in identical chromosomes, but vastly different cell types evolve from this common endowment. Not only do cells assume innumerable different properties, but cells of a single type—lymphocytes—can produce multiple different products. A population of lymphocytes possessing initially identical chromosomes can produce millions of uniquely structured antibody molecules. Studies over the past decade have revealed molecular events that offer a plausible explanation for observed immunologic diversity.

GENETIC LIBRARIES

The undifferentiated genome contains much information that is never used. Sequences of nucleotide triplets in deoxyribonucleic acid (DNA), called **codons,** determine the selection of amino acids for polypeptide chains. There is one-to-one correspondence between codons and the sequence of amino acids in the manufactured protein, but many DNA segments exist that are never translated into protein-synthesizing events. The pattern for synthesis of a specific protein is assembled from a pool of many codon sequences, any of which could direct synthesis of that polypeptide. The full array of DNA sequences that exists before selection for specific manufacture is called the **germ line** sequence.

The H-chain, kappa-chain, and lambda-chain loci (on chromo-

DNA REARRANGEMENT

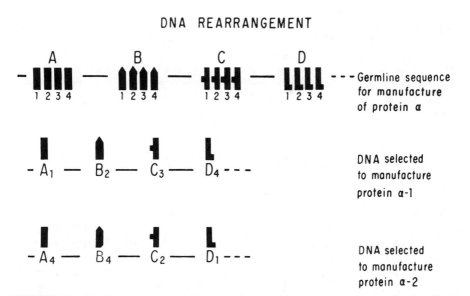

FIGURE 6–6. The top panel depicts the germline sequence in which all alternative sequences in each library are available for selection. In productive rearrangement, one sequence from each library is selected for expression and the others are deleted. The two lower panels show rearrangements by which two cells can produce two different versions of the same protein.

somes 14, 2, and 22 respectively) contain many codon sequences, any of which can direct protein assembly. Only one of the potentially usable DNA segments will become operational; the rest are snipped out of the helical chain and disappear. A group of individual genetic segments all dedicated to potential synthesis of the same polypeptide is called a **library**. Only one selection from the library becomes active in any one cell. The amino acid sequence characteristic of the idiotypic portion of Ig variable domains reflects the selection, in individual cells, of individual DNA segments from chromosomal libraries (Fig. 6–6).

Size of Libraries

Several different libraries contribute segments to the genes that direct Ig synthesis in any one cell; these are called V (for variable), J (for joining), and D (for diversity). Light-chain manufacture employs selections only from V and J libraries; H-chain synthesis includes a D-library unit as well. The kappa-chain locus on chromosome 2 has at least 300 different sequences in the V library and 4 in J; the lambda-chain locus on chromosome 22 is even more complex. The H-chain locus on chromosome 14 includes hundreds of V segments, approximately 20 D segments and 4 J segments. Any one of these segments can be linked with any of the others, in what appears to be random selection. Enzymes cleave the DNA chain between codons and link the selected units to segments from adjacent libraries; the unused intervening material is degraded, leaving the active, rearranged sequence much shorter than the original, unmodified germ line sequence.

JUNCTIONAL EVENTS

Cutting, rearranging, and rejoining DNA segments is subject to random error. When a V segment links with a J segment, a few nucleotides may fail to pair off precisely. This can occur unpredictably at either end of either segment. Thus, even if the same V segment and same J segment are selected in two different cells, slightly different final sequences will be seen, expanding still further the number of possible DNA sequences that can develop. The effects of imprecise joining are called **recombinatorial diversity;** this occurs only once in L-chain manufacture, because only the single splice between V and J takes place. For H chains, V combines with D and D combines with J, providing two opportunities for recombinatorial diversity.

H Chains Are More Diverse

In H-chain construction, yet another event occurs; not only are nucleotides randomly lost through recombinatorial diversity, but new nucleotides are added. At the V-D and D-J splice points, the enzyme terminal deoxynucleotidyl transferase (TdT) inserts randomly selected nucleotides in a brief sequence called an N region. Thus, the DNA pattern for the H-chain variable domain has the sequence V-N-D-N-J. These N regions of unpredictable length and composition further increase the number of possible sequence combinations. TdT is present in the nucleus only at the very early maturational phase when the H-chain gene undergoes rearrangement. By the time L-chain genes rearrange, TdT has disappeared, and L-chain genes do not express N regions.

An Estimated Total

The potential number of different sequences available for Fab construction has been calculated from data obtained with mice, using rather conservative estimates for effects of recombinatorial diversity and insertion of N regions. These figures are 4×10^3 for L chains and 2.4×10^7 for H chains. Because any L chain can link to any H chain, the number of potential Ig molecules is the product of these two numbers. The staggering final figure is 10^{11} different Fab configurations—more than enough to recognize all the past, present, and future antigens an individual might encounter.

ALLELIC EXCLUSION AND FAILURE TO REARRANGE

Each cell contains two sets of chromosomes, each with complete genetic information. For many characteristics, such as blood group antigens and MHC products, genes on both chromosomes are active and direct synthesis of a protein, a biologic phenomenon described as **codominance**. If the immunoglobulin genes were codominant, each cell would produce two H chains, two kappa chains, and two lambda chains, which could associate with one another in random combinations. This does not happen. In any cell, only one H-chain gene is expressed and only one L-chain gene, which will be either kappa or lambda.

If DNA rearranges from germline sequence to a form that directs protein synthesis, this is described as **productive rearrangement**. In a manner incompletely understood, productive rearrangement of the locus on one chromosome for chain production inhibits the other chromosome from rearranging. This inhibitory effect is called **allelic exclusion**. On chromosome 14, this means that only one H-chain variable region develops. On chromosome 2, productive rearrangement of kappa-chain DNA not only inhibits the other chromosome 2 but also inhibits rearrangement of either chromosome 22 at the lambda-chain locus. Some rearrangements of chromosome 2, however, prove nonproductive. If kappa-chain rearrangement has been nonproductive, the lambda-chain locus on chromosome 22 can then rearrange. Cells with lambda-locus rearrangement always have a rearranged but nonproductive chromosome 2; cells producing kappa L chains retain the germline configuration on chromosome 22.

DIVERSITY OF CLASSES

These genetic gymnastics affect only the variable regions. All Ig molecules within an isotype have the same amino acid sequences in their constant portions, so gene rearrangement need not occur for the constant-region portion of the gene locus. Antibodies of a single specificity, however, often show diversity of Ig class. The same Fab site can be found on antibody molecules with different H-chain isotypes. A given idiotype reflects gene rearrangement in a single cell before activation; after that cell encounters its antigen and undergoes clonal expansion, individual daughter cells encounter different mediating events. Suitably stimulated by postactivation events, different daugh-

ISOTYPE SWITCHING

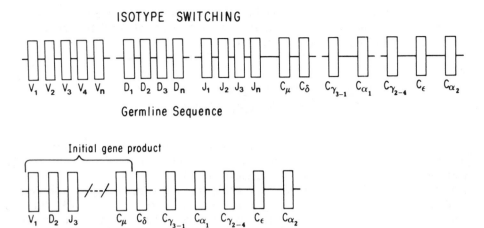

Germline Sequence

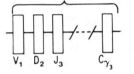

Initial gene product

Variable Region has Rearranged, Spliced with Heavy-chain Gene

Same specificity, different heavy chain

Attachment to Different C Locus
Gives New Isotype

FIGURE 6–7. In the germline sequence for manufacturing heavy chains, libraries for the variable region lie adjacent to numerous sequences for the constant region, as shown in the top panel. After selection from the libraries necessary to determine the variable portion, the productive sequence attaches to the constant-region segment for mu and/or delta heavy chains, as shown in the middle panel. Unstimulated B cells synthesize these isotypes. Heavy-chain segments can be deleted, as shown in the bottom panel, allowing attachment of the variable-region sequence to the constant-region sequence for other chain types.

ter cells manufacture antibody molecules with the same specificity of the Fab portion but different H-chain constant regions.

Switching Isotypes

On chromosome 14, the DNA sequence for the variable region lies adjacent to the sequence that determines the constant-region sequence for the mu chain. After the variable-region sequence has been productively rearranged, it combines with the constant-region sequence for the mu chain; the Ig that contains this chain is IgM. Deoxyribonucleic acid sequences for other H-chain isotypes are downstream from the mu-chain segment. Suitably stimulated, a daughter cell can detach the entire variable-region sequence from one H-chain sequence and attach it to another (Fig. 6–7); the signals controlling this switch are incompletely understood. Unstimulated B lymphocytes can manufacture IgM and IgD simultaneously, and many virgin B cells have as membrane receptors both IgM and IgG molecules of a single idiotype. Once activation and clonal expansion occur, only IgM is secreted. Daughter cells in a single clone subsequently encounter and respond to different regulatory messages; cells exposed to different cytokines subsequently secrete antibody of different classes. Memory cells seem to develop only from cells that have switched isotype away from mu-chain production; anamnestic stimulation does not provoke accelerated IgM synthesis.

A NOTE ON THE T-CELL RECEPTOR

Genetic rearrangement occurs in T cells to determine idiotypic specificity of the heterodimer that contributes antigenic specificity to the CD3 complex. Genes for these chains reside on chromosomes 7 and 14 and, like those for immunoglobulins, have libraries of V, D, and J segments as well as constant-region sequences. Genetics of the T-cell receptor are further complicated by the fact that three different loci—designated alpha, beta, and gamma—all undergo rearrangement. The alpha and beta sites determine the alpha and beta chains of the membrane receptor. The gamma locus occupies a separate site on chromosome 7. It does not participate in the variability that determines idiotype but appears to be associated with the T3 part of the complex, which is common to all cells of a single individual.

———— IMMUNOGLOBULIN ALLOTYPES ————

It is not strictly correct to describe the constant regions of all antibodies in a single isotype as identical. Immunoglobulin molecules produced by different individuals exhibit short segments of amino acid sequences that differ from one person to another according to which alleles they possess. Constant-region genes for several Ig chains manifest several allelic forms within the population. In a single individual, all IgG1 molecules will have the same amino acid sequence, but IgG1 molecules from a different individual may have different amino acids in a limited segment of the chain. These amino acid configurations can elicit antibodies specific for one sequence if introduced into an individual whose Ig chains have a different sequence. The molecular feature defined by these antibodies is the **allotype** of the Ig.

Allotypes reside in the constant region of the Ig chain; they are

TABLE 6–3. Ways of Classifying Immunoglobulins

Discriminator	Identifying Feature
Idiotype	The unique amino acid sequence in the variable regions of L and H chains, through which antibody interacts with a specific antigen. All antibodies that react with the same antigen have the same idiotype, regardless of class.
Isotype	The features of the antibody molecule determined by distinctive constant regions of H-chain class or subclass and L-chain class. All antibodies possessing those chains possess those features, regardless of antigenic specificity or the genome of the person producing the antibody.
Allotype	Genetically determined amino acid sequence at specific sites in constant regions, present in Ig molecules from individuals who possess that allele, regardless of idiotypic specificity of the antibody.

not affected by idiotypic specificity and do not seem to affect the biologic properties of the Ig molecule. Humans occasionally develop antibodies against Ig allotypes to which they have been exposed by transfusion or pregnancy, but such antibodies have no adverse clinical effects. Allotypes, as best as we know, are significant only as genetic traits that differentiate individuals from one another.

Allotypic distinctions are most prominent in gamma H chains and kappa L chains. Gamma chains of subclasses 1, 2, and 3 manifest allotypic differences that have been named **Gm groups**. The allotypic distinctions on kappa chains were called **Inv** groups when first discovered, but are now called **Km** groups. The alpha 2 chain exhibits **Am** groups and a recently discovered polymorphism in the epsilon chain is called **Em**.

Table 6–3 summarizes the features that distinguish Ig molecules from one another.

SUGGESTIONS FOR FURTHER READING

Burdette S, Schwartz RS: Idiotypes and idiotypic networks. NEJM 1987; 317:219–24

Kieber-Emmons T, Kohler H: Towards a unified theory of immunoglobulin structure-function relations. Immunol Rev 1986; 90:29–48

Kishimoto T, Hirano T: Molecular regulation of B lymphocyte response. Ann Rev Immunol 1988; 6:485–512

Köhler G: Derivation and diversification of monoclonal antibodies. Science 1986; 233:1281–86

Radbruch A, Burger C, Klein S, Müller W: Control of immunoglobulin class switch recombination. Immunol Rev 1986; 89:69–83

Rees AR: The antibody combining site: retrospect and prospect. Immunol Today 1987; 8:44–5

Teale JM, Abraham KM: The regulation of antibody class expression. Immunol Today 1987; 8:122–26

Williams AF, Barclay AN: The immunoglobulin superfamily—domains for cell surface recognition. Ann Rev Immunol 1988; 5:381–405

CHAPTER 7

Cytokines, Cellular Cooperation, and Cell-Mediated Immunity

Immune reactions go far beyond the interaction between antigen and a membrane receptor of complementary configuration. Many populations of cells act to enhance, to suppress, to modulate, and otherwise to orchestrate the events we identify as a detectable immune response. This chapter discusses some of the ways that cells and their products interact after antigenic exposure stimulates an immunocompetent host.

106

CYTOKINES: LYMPHOKINES AND OTHERS

Cell products that influence activities of other cells are called **cytokines**. If synthesized by a lymphocyte, the product is called a **lymphokine**. Monocyte products can be called **monokines,** but products of monocyte/macrophages are more often named descriptively for the functions they subserve.

INTERLEUKIN 1

One broadly reactive group of macrophage products is called **interleukin 1** (IL-1), which comprises several small (MW 15–17 kD) thermostable peptides. When first discovered in the late 1970s, this substance of monocyte origin was seen to affect lymphocyte proliferation and reactivity and was called **lymphocyte activating factor** (LAF). Further investigation has revealed numerous additional functions.

Almost anything that perturbs its cell membrane stimulates the macrophage to produce IL-1; perhaps the most potent stimulating event is incorporation of antigenic material, with subsequent processing and presentation. IL-1 has both local and systemic effects on

---

TABLE 7–1. Actions of IL-1

On Lymphocytes
   Induces IL-2 production and Tac expression in T cells
   Influences suppressor-cell activity
   Increases mIg expression in pre-B cells
   Promotes proliferation and differentiation of B cells
   Enhances NK-cell activity
On Inflammatory Events
   Mobilizes neutrophils from marrow into circulation
   Attracts neutrophils, lymphocytes, monocytes to affected sites
   Increases systemic breakdown of proteins
   Stimulates hepatic production of C-reactive protein, "acute-phase reactants," amyloid A, metal-binding proteins, and so forth
   Reduces hepatic synthesis of albumin
On Other Cellular Events
   Increases bone resorption by osteoclasts
   Increases production of proteolytic enzymes by cells of cartilage, synovium, and many epithelial sites
On Central Nervous System
   Leads to elevated body temperature
   Depresses appetite
   Promotes slow-wave sleep

many different cells, affecting metabolic and neurophysiologic events as well as immune and inflammatory reactions. Table 7–1 lists the major actions of IL-1. Systemic effects occur only when a large-scale stimulus induces secretion of IL-1 into the bloodstream. Local effects, especially those on nearby lymphocytes, can occur after limited macrophage activity. Interleukin 1 provokes membrane changes in B cells, T cells, and natural killer (NK) cells, leading to enhanced sensitivity to other immunostimulating events. Interleukin 1 causes T cells to produce the lymphokine IL-2 (see later section) and to express receptors for IL-2 (the Tac antigen, see chapter 5); B cells display increased levels of membrane immunoglobulin and express receptors for IL-2. Macrophages produce IL-1 without regard to antigenic specificity, and its effects on target cells are not antigen restricted; IL-1 induces conditions that increase the immunogenicity of whatever antigen is present.

INTERFERONS

Interferons (IFN) are small (MW 16–25 kD) proteins produced by several different kinds of cells. Initially considered antiviral mediators, IFNs have been shown to elicit diverse effects on a variety of targets. Interferons were initially separated into naturally occurring (type I) or immune-stimulated (type II) products; current classification is by cell of origin. Macrophages, lymphocytes, and fibroblasts produce interferons after exposure to many inducers: viral antigens, mitogens, cells with foreign major histocompatibility complex (MHC) antigens, or certain kinds of ribonucleic acid (RNA). Antigenically specific T cells produce the interferon sometimes called "immune interferon" after encountering either their predestined antigen or an appropriate mitogen. Viral exposure can stimulate T cells that recognize the viral antigens, but viral infection per se does not cause T cells of other idiotypes to produce IFN. T cells produce interferon after their receptors combine with antigen of any type, not just of viral origin. In current terminology, **IFN-alpha** and **IFN-beta** are the types produced by non-T cells after viral infection; **IFN-gamma** is the product of antigenically activated T cells. See Table 7–2.

Physiologic Effects

Interferon receptors mediate the effects of interferons on target cells. One type of receptor serves for both alpha and beta interferons; IFN-gamma has its own receptors. Interferons promote many target effects; experiments and observations on these effects have produced confusing and sometimes contradictory results. In general, IFNs suppress proliferation but enhance differentiation and level of activity in most inflammatory and immune cells; they inhibit the differentiation of fibroblasts, monocytes, and some bone marrow cells. Interferon-

TABLE 7–2. Human Interferons

	IFN-α	IFN-β	IFN-γ
Former designation	Type I, leukocyte	Type I, fibroblast	Type II, immune
Major producing cells	B lymphocytes, macrophages, large granular lymphocytes	Fibroblasts	T lymphocytes
Major inducing stimulus	Viruses, RNA (double-stranded), B-cell mitogens, allogeneic cells	Viruses, RNA (double-stranded), B-cell mitogens, allogeneic cells	Specific antigens, tumor cells, T-cell mitogens
Functional types	At least 8	1	1
Locus for production on chromosome	9 (various loci)	9	12

gamma stimulates the phagocytic and degradative capacity of macrophages. The target cells secrete larger quantities of IL-1 and increase their expression of Fc receptors, MHC-II products, and membrane molecules that promote intracellular adhesion. Interferon-gamma enhances MHC-I expression on all types of cells, making them better targets for cytotoxic CD8 cells.

Interferons variably stimulate and suppress antigen recognition and immune responses of different populations of lymphocytes in different circumstances. Interferon-alpha and IFN-beta, which are produced at an early stage of viral illness, seem to enhance generalized reactivity and promote a more effective immune response to the virus. Interferon-gamma, which appears after activation of specific T-cells, modulates the nature and intensity of both the inflammatory and the immune responses.

INTERLEUKIN 2

Interleukin 2 (IL-2) was originally called **T-cell growth factor**. Its major function is to enhance proliferation of activated T lymphocytes, but it also affects B lymphocytes, NK cells, and macrophages. Interleukin 2 binds to a membrane receptor, the Tac antigen (see chapter 5), that is not expressed on resting cells. Tac develops after contact with specific antigen; if the antigen disappears, Tac diminishes or disappears. Interleukin 2 promotes the expression of its own receptors, especially on cells other than T lymphocytes; IL-1 also enhances expression of Tac.

After contact with antigenic material, a macrophage releases IL-1 at the same time that its MHC-II-positive membrane presents the antigen. Interleukin 1 stimulates T cells to produce IL-2 and modifies the T-cell membrane to enhance its reactivity with antigen. Receptors for IL-2 develop after contact with antigen presented in the context of MHC-II. Secretion of IL-2 and expression of IL-2 receptors enhance the activation initiated by contact with antigen and IL-1. Several events can inhibit T-cell activation: agents that inhibit synthesis of IL-2, like adrenal steroids and certain neurohormones; reduction in expression of Tac, if antigen level diminishes; and reduction in IL-1 concentration, which causes IL-2 production to diminish.

Effects on Non-T Cells

Interleukin 2 has less striking but still significant effects on cells other than T lymphocytes. It enhances NK activity of large granular lymphocytes, which express IL-2 receptors after stimulation by IL-1. Antigen specificity does not restrict the targets that NK cells attack, but specific antigens stimulate T cells to generate IL-2, which enhances the activity of non-specific NK cells. Interleukin 2 enhances proliferation of B cells that have undergone activation and immunoblast transformation, but B-cell stimulation requires much higher concentrations than T-cell proliferation. With very high concentrations of IL-2, macrophages already in an activated state may acquire tumor-killing capacity. Table 7–3 lists the major actions of IL-2.

TABLE 7–3. Actions of IL-2

On T Cells
    Induces Tac expression
    Enhances clonal expansion of antigen-stimulated cells
    Promotes production of IL-2
    Increases production of interferon and other lymphokines
    Increases cytotoxicity of antigen-stimulated T8 cells
On Non-T Cells
    Enhances proliferation and differentiation of antigen-stimulated B
        cells
    Promotes tumoricidal properties of large granular lymphocytes
    Increases cytotoxic actions of NK cells

OTHER LYMPHOKINES

Activated T cells produce an impressive array of peptides that influence other cells. These products were initially identified by effects observed on target cells, and they were named for these activities. Lymphokines have subsequently been intensively characterized; some have been prepared in pure form by recombinant genetic techniques, but the descriptive names persist. **Macrophage-inhibiting factor** (MIF), **macrophage-activating factor** (MAF), and **B-cell growth factor** (BCGF) were some of the materials described. It is now clear that these actions are mediated by many different T-cell products, and a bewildering array of initials and numbers is used to define the T-cell products that enhance, suppress, and modify cell behavior. Table 7–4 lists some of the more important lymphokines and their biologic effects.

TABLE 7–4. Major Categories of Lymphokine Activity

Attraction of Cells
    Macrophage chemotactic factor
    Granulocyte chemotactic factors
        Neutrophil
        Eosinophil
        Basophil
    Lymphocyte chemotactic factors
        B cells
        T cells
    Fibroblast chemotactic factor
Inhibition of Cell Movement
    Macrophage inhibitory factor
    Inhibitor of endothelial cell migration
    Leukocyte inhibiting factor
Promotion of Inflammation
    Skin reactive factor
    Platelet aggregating factor
    Procoagulant of ? type
Promotion of Cell Growth and Differentiation
    Interleukin 2 (IL-2): T cells, some effect on B cells
    Interleukin 3 (IL-3): T cells, B cells, multiple hematopoietic cell lines
    Interleukin 4 (IL-4): T cells, B cells, mast cells
    Interleukin 5 (IL-5): Eosinophils, activated B cells
    Colony stimulating factors for various cell lines
Enhancement of Cellular Activities
    Macrophage activating factor
    Interleukin 2 (IL-2)
    Interferon-gamma
    Osteoclast stimulating factor
    Antigen-specific helper and suppressor factors

CELLULAR ADHESION

Cells interact through direct membrane contact as well as, or instead of, through secretion and recognition of soluble mediators. Certain membrane receptors are present only in certain states of cellular activation, but many molecules that participate in cell-to-cell interactions are a permanent part of cell membranes.

THE LEUKOCYTE FUNCTION-ASSOCIATED ANTIGEN 1

One major contact system requires combination between a molecule on the leukocyte membrane and a complementary ligand on target cells. Granulocytes, lymphocytes, and some macrophages express a heterodimer called **leukocyte function-associated antigen 1** (LFA-1 or CD11a), which binds intimately to reciprocal material called **intercellular adhesion molecule 1** (ICAM-1), which exists on endothelial cells, certain antigen-presenting cells, and many mucosal cells. Association of these molecules can be blocked by antibodies against either LFA-1 or ICAM-1; this blockage inhibits several contact-mediated events, notably T-cell cytotoxicity, NK-cell toxicity, and antibody-dependent cell-mediated cytotoxicity (see later section). These three forms of cytotoxicity arise from different mechanisms: Cytotoxic T cells recognize specific antigens on the target cell; NK cells attack target cells without antigen restriction; and antibody-dependent cell-mediated cytotoxicity requires prior combination of antibody with specific antigen. The common feature is that the effector cell must engage the membrane of the target cell.

Leukocyte function-associated antigen 1 is expressed on all circulating leukocytes, on developing B cells at the pre-B or later stages, and on macrophages stimulated by interferon-gamma and other mediators. It does not occur on non-hematopoietic cells. Expression of ICAM-1, the ligand for LFA-1, is increased by acute inflammatory events and by the products of activated lymphocytes and macrophages, notably IL-1 and INF-gamma. These cellular interactions potentiate and focus immune and inflammatory defense mechanisms that would otherwise be less intense and less specifically targeted.

CD2 AND LFA-3

One of the first properties observed in T cells was formation of rosettes with sheep red blood cells. Thymocytes at the earliest recognizable stage have the surface molecule that promotes this interaction, and this marker persists throughout all phases of T-cell differentiation and function. The responsible molecule, originally called the **sheep-cell receptor,** has been characterized as the T-11, or Leu-5, antigen and is now increasingly designated **CD2;** it is also designated LFA-2. CD2 has a receptor-ligand relationship with a glycoprotein present on many epithelial, endothelial, and connective tissue cells. The reciprocal molecule, although designated **leukocyte function-associated antigen-3** (LFA-3), is not a leukocyte characteristic. Interference with the CD2/LFA-3 interaction abolishes cytotoxic T-cell activity and prevents formation of sheep-cell rosettes but does not affect NK-cell activity. Interventions that block both the LFA-1/ICAM-1 interaction and the CD2/LFA-3 interaction have an additive effect, indicating that the two contact systems act independently of one another.

MHC RECEPTORS

We have already seen that MHC products affect intercellular recognition. T cells interact with their specific antigens only if they are on a surface that expresses MHC properties. T cells recognize these properties through both the T3 portion of the CD3 complex and the CD4 and CD8 membrane molecules. Physical interaction between MHC products on the target cell and recognition receptors on the effector cell brings antigenic material into the closest possible contact with the idiotypic receptor. Cells positive for CD4, involved principally in immune stimulation and in tissue reactions of the delayed hypersensitivity type (see section on Types of Cell-Mediated Immunity, below), require MHC class II (MHC-II) products; CD 8-positive cells perform suppressor and cytotoxic activities and require MHC class I (MHC-I) products. B lymphocytes and the cells that process and present antigen consistently express both class I and class II material and can interact with both T-cell populations. Somatic cells express class I but not class II products; they are thus potential targets for cytotoxic attack. Immune or inflammatory activation, however, may stimulate many cells to manifest class II reactivity; this expands the range of cells and surface properties that can initiate immune reactions.

ADHERENCE TO ENDOTHELIUM

Receptor-ligand interactions also regulate recirculation of lymphocytes. Lymphocytes of all types move in predictable and repetitive patterns from bloodstream to lymphoid tissues to lymphatics and back to bloodstream. Peripatetic cells return time and again to the same lymphoid region, whether lymph node, spleen, or mucosa-associated lymphoid tissue. Lymphocytes migrate from the bloodstream into lymphoid tissue across specialized vascular structures called **high endothelial venules** (HEV). It is thought that individual HEV sites express unique membrane molecules that differentiate each location from all others. These interact with adherence molecules on circulating T and B lymphocytes and direct their preferential return to specific locations. The nature of these recognition structures and the manner in which lymphocytes acquire individualized receptors remain under investigation.

——— TYPES OF CELL-MEDIATED IMMUNITY ———

Cell-mediated immunity (CMI) is not a single entity. Any activity that requires viable cells and is targeted to specific antigens can be considered CMI. This contrasts with the humoral response, in which antibody molecules exert serologic and biologic effects independent of the immunoglobulin-producing cells; and with the actions of macrophages and NK cells, which do not exhibit antigenic recognition. The major types of cell-mediated immune reactions are (1) **delayed (or tuberculin) type hypersensitivity** (DTH); (2) the effects of **cytotoxic T lymphocytes** (CTL); and (3) a combined cellular and humoral event called **antibody-dependent cell-mediated cytotoxicity** (ADCC). Delayed, tuberculin type hypersensitivity was the first form of CMI recognized. In DTH, antigen-restricted T cells interact with their specific antigen and produce lymphokines, which activate effector macrophages and other cells that are not antigen-restricted. In T-cell cytotoxicity, the CD8-positive effector T cells exert direct cell-to-cell effects on targets that display the appropriate antigen specificity. In antibody-dependent cell-mediated cytotoxicity, antigenic specificity resides in antibody, which is synthesized by cells of B lineage. Antibody attaches to the antigen-bearing target cell. The effector cytotoxic cell interacts with the Fc of attached antibody; it does not respond to characteristics of the underlying cell. The actions of NK cells and of lymphokine-activated killer (LAK) cells are not antigen directed and must be considered separately.

DELAYED HYPERSENSITIVITY

In delayed-type hypersensitivity (DTH), antigen-specific T cells encounter an antigen, undergo activation, and acquire memory for the activation. They respond to subsequent contact with the antigen by elaborating lymphokines that affect other cells and tissues (Fig. 7–1). Major effects are accumulation of macrophages and enhancement of macrophage activity, increased blood flow and increased permeability of small blood vessels, and initiation of the coagulation and contact-activation kinin cascades. Tissue undergoing a DTH reaction is often somewhat swollen because increased fluid and protein accumulate in the interstitium. Early in the reaction, vascular congestion causes reddening, but if tissue changes are intense, necrosis and later scarring renders the tissue pale or grayish white. Some of the protein that accumulates is fibrin, generated by the coagulation cascade; some proteins escape from the serum, notably antibodies, complement components, and albumin; and some proteins are synthesized by activated macrophages. The most conspicuous tissue change is accu-

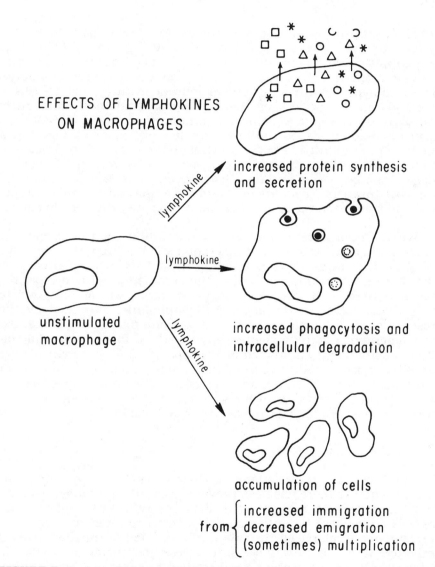

FIGURE 7–1. Lymphokines, produced after antigen-specific stimulation of T cells, affect many aspects of macrophage function and replication. Activation of only a few antigen-restricted lymphocytes can influence large numbers of non-specific effector cells.

mulation of macrophages, often manifesting the altered appearance characteristic of heightened activation. The reaction is called "delayed" hypersensitivity because many hours elapse between contact of sensitized T cells with antigen and the development of these vascular, protein, and cellular changes.

Specificity and Cross-reactivity

The antigen-specific cells responsible for DTH are CD4 positive. Delayed hypersensitivity develops only if MHC-II positive cells present antigen initially and if sensitized memory cells encounter later examples of antigen in the context of MHC-II products. Effective stimulants to delayed hypersensitivity include membrane features of viable tissue cells and complex organisms that are ingested but not immediately destroyed by macrophages. *Mycobacterium tuberculosis,* the etiologic agent of tuberculosis, is the most familiar organism that provokes this form of immunity. Other organisms that elicit DTH are *Mycobacterium leprae,* which causes leprosy; many fungi that elicit a macrophage response, like *Candida, Histoplasma,* and *Blastomyces;* the protozoal invaders *Toxoplasma gondii* and several leishmania species; and such bacteria as *Listeria monocytogenes* and certain salmonellae.

When T cells secrete lymphokines after stimulation by specific organisms, there is activation of macrophages that are not specific for antigens; this leads to apparent cross-reactivity. The CD4-positive cells that recognize and respond to the organism are highly specific; cells sensitized to *M. tuberculosis,* for example, will not respond to the presence of *L. monocytogenes.* Lymphokines provoked by the presence of *M. tuberculosis,* however, activate macrophages that exhibit heightened activity against any invaders. In experimental settings, macrophages stimulated after exposure to *M. tuberculosis* are more than normally effective in killing *L. monocytogenes* or any other intracellular invader. This kind of cross-reactive immunity is less apparent in clinical settings, although it may well have physiologic consequences that are difficult to observe or to measure.

The Tuberculin Test

The tuberculin test is a familiar example of DTH. It is done to determine whether there has been previous immunizing exposure to the tubercle bacillus *(M. tuberculosis)* and gives a positive result if memory cells are present for antigens of this organism. A small amount of antigenic material, called the **tuberculin** antigen or **purified protein derivative** (PPD), is introduced into an easily observed skin site. No viable organisms are present, so there is no danger of causing infection, and the quantity of antigen is too small to elicit primary immunization. If sensitized memory cells are present, tissue changes develop where the antigen was injected. Within 48 hours the skin becomes reddened, firm, and somewhat swollen, owing to vascular

TUBERCULIN REACTION

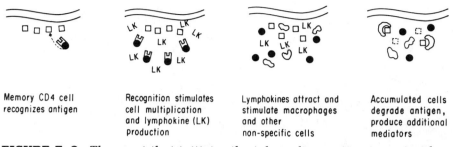

| Memory CD4 cell recognizes antigen | Recognition stimulates cell multiplication and lymphokine (LK) production | Lymphokines attract and stimulate macrophages and other non-specific cells | Accumulated cells degrade antigen, produce additional mediators |

FIGURE 7—2. The event that initiates the tuberculin reaction is contact between injected antigen and antigen-specific CD4 cells that have memory of previous activation. The anamnestic response stimulated by injected antigen promotes clonal expansion and subsequent production of lymphokines that induce vascular changes and cellular accumulation. An individual who has never before encountered the antigen will have no memory cells capable of promoting these changes.

changes and macrophage accumulation induced by the lymphokines. The tissue events act to degrade the antigen within a few days, eliminating the immune stimulus and allowing the tissue to return to normal (Fig. 7—2). If the individual does not have immune memory for the organism, no tissue changes occur at the injection site.

This procedure is used to demonstrate delayed hypersensitivity to various antigens in a variety of circumstances. It is used to diagnose previous or present infection with various fungi, to demonstrate memory-cell function against commonly encountered environmental antigens, and to investigate whether a patient has sufficient cell-mediated immune capability to mount a response after deliberate exposure to an unfamiliar antigen.

CYTOTOXIC T LYMPHOCYTES

Several populations of lymphocytes express the CD8 antigen. CD8-positive cells are sometimes described as the **suppressor/cytotoxic** population, but different populations exist, performing different functions although sharing expression of the CD8 antigen. **Suppressor T** cells are immunoregulatory cells that inhibit or down-regulate effector actions of B cells or other T cells. **Cytotoxic T** cells engage in lethal membrane interactions with target cells that express specific antigen.

A notable example of cytotoxic action is attack on virus-infected cells. In a cell that harbors virus, the membrane often expresses viral antigens in addition to intrinsic cellular characteristics. Virtually all cells express MHC-I products, so any cell displaying viral antigens can

ACTION OF CYTOTOXIC T CELL

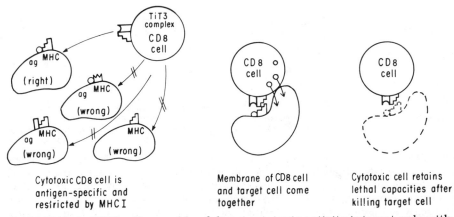

Cytotoxic CD8 cell is antigen-specific and restricted by MHC I	Membrane of CD8 cell and target cell come together	Cytotoxic cell retains lethal capacities after killing target cell

FIGURE 7–3. CD8 cells capable of direct cytotoxic activity interact only with target cells expressing both antigen and the appropriate MHC class I product. MHC restriction is significant only in experimental settings because, in an intact individual, all cells have the host's MHC I products. The CD8 cell lethally damages the target cell without damaging itself and can move on to additional cells that express the right combination of membrane attributes.

be attacked by CD8 cells specific for the viral products. The cytotoxic T cell binds to the infected cell and introduces its lethal material across the membrane (Fig. 7–3). The nature of the injury is unclear. The T cell may inject material that lyses the cell or paralyzes certain functions, the adhesion process may disrupt membrane integrity, or the physical interaction may damage internal structures or interfere with intracellular transmission of messages. The effector cell is not destroyed. A cytotoxic cell can experience lethal engagements with several successive targets. The lethal effects need not be immediate; target-cell death has been observed at intervals ranging from 10 minutes to 3 hours after the event.

Usual Targets

Because CD8 cells are MHC restricted, they do not attack isolated viruses, bacteria, or parasites. Activity of cytotoxic T lymphocytes (CTL) occurs only if antigenic material adheres to a cell membrane, or if infection or metabolic damage causes the membrane to express new antigens. The beneficial effects of CTL are to halt intracellular multiplication of pathogens and to eliminate partially degraded foreign material. The adverse effect is death of the affected cell. Cytotoxic T lymphocyte immunity is most conspicuous against agents that alter membrane characteristics in the affected cell and against organisms that invade and multiply in cells that lack MHC-II products. Organisms that invade cells with MHC-II characteristics elicit immunity in CD4-positive cells, as described in the preceding section. Non-specific inflammatory events enhance antigen-specific CTL because stimulated macrophages secrete IL-1. Interleukin 1 not only promotes the cytotoxic properties of CD-8 cells, but also stimulates expression of MHC-I products in many target cell populations.

ANTIBODY-DEPENDENT CELL-MEDIATED CYTOTOXICITY

Antibody-dependent cell-mediated cytotoxicity (ADCC) differs from other forms of cell-mediated immunity in that the effector cell does not recognize antigen. The cellular aspect is the interaction between a receptor on the cell membrane and the Fc of antibody bound to the target cell or particle. Antigenic specificity resides in the interaction between antibody and surface antigen. Antibody-dependent cell-mediated cytotoxicity is not opsonization. The effector cell does not phagocytize the coated cell; it exerts lethal injury after cell-to-cell binding occurs. Large granular lymphocytes, which have virtually no phagocytic capability, are the cells most conspicuous in ADCC, although macrophages and granulocytes sometimes destroy an antibody-coated target instead of engulfing it. The large granular lymphocytes recognize the target cell through the immunoglobulin Fc and bind it to it through the LFA-1/ICAM-1 combination. Once bound, the effector lymphocyte releases lethal materials from its cytoplasmic granules.

Early workers divided large granular lymphocytes into two categories: **K cells,** which engaged in ADCC; and **NK cells,** which were cytotoxic for cells in their native state. It appears that a single population, now designated NK cells, can engage in either form of target-cell damage, so the distinction between K and NK cells is no longer germane.

Role of Antibody

The antigen-specific immune event in ADCC is interaction between antibody and cell-surface antigen. Before ADCC can occur, primary immunization must generate plasma cells that secrete specific antibody, and antibody molecules in body fluids must combine with antigen molecules on the target cell (Fig. 7–4). Targets of ADCC include bacteria, autologous cells coated with autoantibodies, and allogeneic cells introduced through transplantation. Antibody-dependent cell-mediated cytotoxicity is restricted by immunoglobulin isotype. Macrophages, granulocytes, lymphocytes, and other antibody-directed cells express Fc receptors that recognize individual immunoglobulin classes. Fc receptors for the gamma chain of IgG are most often involved in ADCC; on mucosal surfaces, IgA antibodies and Fc-alpha receptors may be significant.

ANTIBODY-DEPENDENT
CELL-MEDIATED CYTOTOXICITY

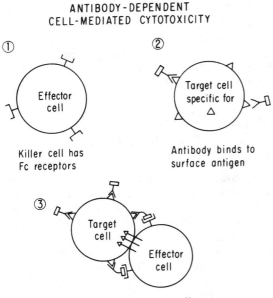

Killer cell has
Fc receptors

Antibody binds to
surface antigen

Fc receptor brings Killer cell
into intense interaction with
cell coated by specific antibody

FIGURE 7–4. The large granular lymphocytes that perform antibody-dependent cell-mediated cytotoxicity do not recognize specific antigens. They have membrane receptors with high affinity for the Fc of immunoglobulin molecules, as shown in 1. When the Fab sites of antibody combine with cell-surface antigen, the Fc portion remains accessible, as shown in 2, offering a ligand through which the effector cell can bind to the target cell and lethally damage it, as shown in 3. These effector cells will not react with target cells that have not first been coated with antibody.

NATURAL KILLER CELLS AND LYMPHOKINE-ACTIVATED KILLER CELLS

In chapter 5, we described the cell population called **natural killer** (NK) cells. These cells, which are large granular lymphocytes with rather sparse and ambiguous markers for lineage, adhere to their target cells without regard to MHC characteristics or antigenic specificity. Natural killer cells constitute approximately 5 percent of circulating lymphocytes in normal individuals; their concentration in tissues is harder to quantify. Cells described as **lymphokine-activated killer** (LAK) cells do not occur naturally. These are cells exposed, in the laboratory, to very high concentrations of IL-2. They exhibit enhanced cytolytic capacities, especially against tumor cells and cells with growth properties transformed by viral infection or neoplastic events. Lymphokine-activated killer cells are predominantly large granular lymphocytes; before exposure to IL-2, they may have been NK cells, but this relationship is not fully established.

NATURAL KILLER CELLS

Although they do not recognize specific antigens, NK cells are not indiscriminate in their actions. Receptor-ligand restriction appears to

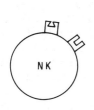
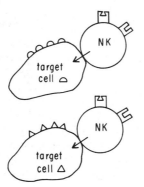
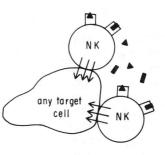

NK cells have receptors for IFN-γ, IL-2 but not for specific antigens

NK cells can attack target regardless of antigens expressed

IFN-γ and IL-2 generated by immune-stimulated T cells enhance NK cell activity

UNMODIFIED vs IMMUNE-ENHANCED
NK CELL ACTIVITY

FIGURE 7–5. Although NK cells can interact with target cells independent of antigenic specificity or state of immune activation, an ongoing immune response heightens NK cell activity. Lymphokines secreted by antigen-stimulated T cells increase the lethal effects that NK cells exert but do not influence selection of the target against which they act.

exist, but neither participant has been fully characterized. Antibodies against the LFA-1/ICAM-1 adhesion system abolish NK-mediated cytolysis, but this may not be the primary recognition system. Tumor cells and other immature cells are especially susceptible to NK action. ICAM-1 expression is enhanced on cultured cells stimulated by mitogens or transformed by Epstein-Barr virus, but this laboratory observation may not reflect physiologic events. Natural killer cells are active against fibroblasts, virus-infected cells, and many hematopoietic precursors, a diverse target population for which no unifying membrane property has been identified.

Immune events affect NK-cell activity through cytokines secreted in response to antigenic exposure. Interferon-gamma, produced by T cells after specific antigenic stimulation, directly stimulates NK activity and also increases expression of Fc receptors on the NK-cell membrane, thereby enhancing ADCC. Interleukin 2, secreted by T cells after stimulation by IL-1, also heightens NK activity (Fig. 7–5). These effects have been demonstrated under experimental conditions; the physiologic role of NK cells is by no means clear.

LYMPHOKINE-ACTIVATED
KILLER CELLS

Lymphokine-activated killer cells are large granular lymphocytes incubated, *in vitro*, with large amounts of IL-2. This is an example of the anticancer strategy called **adoptive immunotherapy,** which exploits immune mechanisms active against abnormally multiplying cells. Adoptive immunotherapy involves artificial introduction of immunologically reactive materials. Several adoptive approaches have been tried: injection of antibodies directed against generalized or specific tumor antigens; administration of cytotoxic drugs coupled to antigen-targeted carriers; injection of lymphokines, especially IL-2; and introduction of cytotoxic cells preferentially or specifically active against tumor cells. Injecting IL-2 alters circulating lymphocytes and affects immune reactivity, but effects on tumor behavior have been disappointing, and troublesome side effects occur consistently. Injecting cells with specific antitumor action has had promising effects on experimental tumors, but it has been difficult to develop human cells targeted against human tumors.

Natural killer cells in their native state have lytic capacity only against cultured tumor cells, not against fresh tumor cells. When lymphoid cells are cultured for 3 to 5 days in a high concentration of IL-2, a population acquires the capacity to lyse fresh, unmodified tumor cells. These LAK cells do not affect freshly prepared, unmodified normal cells but do inflict damage on normal cells maintained in culture and on previously normal cells subjected to alterations of the membrane surface. Without continuing IL-2 stimulation, however, LAK cells lose their tumoricidal characteristics, and administering LAK cells to patients whose immune status is unmodified has given disappointing results. The most promising protocol at present is *in vitro* generation of LAK cells and simultaneous infusion of high-dose IL-2 along with the LAK cells. The mechanisms whereby antitumor activity is enhanced and maintained are under intense investigation.

SUGGESTIONS FOR FURTHER READING

Braquet P, Rola-Pleszczynski M: Platelet-activating factor and cellular immune responses. Immunol Today 1987; 8:345–52

Cohen S: Physiologic and pathologic manifestations of lymphokine action. Hum Pathol 1986; 17:112–21

Dinarello CA, Mier JW: Interleukins. Ann Rev Med 1986; 37:173–78

Dinarello CA, Mier JW: Lymphokines. NEJM 1987; 317:940–45

Goldfarb RH: Cell-mediated cytotoxic reactions. Hum Path 1986; 17:138–45

Gordon J, Guy GR: The molecules controlling B lymphocytes. Immunol Today 1987; 8:339–43

Herberman RB: Lymphocyte-mediated cytotoxicity. In: Marchalonis JJ, ed: The Lymphocyte: Structure and Function, 2nd ed. New York: Marcel Dekker, 1988:95–119

Paul, NL, Ruddle NH: Lymphotoxin. Ann Rev Immunol 1988; 5:407–38

Romain PL, Schlossman SF: The T cell circuit: clinical and biological implications. Adv Int Med 1986; 31:1–16

Springer TA, Dustin ML, Kishimoto TK, Marlin SD: The lymphocyte function-associated LFA-1, CD2, and LFA-3 molecules: cell adhesion receptors of the immune system. Ann Rev Immunol 1987; 5:223–52

Young JDE, Cohn ZA: Cellular and humoral mechanisms of cytotoxicity. Structural and functional analogies. Adv Immunol 1987; 41:269–332

CHAPTER 8

The Complement System

The 14 effector proteins and 7 control proteins that constitute the complement system circulate in normal blood, either in active or precursor form. As far back as the 1890s, serologists observed that adding normal, non-immune serum changed the consequences of many antigen-antibody reactions. This effect, which disappeared if the serum was heated, came to be known as **complement,** because it complemented immune activity that had developed independently. Complement activity evolves only after the constituent proteins interact in an obligatory sequence; antigen-antibody reactions often initiate the sequence, but other stimuli can also promote these interactions. Antigen-antibody reactions trigger the **classical pathway** of complement activation; other substances and events can initiate the **alternative pathway** of complement activation (Fig. 8–1). Biological systems that require a stringent sequence of interactions are often described as **cascades**. Other physiologic cascades include the reactions that lead to coagulation activity, and the kinin system, which mediates many vascular events.

COMPLEMENT ACTIVATION

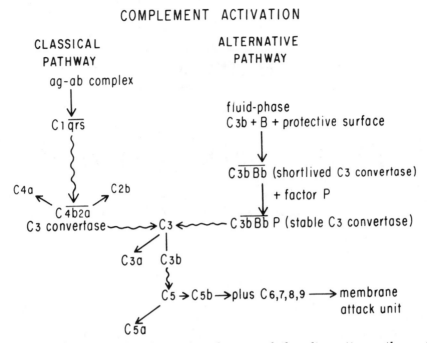

FIGURE 8–1. Both the classical pathway and the alternative pathway induce cleavage of C3, and the late-stage consequences are the same for both routes of activation. These consequences are generation of anaphylatoxic cleavage fragments, promotion of opsonic activity through attachment of C3b to surfaces, and generation of the membrane attack unit.

GENERAL PROPERTIES OF COMPLEMENT

Complement was first discovered in experiments with antibacterial antibodies. Native antibody would agglutinate suspended microorganisms into coarse clumps, but in the presence of complement, the antibody caused dissolution, or **lysis,** of the organisms. Antibodies against a variety of antigen-bearing cells may lyse their target when active complement is present. Lysis is especially conspicuous when the target is the red blood cell, because hemoglobin escapes from the cytoplasm and discolors the suspending medium.

MAJOR ACTIONS

Lysis is a commonly employed end point for laboratory observations but is probably not the major role that complement plays in the living body. As the cascade progresses, enzyme activities evolve, proteins are cleaved, and polypeptide fragments accumulate. The major physiologic consequences of complement activation are opsonization, immune adherence, and anaphylatoxic activity, which influences inflammatory events.

Interaction with Cells

Fragments of complement molecules adhere to the surface of cells or particles at sites where activation occurs. Macrophages and neutrophils, the principal phagocytic inflammatory cells, have receptors for complement fragments; coated cells or particles are engulfed and attacked much more effectively than uncoated targets. Enhancement of phagocytosis is called **opsonization**. Opsonization also results from attachment of IgG antibodies to surfaces. Phagocytic cells have receptors for the Fc portion of IgG; these receptors are completely different from those for complement fragments.

Non-phagocytic cells also have receptors for complement fragments. B lymphocytes, red blood cells, and many endothelial and epithelial cells express receptors for various complement fragments. Protein aggregates that include complement or particles coated with complement may combine with receptors on cell membranes in a process called **immune adherence**. This interaction intensifies the contact between a reactive cell and the antigen, particle, cell, or immune complex that provokes the reaction. Events in which complement-mediated immune adherence participates include modulation of B-cell responses to antigen, degradation of cells and proteins, and regulation of inflammation and cell regeneration.

Effects on Inflammation

Complement exerts potent actions in enhancing inflammation. Several fragments generated by the complement sequence are called **anaphylatoxins;** these mediators promote vascular and cellular events in acute inflammation and stimulate basophilic and eosinophilic granulocytes and platelet granules to release stored materials that exert powerful effects on blood vessels, cellular synthetic processes, and coagulation sequences. Complement-derived anaphylatoxins attract neutrophils and macrophages, an action called **chemotaxis,** and affect endothelial cells and the permeability of small blood vessels. Complement products directly affect actions of macrophages, which are, in addition, secondarily stimulated by a variety of inflammatory and immune events.

Enzyme Activity

During sequential activation, many complement proteins acquire enzyme activity of the type described as **serine protease;** serine proteases active in other contexts include trypsin, plasmin, thrombin, and elastase. All these serine proteases are powerful enzymes essential in restricted reactions but highly destructive if they manifest excessive, inappropriate, or misplaced activity. Serine proteases that evolve during the complement cascade generally lose their activity within a short time, but, while active, they may cleave protein substrates additional to those targeted in the complement sequence.

TERMINOLOGY

Combination of antibody with antigen initiates the first step in the classical complement pathway; contact with protein aggregates or with materials of appropriate surface characteristics initiates the alternative pathway. These pathways converge, as shown in Figure 8–1. Proteins of the classical pathway and of the later common phase are called **components** and are identified by numbers. Proteins of the alternative pathway are described as **factors** and are identified by letters. As interactions occur and inactive precursors become active, the state of activation is sometimes denoted by a bar above the letter or number. In the early activation phases, inactive precursor proteins are cleaved into fragments with various activities. The fragments are identified by lowercase letters; with one exception (C2), the "a" fragment is a small soluble molecule that enters the fluid medium, and the "b" and later fragments accumulate at the site of activation and participate in the cascade. As enzyme activity is generated, the active protein complex is called a **convertase,** because it converts the next protein in the sequence into the active form.

CLEAVAGE OF C3, THE PIVOTAL EVENT

The most abundant complement component is C3; both the classical and the alternative pathways have the same end point, namely, cleavage of C3 into C3a and C3b. This event has three major consequences: (1) the small, free C3a fragment has significant anaphylatoxic effect; (2) C3b and several of its evolutionary products have potent activity as opsonins and in immune adherence; and (3) suitably complexed C3b is the convertase necessary to perpetuate the cascade. Not every activation event precipitates the entire complement cascade; many physiologic effects occur following cleavage of C3, whether or not the later steps proceed. The liver synthesizes most of the 1200 to 1600 micrograms/ml of C3 present in the serum, although activated macrophages may elaborate this and other complement components under localized conditions.

Consequences of C3 Cleavage

C3b perpetuates the complement cascade by serving as **C5 convertase,** cleaving native C5 into C5a and C5b. C5a is a potent anaphylatoxin, with particularly striking effects on neutrophils. Accumulated C5a attracts neutrophils and activates them to heightened enzyme production and intracellular bacterial killing. C5b participates in the cascade, assembling the later numbered components into the **membrane attack unit,** which lethally damages cell membranes. C5 cleavage is the last protein-splitting event in the complement cascade; later steps involve association and rearrangement of proteins. C5b causes C6 and C7 to form a stable C5b67 complex, and this, in turn, attracts and gives structure to C8 and C9, the elements that actually penetrate the membrane. Association of C5b, 6, 7, 8, and 9 initiates the membrane attack unit without generating any independently active fragments. The classical and the alternative pathways are identical in their effects on C5 and later assembly of the membrane attack unit.

THE CLASSICAL PATHWAY

Unfortunately for ready comprehension and recall, components of the classical pathway do not interact in orderly numerical sequence. Numbers were assigned as the proteins were identified, before their interactions were clarified. The two phases of the classical pathway that lead to cleavage of C3 are called **recognition** and **activation**. C1 is involved in the recognition phase; C4 and C2 participate, in that order, in the activation phase that initiates C3 convertase activity.

RECOGNITION

The recognition aspect of the recognition phase is the association of antibody with specific antigen; if the antibody is one that possesses a complement-binding domain in its heavy chain, C1 binds to the antibody molecule as it participates in the antigen-antibody complex. Classical-pathway activation requires the previous occurrence of an immunizing event that generates antibody. Only after antibody has combined with antigen does complement activation begin, a process that takes place only at the site of antigen-antibody interaction. IgM antibodies are more effective than any IgG subclass in activating the classical pathway. Of the IgG subclasses, IgG1 and IgG3 are moderately effective; IgG2 is weakly active, and IgG4 is ineffective.

Physiologic Consequences

The greater efficiency of IgM has beneficial physiologic consequences. IgM antibodies, which develop early in the primary immune response, do not promote opsonization because phagocytic cells lack receptors for the mu chain. The combination of IgM with antigen, however, serves to attract and to stimulate inflammatory cells by generating anaphylatoxic complement fragments, and to promote immune adherence and phagocytosis through deposition of C3b. Immune adherence brings the complement-coated antigenic material into contact with macrophages, the cells best capable of presenting it to additional antibody-producing cells. Antibodies that develop later in the immune response tend to have greater affinity for antigen than early-appearing immunoglobulins and often express specificity against additional epitopes. As the immune response progresses, IgG antibodies predominate; these promote opsonization and immune adherence through their own properties, with less need for complement.

When immunoglobulin attaches to antigen through its Fab sites, the rest of the molecule undergoes a configurational change that exposes the complement-binding site in the constant region. Complement does not bind to immunoglobulin molecules that have not first combined with antigen. Complement binds only when constant domains from two separate monomers lie close to one another; it does not unite with the symmetrical parts of a single Fc portion.

THE C1 COMPLEX

C1 consists of three separable proteins that remain associated only if ionized calcium is present. The three constituents are called **C1q, C1r,** and **C1s;** it is C1q that attaches to the immunoglobulin heavy chain. After C1q binds to two immunoglobulin monomers, C1r and C1s undergo a configurational change that generates enzyme activity. C1q is a remarkable protein, consisting of 18 polypeptide chains and 6 globular protein masses, as shown in Figure 8–2. Each globular mass is attached to three chains that twine into a triple helix; the complex resembles a bunch of flowers, with six blooms, each supported by a triple-helical stem. The six "blooms" are grouped into three pairs by disulfide bonds that link adjacent stems. Combination with immunoglobulin occurs through the globular heads; the stalks form a central support around which C1r and C1s enfold, as shown in Figure 8–3.

Protein Interactions

At least two globular C1q heads must interact with constant domains of separate monomers. A single bound IgG molecule will not initiate the process; there must be at least two IgG monomers sufficiently close together that two heads of a single C1q molecule can attach. IgM antibodies activate complement more effectively than IgG antibodies, because the IgM pentamer presents a simultaneous array of five different sites for C1q attachment. When IgM reacts with surface antigens, a single antigen-antibody event can initiate the complement cascade; if IgG is to activate complement, antigen sites must be closely enough spaced that two different antibody molecules can react

STRUCTURE OF C1q

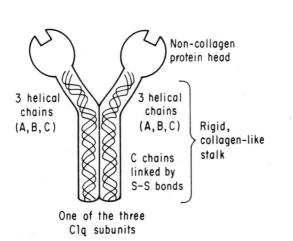
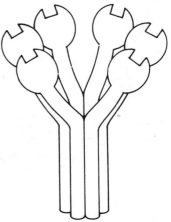

FIGURE 8–2. C1q consists of 6 globular masses of non-collagen protein plus strands of collagenlike protein twined into 18 helical chains. Each globular "head" has a "stalk" of 3 entwined chains, designated A, B, and C. Disulfide bonds link adjacent C chains to form paired units. Interaction with the heavy chain of bound immunoglobulin occurs through the globular protein heads. The collagenlike stalks provide the structural framework on which C1r and C1s interact.

STRUCTURE OF C1qrs

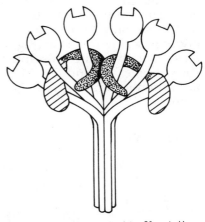

FIGURE 8–3. C1r and C1s are dimeric polypeptides that require the presence of ionized calcium to associate with one another and with the stalks of C1q. If ionized calcium is removed, C1r and C1s dissociate from C1q and the classical-pathway cascade cannot occur.

C1r dimer is attached to C1q stalks.
C1s dimer is attached to C1r.

ACTIVATION OF C1$\overline{qrs}$

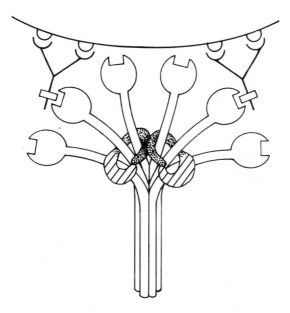

Attachment of Clq changes molecular shape, allows activation of Clrs.

FIGURE 8—4. When two or more globular heads of C1q attach to bound immunoglobulin molecules, the collagenlike stalks change their configuration. The resulting shape change causes C1r to evolve into a serine protease, which cleaves a small fragment off C1s. This uncovers the C1$\overline{s}$ serine protease, whose sole targets are C4 and C2.

independently within a small area. It has been estimated that at least 800 IgG molecules must attach to a red-cell membrane before complement-mediated lysis will occur.

After C1q attaches, C1r undergoes a change in shape that uncovers serine protease activity. Active C1$\overline{r}$ is an enzyme of exquisite specificity; its only known substrate is C1s, which it cleaves to reveal another serine protease (Fig. 8—4). Activated C1$\overline{s}$ also has highly restricted activity; its only substrates are the next two components in the cascade, C4 and C2. The recognition phase of classical-pathway activation generates the C1$\overline{qrs}$ complex, which then initiates the later events.

Inhibitory Actions

Factors that limit or modify the recognition phase are: the specificity of antibody for antigen, the presence of appropriate domains on the Ig heavy chain, the density of Ig monomers present, and absence of interference with the actions of C1$\overline{r}$ on C1s and of C1$\overline{s}$ on other proteins. An inhibitor called **C1INH,** described later in more detail, interrupts this process if only small amounts are present, but massive accumulation of activated C1$\overline{qrs}$ overcomes the inhibitory effects. Absence of ionized calcium causes C1r and C1s to dissociate from C1q, so plasma anticoagulated with chelating agents like citrate or oxalate cannot manifest complement activity. Heating serum to 56°C or above inactivates all elements of the C1 complex.

THE ACTIVATION PHASE

C1$\overline{s}$ exerts proteolytic action on the next protein, the large beta-1-globulin called **C4**. C4 is the second most abundant complement protein, with a serum concentration of approximately 600 μ/ml, as compared with approximately 1600 μg/ml for C3 and concentrations below 100 μg/ml for the other classical-pathway components (see Table 8–1). Cleavage by C1$\overline{s}$ generates a small free-floating fragment, C4a, which has modest anaphylatoxic effect, and a large C4b fragment that possesses a high reactive binding site (Fig. 8–5). This binding site is short lived; unless C4$\overline{b}$ binds to a substrate within a few seconds, it loses its ability to do so.

TABLE 8–1. Proteins of the Complement System

Designation	Mol. Wt. in kD	Electro-phoretic Mobility	Inactivated by 56°C Incubation	Approximate Serum Concentration (μg/ml)
Classical Pathway				
C1q	385–400	γ2	Yes	70
C1r	190	β	Yes	34
C1s	87	α	Yes	31
C4	206–209	β1	No	450–600
C2	117	β1	Yes	25–30
C3	180–185	β1	No	1300–1600
Alternative Pathway				
Factor B	93–100	β2		200–240
Factor D	23–24	β2		1–2
Factor P (properdin)	220	γ2		25
C3	180–185	β1		1300–1600
Terminal Sequence				
C5	190–206	β1	Yes	70–75
C6	120–128	β2	No	60–65
C7	110–121	β2	No	55
C8	150–153	γ1	Yes	55–80
C9	71–79	α	Yes	60–160

CLEAVAGE OF C4

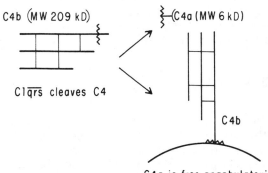

C4b (MW 209 kD)

C4a (MW 6 kD)

C1qrs cleaves C4

C4b

C4a is free anaphylatoxin.

C4b binds to membrane.

FIGURE 8–5. C4 is a large protein with 3 chains. The C1s̄ protease cleaves a small fragment from the longest chain, uncovering a short-lived binding site through which the large fragment can attach to a membrane or surface. The small cleavage fragment, C4a, remains in the fluid phase and has anaphyla-toxic activity.

One C1s̄ unit cleaves many molecules of C4, generating many activated C4b fragments, of which only a few actually attach to substrate. The rest are inactivated by a control protein (**factor I,** formerly called C3bINA), in a reaction discussed more fully in a later section. C4b̄ does not bind to the C1qr̄s̄ complex or to the immunoglobulin molecule; it attaches to the cell membrane or bacterial wall at a separate site near the antigen-antibody reaction. C1 is the only complement protein that reacts directly with the immunoglobulin molecule.

C2 and Its Actions

Besides its action on C4, C1s also cleaves **C2,** a single-chain protein present at low serum concentration. Cleavage generates a small free fragment that enters the fluid phase and a larger fragment that adheres to the active surface. The nomenclature for the C2 fragments is anomalous; the large fragment that perpetuates the cascade is called "a," and the small fluid-phase fragment is 2b. C1s̄ has only weak action against free C2 molecules, but C2 that has united with C4b is powerfully affected. C1s̄ thus promotes accumulation on the antigen-bearing surface of C4b2a, which possesses potent but short-lived convertase activity against free C3 molecules (Fig. 8–6). If it does not encounter its substrate, C4b2a decays within a few minutes.

C4b2a divides the C3 molecule into the small, fluid-phase C3a, which has anaphylatoxic activity, and the much larger C3b, which expresses an active binding site (Fig. 8–7). Each C4b2a complex cleaves many C3 molecules, generating many anaphylatoxic C3a fragments and many C3b residues that must either bind promptly to a surface or be degraded by factor I. When C3b combines with C4b2a, the resulting C4b2a3b complex is a potent C5 convertase. Many C3b mole-

CLEAVAGE OF C2

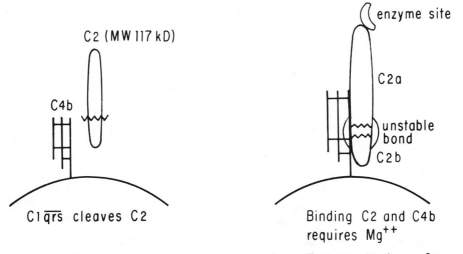

C2 (MW 117 kD)

C4b

C1$\overline{qrs}$ cleaves C2

enzyme site

C2a

unstable bond

C2b

Binding C2 and C4b requires Mg^{++}

Enzyme site is on C2a, half-life a few seconds

FIGURE 8–6. C2 is a single-chain protein susceptible to cleavage by C1$\overline{s}$. C2 can attach, through an unstable bond, to C4b present on a membrane. C1$\overline{s}$ has stronger proteolytic activity against C2 molecules associated with C4b than against free C2. Cleavage of C2 by C1$\overline{s}$ generates a small fluid-phase fragment, designated C2b, and a large fragment, designated C2a, which joins the C4b complex and expresses an enzyme site capable of perpetuating the cascade.

cules bind independently to the membrane surface; these fragments do not propagate the complement cascade, but they do promote the immune adherence and opsonizing effects described earlier.

Effects of Activation

Activation of the classical pathway results in an antigen-bearing surface that exhibits numerous attached C3b molecules and in the C$\overline{4b2a3b}$ complex, which has potent C5 convertase activity. Activation also generates moderate numbers of C4a fragments and larger numbers of C3a fragments free in the surrounding medium. After C$\overline{4b2a}$ forms, the immunoglobulin molecules and attached C1 are no longer necessary; antibody can elute from the antigen-bearing surface without affecting later complement-mediated events.

CLEAVAGE OF C3

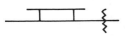

C3 (MW 190 kD)

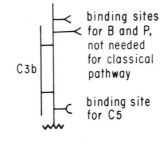

⅃— C3a (MW 9 kD)

C4b2a cleaves C3

C3b

binding sites
for B and P,
not needed
for classical
pathway

binding site
for C5

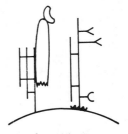

C3a is free anaphylatoxin.

C3b has short-lived ability
to bind on surface

C3b binds
independently
to membrane

FIGURE 8–7. The C4b2a complex is a C3 convertase. It cleaves a small fragment from the larger of the two C3 chains; the small C3a fragment remains in the fluid phase as an anaphylatoxin. The large C3b fragment binds to the membrane near, but not in, the C4b2a complex. One C4b2a complex can generate large numbers of C3b units, which exert powerful opsonic effects. Membrane-bound C3b also serves as the C5 convertase, which perpetuates the cascade.

THE ALTERNATIVE PATHWAY

Like the classical pathway, the alternative pathway generates fluid-phase C3a and surface-bound C3b and eventuates in C5 convertase, but the initiating events are very different. Alternative-pathway activation is surface dependent; the plasma proteins interact and accumulate exclusively on surfaces displaying the required characteristics. No antigen-antibody reaction is necessary, and the host need have had no previous exposure to foreign material or pathogenic microorganisms. The necessary proteins are already present in plasma; the critical element is a spatial configuration that permits accumulation.

THE PROTEINS INVOLVED

Proteins of the alternative pathway perform activities roughly comparable to those in the classical pathway. **Factor D,** a small protein present in very low concentration, corresponds to C1s; and **fac-**

tor B, present at approximately 240 μ/ml, is analogous to C2. C3 participates in the early interactions of the alternative pathway as well as in the later C5 convertase complex. Another major participant is **properdin** (factor P), a large molecule present in serum at approximately 25 μ/ml, which serves to stabilize the evolving molecular complex. The alternative pathway was originally called the **properdin system,** based on the enhancing effects noted for this large serum protein.

It is important to understand that plasma proteins continually undergo low-level cleavage. Precursor proteins in many mediator systems spontaneously evolve into activated forms, but unless they accumulate to a critical concentration, the randomly activated molecules have no biological effect. Alternative-pathway activation results from this continuous generation of C3b in normal body fluids and plasma.

INTERACTIONS IN FLUID

The major C3 convertase of the alternative pathway is the C3bBb complex, of which small amounts accumulate through spontaneous cleavage events. C3 is cleaved to C3b, generating slight activity as a C3 convertase and modest proteolytic action against the alternative-pathway protein called **factor B**. The enzyme principally responsible for cleaving factor B into Bb is not C3b, however, but **factor D**. Factor D circulates as an active protease in native plasma, but at very low concentrations; it does not degrade plasma proteins in an uncontrolled fashion because it is highly restricted as to substrate. Its only target is factor B, specifically factor B that has bound to C3b (Fig. 8–8). Factor B binds in a random fashion to available C3b and thus becomes subject to factor D action, but very little C3bBb accumulates. Under normal conditions, little C3b is available because it is degraded by the control protein, **factor I;** and interaction of factor B with C3b is inhibited by another control protein, **factor H** (see later section). Consequently there is little C3bB complex on which factor D can act.

INTERACTIONS ON SURFACES

These limiting conditions change if the plasma proteins interact on certain surfaces with appropriate properties; these include cell-wall polysaccharides of yeasts and some bacteria, aggregated protein complexes, bacterial endotoxins, and products of trypsin and other enzymes. The effect of these surfaces is to shelter C3b, B, and C3bBb complexes from the dissociative effect of factor H and the degradative actions of factor I (Fig. 8–9). This protection allows factor B to bind to C3b in quantities sufficient for factor D to generate abundant C3bBb. Accumulating C3bBb serves as a C3 convertase that generates additional C3b, which attracts and cleaves additional factor B, which is

INTERACTIONS IN ALTERNATIVE PATHWAY

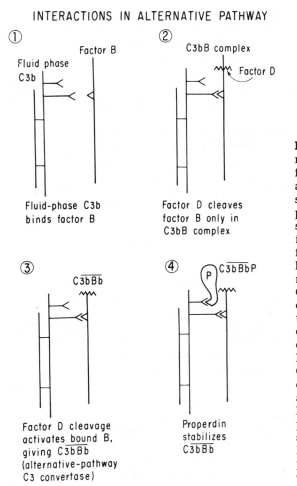

① Fluid phase C3b

Factor B

Fluid-phase C3b binds factor B

② C3bB complex

Factor D

Factor D cleaves factor B only in C3bB complex

③ C3bBb

Factor D cleavage activates bound B, giving C3bBb (alternative-pathway C3 convertase)

④ C3bBbP

Properdin stabilizes C3bBb

FIGURE 8–8. The alternative pathway comprises four interactions. Small amounts of C3b evolve spontaneously in the fluid phase and bind factor B, shown in 1. Bound factor B is the target for cleavage by factor D, as shown in 2, leaving the large Bb fragment bound to C3b. The C3bBb complex is a C3 convertase, cleaving additional C3 molecules to generate additional C3b which can bind additional factor B, as shown in 3. The C3bBb complex retains C3 convertase activity for only a short time, unless stabilized by combination with properdin (factor P), as shown in 4. Factors I and H, in plasma, inhibit fluid-phase interactions among C3b, factor B, and factor D.

the target of additional factor D activity, and so on. This autocatalytic process does not exhaust serum C3 because C3 is present at serum concentrations more than adequate to perpetuate the process (see Table 8–1). The C3bBb complex has a short half-life—approximately 5 minutes. The function of **properdin** is to bind to C3bBb and to prolong its half-life to 30 minutes, much amplifying its physiologic effects. Properdin does not initiate the sequence, but it enhances the accumulation and reactivity of C3bBb (See Fig. 8–8).

C5 is cleaved by molecular complexes that contain C3b. Surface-bound C3b generated by the alternative pathway has the same convertase effect as C3b produced by the classical pathway (Fig. 8–10). Both pathways achieve the same effects: (1) coating of the cell, particle, bacterium, or aggregate by opsonic C3b; (2) generation of the

FIGURE 8–9. Effective generation of alternative-pathway activity requires a protective surface so that protein interactions can occur without inhibition by factors I and H. Alternative-pathway surfaces provide a sheltered location on which the C3bB complex can accumulate, allowing cleavage by factor D into the C3bBb complex, which then promotes additional C3b accumulation. Stabilization of the evolving C3bBb complexes by properdin enhances the capacity to cleave C3 and to generate activated products.

ROLE OF SURFACE
IN ALTERNATIVE PATHWAY

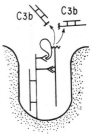

Surface attachment
protects fluid-phase
C3b from degradation

Properdin-stabilized
C3bBb accumulates,
cleaves C3, generates
additional C3b

anaphylatoxins C3a and C5a; and (3) generation of C5b, which mobilizes C6, 7, 8, and 9 into the membrane attack unit.

─────────── **THE MEMBRANE ATTACK UNIT** ───────────

Cleavage of **C5** generates the small fluid-phase C5a fragment and the larger residual molecule, C5b. C5a is a potent anaphylatoxin. C5b is a highly active molecule with a very short life. It decays spontaneously in 0.1 second if binding does not occur, but it can interact with soluble complement proteins or can bind to nearly any membrane or surface. C5b does not cleave other proteins; its effect on later components is one of steric rearrangement (See Fig. 8–10). C5b attracts **C6,** which forms a soluble C5b6 complex to which **C7** subsequently attaches. C5b67, during its period of reactivity, will cling tightly to any cell membrane it touches. Fluid-phase C5b67 complex can deposit on any nearby cell or membrane, independent of the nature or location of the initial activating event. This is called the **innocent bystander** phenomenon, because the site where the complex settles may be totally uninvolved in ongoing immune or inflammatory activities. Instead of attaching to membrane, the C5b67 complex may cohere into a free-floating spherical unit called a **micelle,** which can exert an independent destructive effect on viral proteins.

Association of C6 and 7 with C5b is followed by gradual accretion of **C8** and later of **C9**. When C8 combines with C5b67 on a mem-

C3b IS C5 CONVERTASE

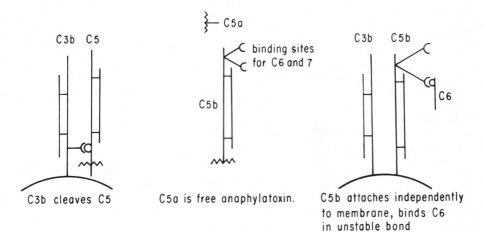

C3b cleaves C5

C5a is free anaphylatoxin.

C5b attaches independently to membrane, binds C6 in unstable bond

FIGURE 8–10. C3b, whether generated by the classical or the alternative pathway, acts as a C5 convertase. It cleaves a small fragment from the larger of the two C5 chains, generating fluid-phase C5a, which is a potent anaphylatoxin, and the larger C5b, which binds independently to membranes. C5b interacts with C6 to form a loosely bound, unstable complex.

EVOLUTION OF MEMBRANE ATTACK UNIT

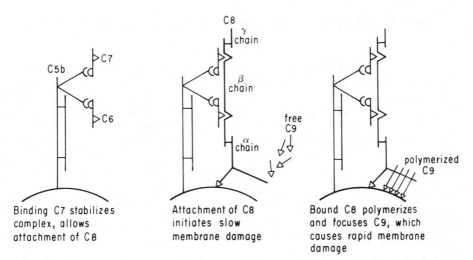

Binding C7 stabilizes complex, allows attachment of C8

Attachment of C8 initiates slow membrane damage

Bound C8 polymerizes and focuses C9, which causes rapid membrane damage

FIGURE 8–11. The unstable complex of C5b and C6 becomes permanent when C7 enters a steric bond with C5b. The C5b67 complex enters a steric interaction with the 3-chained C8 molecule. The C5b678 complex initiates a slow attack on membrane integrity, and also provides a setting on which individual C9 molecules can polymerize. Polymerized C9, in this membrane-bound complex, rapidly generates a discrete defect in the cell membrane.

brane, it disturbs the membrane in a way that slowly damages osmotic regulation and gradually destroys the cell. Attached C8 provides a site on which C9 units can polymerize; polymerized C9 generates a discrete tubular structure that penetrates the membrane and causes rapid osmotic disruption of the cell (Fig. 8–11). Complement-mediated membrane dissolution lyses the target cell, whether the process was activated by the cell in question or resulted from innocent-bystander involvement.

Table 8–2 lists the numbered complement components and summarizes their interactions.

--------------- **CONTROL OVER THE SYSTEM** ---------------

Ordinarily, complement activity remains where the initiating event occurs, so only the antigen-bearing surface or the localized fluid environment sustains the potent biologic consequences. Uncontrolled or widespread complement activity could cause dangerous inflammatory and cytolytic effects. Two control mechanisms exist: (1) individual protein molecules have a relatively short half-life, and (2) numerous control proteins, some free in plasma and others on cell membranes, prevent excessive accumulation of activated elements. Every 24 hours, approximately half the plasma complement molecules undergo replacement. Although macrophages and other cells are capable of synthesizing many complement proteins, most of the circulating elements derive from the liver. Plasma complement levels rise if systemic events enhance hepatic protein synthesis; in severe liver disease, complement levels fall because reduced protein production cannot compensate for continuous degradation.

C1 INHIBITOR

The control protein that acts earliest is C1 inhibitor, also called alpha-2-neuraminoglycoprotein or **C1INH,** which interferes with activation of C1r and C1s. The C1 inhibitor combines irreversibly with C1q that has bound to immunoglobulin, forcing C1r and C1s to dissociate. C1q remains bound to the immunoglobulin, but no C1s esterase activity evolves to cleave C4. C1INH has other targets besides C1r and C1s; it inhibits the actions of the proteases: plasmin, kallikrein, activated factor XII (Hageman factor), and activated factor XI. Normal activity of the coagulation and inflammation systems depends upon precisely adjusted concentrations of active materials; these proteases are intimately interrelated in maintaining suitably balanced

TABLE 8–2. Evolution of Complement Activities

Original Protein	Active Protein	Physiologic Activities
C1q	Bound C1q	Binds to Ig heavy chain, activates C1r
C1r	C1r̄	Cleaves C1s
C1s	C1s̄	Cleaves C4 and C2 (more effective on C2 bound to C4b than free C2)
C4	C4a	Anaphylatoxin; provokes histamine release
	C4b̄	Binds to C2; has weak opsonic effect
C2	C2a	When bound to C4b, cleaves C3
C3	C3a	Anaphylatoxin; provokes histamine release
	C3b	Bound monomers are opsonic
		When bound to C4b2a complex, cleaves C5
C5	C5a	Potent anaphylatoxin; attracts and activates PMNs; promotes release of oxygen species, inflammatory mediators (also provokes histamine release)
	C5b	Promotes association of C6–9
		Binds to any available membrane
C6, 7	C5b67	Forms micelles; promotes attachment of C8 and C9
C8	C8	In C5b678 complex, causes slow membrane leak
C9	Polymerized C9	In C5b6789 complex, produces transmembrane tubule, acute osmotic lysis

levels of activated proteins. C1INH, which is widely distributed in plasma, helps regulate these proteases and maintain adequate but not excessive levels of active products. In C1INH deficiency, a relatively rare genetic abnormality, these complex interactions are significantly distorted.

Congenital Deficiency

C1INH is the only material that inhibits activation of C1qrs. With deficiency of C1INH, excessive C1s accumulates, large amounts of C2 are cleaved, and excessive levels of C2b develop. After contact with plasmin and other enzymes of the inflammatory and coagulation systems, C2b is converted into a protein that is inactive in the complement cascade but has massive effects on vascular permeability. Patients with C1INH deficiency suffer from excessive and inappropriate enhancement of vascular permeability, in a condition called **hereditary angioedema**. Complement dysfunction is not conspicuous in this condition, presumably because the alternative pathway compensates for defective classical-pathway activation.

FACTOR I

The most broadly reactive control protein is **factor I,** formerly called C3b inactivator or C3bINA. Because it modifies the reactive portions of both C4b and C3b, it affects both the classical and the alternative pathways. Factor I cleaves the large C4b and C3b proteins into a small, biologically inert free fragment designated "c" and a residual large fragment called "d" that remains bound to the membrane but has no effect on other proteins. Generation of C4d aborts the classical pathway. Generation of C3d leaves cells coated with a protein that has little opsonic effect. Granulocytes and macrophages have receptors for C3b but not for C3d, and cells coated with C3d are not more rapidly phagocytized than native cells or particles. B lymphocytes express C3d receptors, but the immunologic significance of this potential for interaction between C3d-coated material and resting B lymphocytes remains unclear.

Alternative-Pathway Effects

Factor I also affects the alternative pathway. When it interacts with C3b, it occupies the molecular site to which factor B would otherwise attach. During spontaneous evolution of C3b, there is competition between factor B and factor I for this binding site. Attachment of factor I prevents accumulation of the C3bBb complex that initiates the alternative pathway. Factor I attaches more effectively than factor B when the unbound proteins interact in fluid; if C3b accumulates on an activating surface, the equilibrium shifts to favor factor B. Alternative-pathway activators provide a sheltered location in which C3bBb can evolve, allowing accumulation of active elements and protecting the bound C3b from cleavage by factor I.

COFACTOR PROTEINS IN PLASMA

Several cofactors enhance factor I activity against its substrates C4b and C3b. Whereas accumulation on an activator surface shifts the C3b equilibrium toward factor B attachment, combination with the control protein **factor H** gives factor I the competitive advantage. Factor H modifies one chain of fluid-phase C3b, rendering it more receptive to cleavage and degradation by factor I. When sheltered on an activator surface, C3b is not affected by factor H.

A separate protein enhances the interaction of factor I with C4b. Called **C4-binding protein** (C4BP), it acts on either fluid-phase or bound C4b, rendering it susceptible to attack by factor I. If C4BP and factor I predominate in the protein mix, classical-pathway activation will cease. If there is enough C4b to overcome the effects of C4BP, then C3b is generated in its bound form, and this circumvents the

TABLE 8–3. Plasma Proteins that Regulate Complement Interactions

Designation	Other Terms Used	Mol. Wt. in kD	Approximate Serum Concentration (μg/ml)
C1 inhibitor	C1INH, C1 esterase inhibitor	105	150–180
Factor I	C3b inactivator, C3bINA, KAF	88	35
Factor H	C3b inactivator accelerator, B1H	150	360–500
C4 binding protein	C4BP	500–590	400

effect of factor H, allowing the cascade to go on to completion. Table 8–3 lists the serum proteins that regulate complement activity.

CELL-MEMBRANE PROTEINS

In addition to inhibitory proteins in serum, several cell-bound glycoproteins also restrict complement activity. A recently systematized group of proteins called **complement receptors (CR proteins)** have specificity for different fragments of C3 (Table 8–4). Their biologic role in the complement drama remains to be fully clarified, but they have already proved useful as cell-identification antigens (Table 5–4). The most fully characterized is the receptor for C3b, now called CR1. Membrane proteins designated CR2, CR3, and CR4 have also been characterized and their presence determined on different cell populations. The functions of these membrane characteristics in controlling the complement cascade or in other biologic activities are under scrutiny.

CR1, the Receptor for C3b

The gene determining CR1 manufacture resides on chromosome 1 in a cluster that also contains genes for factor H and the C4-binding protein. CR1 glycoprotein acts as a cell-bound cofactor for factor I, affecting bound C3b in a manner comparable to the effect of factor H in the fluid phase; it also accelerates the decay of complexes that would generate more C3b. Cells exhibiting CR1 can form rosettes with cells coated with either C3b or C4b. Most blood cells, including red cells, neutrophils, T and B lymphocytes, and monocyte/macrophages, express the CR1 glycoprotein.

TABLE 8—4. Complement Receptors on Cell Membrane

Receptor	Ligand	Cellular Distribution	Function
CR1	C3b	RBCs, neutrophils, B lymphocytes, T lymphocytes (some), monocytes, macrophages, follicular dendritic cells, glomerular podocytes	Cofactor for degradation of immune complexes
CR2	C3d, C3dg*	B lymphocytes, follicular dendritic cells	Physiologic role not clear Acts as EBV receptor
CR3	iC3b*	Monocytes, macrophages, neutrophils, follicular dendritic cells	Involved in cell-adherence functions, antibody-mediated cellular cytotoxicity Related to lymphocyte function-associated (LFA-1) antigen
CR4	C3dg*	Monocytes, neutrophils	Not clear
C5a receptor	C5a	Monocytes, macrophages, neutrophils, mast cells	?Mediator for anaphylatoxic effects of C5a on inflammatory cells
C1q receptor	C1q	Monocytes, macrophages, platelets, fibroblasts, neutrophils	Function not clear; interacts with collagen-like portion of molecule

*These are intermediate cleavage fragments of C3

A peculiarity of CR1 is that the CR1 molecules of a cell do not act on the proteins bound to the membrane of that cell. CR1 reacts with components bound to the membrane of nearby cells or complexes in surrounding fluid. Rather than protecting its own cell from the complement cascade, it seems to adsorb partially activated complement components or immune complexes present in body fluids or on surfaces. This may serve to remove immune complexes from the blood, because circulating cells have intimate contact with macrophages of the reticuloendothelial system after experiencing intense exposure to material in plasma.

Other Receptors

In contrast to CR1, the membrane protein called **decay-accelerating factor** (DAF) affects only components on its own cell membrane. This glycoprotein, present predominantly on red cells, enhances the activity of factor I on either C3b or C4b. Decay-accelerating factor appears to protect red cells against complement-mediated lysis. Patients with the disease **paroxysmal nocturnal hemoglobinuria** (PNH) have red cells that are excessively sensitive to complement-mediated hemolysis and have significantly reduced levels of DAF. The DAF deficiency, however, appears to develop as a consequence of the condition rather than existing as a constitutional abnormality that renders the individual susceptible to PNH.

Another C3b-binding membrane glycoprotein is called **gp45-70,** but its manner of action and its biologic function are poorly understood. Present on white cells and platelets but not on red cells, it may be another cofactor for factor I.

Table 8–5 summarizes the major controlling materials that affect the complement cascade.

TABLE 8–5. Control Proteins in the Complement System

Control Material	Target	Action
C1INH	C1qrs Other serine proteases	Inhibits activation phase of classical pathway
Factor I (formerly C3bINH)	C4b and C3b, classical pathway	Generation of C4d and C3d, which have little physiologic function
	C3b, in alternative pathway	Prevents interaction with factor B, by occupying binding site
Factor H	C3b free in fluids	Renders protein more susceptible to cleavage by factor I
C4-binding protein (C4BP)	C4b, either bound or free in fluids	Renders protein more susceptible to cleavage by factor I
CR1	C3b bound to surfaces or complexes	Renders protein more susceptible to cleavage by factor I; inhibits C3 convertase action of complexes containing C3b
Decay-accelerating factor (DAF)	C4b or C3b on same cell as DAF molecule	Renders protein more susceptible to cleavage by factor I

SUGGESTIONS FOR
FURTHER READING

Arlaud GJ, Colomb MG, Gagnon J: A functional model of the human C1 complex. Immunol Today 1987; 8:106–10

Bitter-Suermann D: The anaphylatoxins. In: Rother K, Till GO, eds: The Complement System. New York: Springer-Verlag, 1988:367–95

Griffin FM, Jr: Opsonization, phagocytosis, and intracellular microbial killing. In: Rother K, Till GO, eds. The Complement System. New York: Springer-Verlag, 1988:395–418

Rother K, Rother U: Biological functions of the complement system. Progr Allergy 1986; 39:24–100

Rother K, Rother U: The reactivity of the complement system. Progr Allergy 1986; 39:8–23

Whaley K: The complement system. In: Whaley K, ed: Complement in Health and Disease. Norwell, MA: MTP Press, 1987:1–36

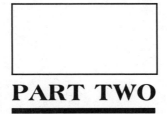

PART TWO

Clinical Applications

CHAPTER 9

Protective Immunity

The immune mechanisms discussed in the preceding section serve protective functions against microbial invasion, and regulatory functions that affect generation, differentiation, and function of many cells and tissues. This chapter considers antimicrobial immune effects. The regulatory actions are most clearly distinguished through the consequences of malfunction; succeeding chapters consider immune deficiencies and dysfunctions.

Immunity can be acquired either actively or passively. **Passive immunization** is transfer of protective material from an individual immune to a specific antigen into another individual with no protection established against that antigen. **Active immunization** is the response made by an immunocompetent individual to antigens of mi-

149

croorganisms or their products. This chapter will discuss the mechanisms of active and passive immunization and the protective effects of such immunity.

PASSIVE IMMUNITY

Passive immunization involves humoral immunity almost exclusively; antibodies can be transferred from one individual to another quite easily, but transfer of viable cells is fraught with difficulties. The only route, in nature, for passive immunization is transfer of maternal antibodies to the child; as a medical intervention, deliberate injection of specific antibodies is a useful therapeutic approach in selected circumstances.

TRANSFER ACROSS THE PLACENTA

The normal fetus develops in an immunologically null environment. No infectious agents should penetrate the amniotic sac, and the intact placenta prevents maternal cells from entering the fetus. Small molecules, including some proteins, do cross the placenta, but these maternal molecules virtually never provoke an immune response in the fetus. Having had little stimulus for immune activity,

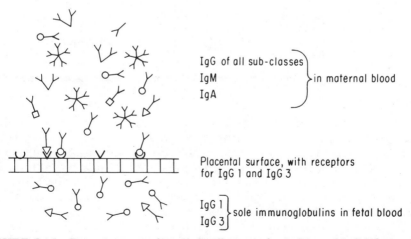

SELECTIVE TRANSFER OF IMMUNOGLOBULINS
ACROSS PLACENTA

IgG of all sub-classes
IgM
IgA
} in maternal blood

Placental surface, with receptors for IgG 1 and IgG 3

IgG 1
IgG 3
} sole immunoglobulins in fetal blood

FIGURE 9–1. Receptors on placental cells transfer IgG1 and IgG3 from maternal to fetal bloodstream; no other maternal immunoglobulins enter the fetus. The receptors are specific for isotype, not for idiotype, so all antigenic specificities in the mother's IgG1 and IgG3 repertory will be present in the fetus.

the infant at birth possesses little functionally mature immune tissue.

The fetal bloodstream does, however, contain antibodies. These are IgG1 and IgG3 molecules that have passed from mother to fetus across isotype-specific receptors on placental cells (Fig. 9–1). There is no selection for antigenic specificity; IgG molecules of those subclasses are transferred indiscriminately from maternal to fetal bloodstream. This transfer may be deleterious, if maternal antibodies have specificity for antigens present on fetal cells. **Hemolytic disease of the newborn** (HDN), discussed more fully in chapter 11, is an example of this event. With this exception, passively transferred maternal antibodies benefit the child. During a lifetime of exposure, the mother will have developed antibodies against a wide range of organisms; the newborn, who suddenly experiences all the pathogens present in the newly encountered environment, has the benefit of the mother's immune history. This protection is not, of course, absolute. A large infecting dose can overwhelm available defenses, and the infant has no protection against organisms for which the mother had no antibodies.

ANTIBODIES IN BREAST MILK

The breast-fed infant ingests, in milk, antibodies and many nonspecific protective materials like complement proteins, interferons, the antibacterial enzyme called **lysozyme,** and an iron-binding protein (**lactoferrin**) that modifies bacterial multiplication. Milk contains antibacterial and antiviral antibodies of the IgA class. When adults ingest antibodies or other complex proteins, digestive enzymes rapidly degrade them, but the newborn alimentary tract has less proteolytic activity, and so ingested proteins retain their function to a considerable extent. Antibodies in breast milk neutralize bacterial toxins and prevent many viruses and bacteria from initiating infection. Breast-fed infants have significantly fewer intestinal infections than bottle-fed infants, especially where hygienic conditions are suboptimal. In part this reflects reduced opportunity for bacterial contamination of breast milk as compared with bottle feeds, but part of the protection parallels the specificity and concentration of antibodies present in the milk. Some workers believe that IgA antibodies in milk modify the ways that proteins cross the infant's highly permeable intestinal mucosa and thereby cause breast-fed infants to have fewer food allergies in later life, but this view is not universally accepted.

INJECTION OF ANTIBODIES

Deliberate injection of antibody-containing serum has been used, both clinically and experimentally, since the turn of the century. Injecting antibodies is less significant as antimicrobial therapy now

TABLE 9—1. Diseases in which Passive Immunization Is Useful

Disease	Product	Source	Indications and Precautions
Botulism	Antibody to specific types of toxin	Horse	Given to patients known to have ingested toxins
Diphtheria	Antibody to bacterial toxin	Horse	Used in established disease, to prevent systemic complications Adverse reactions frequent
Herpes zoster/ varicella	IG* to zoster-varicella virus	Human	Postexposure to varicella (chicken pox) in immunosuppressed children with no history of the disease
Hepatitis A	ISG** preparation containing multiple antibodies	Human	Protection after known specific exposure; prophylaxis for endemic exposure risk
Hepatitis B	IG* specific for hepatitis B virus	Human	Protection after known needlestick or sexual exposure; infants born to mothers carrying hepatitis B virus
Hypogammaglobulinemia	ISG** preparation containing multiple antibodies	Human	Continuous prophylaxis for patients with humoral immunodeficiency
Measles	Antibody to rubeola virus	Human	Postexposure after known specific exposure
Rabies	Antibody to rabies virus	Human	Given as soon as possible after bites, with part of dose directly around injured tissue; active immunization is given at a different site
Rubella	Antibody to rubella virus	Human	Does not prevent viremia; given after specific exposure, to modify symptoms

TABLE 9–1. Diseases in which Passive Immunization Is Useful—*Continued*

Disease	Product	Source	Indications and Precautions
Snakebite	Antibody to venom of snake implicated	Horse	Given after exposure; polyvalent product is effective against pit vipers, rattle-snakes, cop-perheads
Spider bite	Antibody to venom	Horse	Used after bite by black widow, re-lated spiders
Tetanus	Antibody to neuro-toxin of *Clostrid-ium tetani*	Human	Given to non-im-mune individuals after potentially tetanus-contam-inated injury; vac-cine given at sepa-rate site if immunization sta-tus uncertain

*IG: Immune globulin; concentrated preparation containing single antibody
**ISG: Immune serum globulin; see text

than it was before widespread development of effective antimicrobial drugs, but, in selected therapeutic circumstances, passive protection remains extremely important.

Following known exposure to a pathogenic organism, infection can sometimes be prevented or aborted by injecting antibodies against it. In the preantibiotic era, hyperimmune horse serum was used to protect against many infections. Once the infecting agent was identified, the patient could receive serum from animals with high-titered antibodies against the appropriate organism. Unfortunately, the equine protein often provoked an immune reaction, leading to the clinical syndrome called **serum sickness** (see chapter 12).

Use of Globulin Preparations

Injected human antibodies rarely provoke immune reactions. Globulins can be concentrated from whole human serum or plasma to achieve very high levels of specific antibodies or groups of antibodies. Serum preparations with high levels of antibody against such viruses as varicella (cause of chicken pox and shingles) and hepatitis B are used to treat individuals after episodes of known exposure. A concentrate of unselected antibodies, the product called **immune serum globulin** (ISG), can also be useful. Immune serum globulin is prepared from large pools of plasma and contains the wide range of antibodies present in the donor population. The broad-spectrum preparation can be given to individuals with defective humoral immunity. The unselected assortment of antibodies provides generalized immune protection that can be supplemented by antimicrobial drugs and/or specific immunotherapy after episodes of known exposure. Table 9–1 lists many conditions for which passive immunization may be useful.

Until recently, immune globulins could be injected only into muscle because direct introduction into the bloodstream provoked potentially life-threatening problems of immune complex formation and stimulation of the complement and kinin systems. Human globulins are now available in a form suitable for intravascular use; intravenous ISG is used for an expanding list of immunodeficiency and immunodysfunctional conditions.

ACTIVE IMMUNITY

The natural way to acquire immunity is to experience either clinical or inapparent infection, which then stimulates cellular and/or humoral immune activity. Procedures for artificial induction of immunity originated with centuries of observations that persons who survived certain illnesses would never again experience those infections.

EXPOSURE TO NATIVE ORGANISMS

The earliest attempt at immunization was deliberate exposure to the etiologic agent of smallpox, the **variola** virus. Smallpox can range in severity from a relatively mild skin affliction to a rapidly fatal systemic disease. Physicians in China and Asia Minor attempted for centuries to induce protection against the virulent disease by deliberately promoting very mild disease. They injected material from skin lesions of a sick patient into healthy subjects to induce an infection that did, indeed, elicit effective immunity. The problem was the unpredictable severity of the transmitted disease; taking material from a mildly ill patient did not guarantee mild illness in the recipient. When this practice, called **variolation,** was introduced into England in the 18th century, 2 to 3 percent of treated individuals developed fatal illness. However, the natural infection caused 20 to 30 percent mortality, so the practice of variolation remained in use.

The latter part of the 18th century brought a new approach to immunization, arising from the observation that smallpox rarely developed in persons who had had a mild skin disease called cowpox, or **vaccinia**. Cowpox was common in dairy workers; indeed, milkmaids were traditional exemplars of feminine beauty because their lovely complexions were unmarred by disfiguring smallpox scars. In 1796, Edward Jenner injected fluid from a cowpox lesion into a child's arm and 2 months later injected material from a smallpox lesion. The child developed the mild blisters of cowpox but did not succumb to smallpox. Injecting vaccinia material (**vaccination**) provided anti-smallpox protection with much less risk of uncontrolled disease than introducing variola material.

Cross-reactive Immunity

The immunity to variola that follows exposure to vaccinia virus illustrates the principle of **cross-reactivity;** the two viruses have sufficiently similar antigenic composition that antibodies to the one prevent infection with the other (Fig. 9–2). Organisms that differ in clinical respects may share significant epitopes and thus elicit antibodies that react with an agent to which there has been no exposure. Cross-reactivity is not an unmitigated blessing. Antibodies to microbial antigens sometimes cross-react unexpectedly with host tissues or proteins. **Rheumatic fever** is the classical example; antibodies induced by infection with certain strains of streptococcus can react with antigens of human heart constituents and cause a destructive inflammatory process.

EXPOSURE TO MODIFIED ANTIGENS

Immunization attempts to achieve maximum protection with minimum risk to the patient. In the smallpox saga, variolation imposed excessive risk; although unmodified cowpox virus carried less risk, it induced unpredictable protection. Current strategies to induce immunity use a number of techniques to increase protection and to reduce risk, as outlined in Table 9–2. Immunity may develop after injection of **killed organisms,** which retain antigenicity as long as the appropriate epitopes are not denatured. Organisms express a wide range of antigens; antibodies that develop after natural infection react with microbial elements that may or may not participate in the pathologic process. If killed organisms induce antibodies against materials necessary for the organism to cause disease, then a killed preparation can be a safe and effective vaccine. Problems arise if the pathogens are not successfully inactivated or if significant antigens are damaged in processing.

PROTECTION AGAINST SMALLPOX
THROUGH CROSSREACTION WITH COWPOX

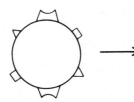 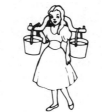 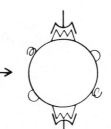

Cowpox virus   Host with no   Antibody against
                      disease experience   cowpox antigen

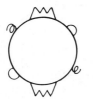 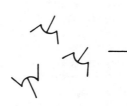

Smallpox virus   Antibody to   Crossreactive antibody
                     cowpox antigen   is adequate to
                                           block infectivity

FIGURE 9—2. Certain antigens of the cowpox and smallpox viruses resemble one another. Infection with cowpox, shown in the upper panel, elicits antibodies for that virus. Because the antigenic configurations are so similar, antibodies to cowpox can block actions mediated by molecules of the smallpox virus, as shown in the lower panel.

Viable Organisms

Some strains of pathogenic organisms do not cause human disease but have the same antigens as more dangerous examples. Such organisms, described as **attenuated,** remain capable of multiplying and of stimulating antibodies but lack properties that significantly damage tissue. Using living but attenuated organisms to induce immunity carries the risk that they may revert to a more virulent state. An associated risk is that other unidentified infectious agents may lurk in a preparation of viable organisms that has not been subjected to inactivation or sterilization.

TABLE 9–2. Preparation of Immunizing Materials

Material Used	Potential Problems
Killed organisms	Damage to epitopes that elicit protective antibodies Failure to inactivate viable pathogens
Living attenuated organisms	During multiplication, non-pathogenic strain may recover virulence During multiplication, organisms may lose epitopes that induce protective antibodies Preparation containing viable organisms may be contaminated with other pathogens
Immunogenic fraction of pathogenic organisms	Difficulty in identifying the specific isolated epitopes that induce desired protective antibodies Difficulty in separating intact epitopes from whole organisms

Antigenic Fractions

Another way to increase the safety of immunization is to identify those epitopes that provoke protective antibodies and to inject only the part of the organism that exhibits the desired antigens. Successfully **fractionated material** induces protection but has no capacity to multiply or to cause disease. This principle was exploited in developing vaccines against hepatitis B. The viral envelope material called hepatitis B surface antigen (**HBsAg**) elicits protective antibody, but purified HBsAg is not alive, does not cause disease, and can be processed to eliminate any other viable organisms. The most recent vaccines for hepatitis B use an HBsAg fraction synthesized by recombinant deoxyribonucleic acid (DNA) technology, which eliminates the need to start with viable virus. Table 9–3 lists many immunization preparations in current use.

PROBLEMS WITH ACTIVE IMMUNITY

Many circumstances conspire against effective immune protection. Some pathogenic organisms, especially viruses, continually change their antigenic features. Several different strains may produce

TABLE 9–3. Immunization Strategies for Specific Diseases

Disease	Nature of Vaccine	Duration of Protection	Booster Schedule	Contraindications
Cholera	Inactivated bacteria	Modest protection for 3–6 months	Every 6 mo, as needed	Severe reactions to previous dose
Diphtheria	Toxoid (denatured toxin)	Approx. 10 yrs.	Repeat dose at age 4; every 10 years	Ongoing febrile illness History of severe allergies
Hemophilus influenzae (b)	Purified capsular polysaccharide	Approx. 4 yrs.	Varies with individual	Age below 18 mo Allergy to vaccine constituents
Hepatitis B	Viral antigen, either fractionated from plasma or prepared by recombinant DNA technology	Approx. 5 yrs.	Probably every 5 yrs.	Allergy to vaccine constituents
Influenza	Killed virus, usually three different strains	One flu season	Yearly, with current strains	Anaphylactic allergy to egg Cancer chemotherapy
Measles	Attenuated live virus	≧15 years	Not necessary	Ongoing pregnancy
Meningococcal infection	Purified capsular polysaccharide	3 years	Only if risk recurs	Allergy to vaccine constituents
Mumps	Attenuated live virus	≧15 years	Not necessary	Ongoing pregnancy Anaphylactic allergy to eggs
Pertussis (whooping cough)	Killed bacteria	4–6 years	Contraindicated in adults	Age over 7 years Ongoing febrile illness Severe allergic history

Plague	Killed bacteria	Not fully characterized	Every 6 mo. to 1 yr. if risk persists	Ongoing pregnancy
Pneumococcal infection	Purified capsular polysaccharides of 23 strains	At least 5 years	Contraindicated	Give before initiating a course of immunosuppressive therapy
Poliomyelitis	Attenuated live virus, given orally	Probably lifelong	Only if high risk is established	Severe allergic history
Rabies	Inactivated virus, grown in human cells	Approx. 2 years	Every 2 years if risk continues	
Rubella	Attenuated live virus	≧15 years	Not necessary	Ongoing pregnancy Ongoing febrile illness
Smallpox	Attenuated live virus	3–10 years	Varies with risk state	Only indication is for laboratory personnel working with virus
Tetanus	Toxoid (denatured toxin)	Approx. 10 yrs.	Every 10 yrs, or after high-risk exposure	Ongoing febrile illness Severe allergic history
Tuberculosis	Live attenuated organism (Bacillus of Calmette-Guerin—BCG)	Partial only; duration varies	Not used	Immunosuppressed state
Typhoid	Killed bacteria	≧3 years	Only if high risk exists	Severe reaction to previous dose
Yellow fever	Live attenuated virus	≧10 years	Every 10 yrs. if risk persists	Immunosuppressed state Anaphylactic allergy to egg

clinically similar disease states, but antibody elicited by one strain may confer no protection against other variants. Some viruses have more variants and are more likely to change their characteristics than others. The influenza viruses and the many agents responsible for "the common cold" are highly heterogeneous and, additionally, mutate frequently into renewably infective strains. The smallpox and measles viruses, by contrast, are antigenically very stable.

Immunity provoked by infection with some organisms may not be protective. Besides the apparent lack of immunity that occurs when antigenically diverse strains all produce identical clinical events, there is the problem that antibodies provoked by some microorganisms genuinely have no effect on limiting disease or preventing subsequent infections. A prominent example is the antibody response to the human immunodeficiency virus (HIV-1); several of the antibodies this virus elicits document the presence of organism but do nothing to eliminate the virus or to protect against clinical illness.

Adverse Effects

Another problem in vaccine development is undesirable side effects. Microbial proteins can elicit local or systemic reactions that are uncomfortable or, in some cases, dangerous. Soreness at the injection site is usually tolerable, but many patients consider malaise and fever acceptable only if the native disease is significantly more dangerous or unpleasant than the reaction to immunization. Still worse are dysfunctional immune reactions that occasionally occur after immunization, especially those that damage the central or peripheral nervous system.

Preparations of live organisms may pose a threat to non-immunized individuals. Attenuated agents that are harmless to normal subjects can cause significant disease if they spread to immunologically compromised individuals. This can occur if live virus given to a pregnant woman crosses the placenta, or if immunodeficient individuals acquire organisms excreted by recently immunized contacts.

EVENTS THAT PROVOKE IMMUNE RESPONSES

Immune activation requires exposure of a certain minimum intensity and duration. Immune response may not occur to very small doses of the microorganism, very transient contact, very superficial infection, or multiplication in a non-accessible body site. Conversely, otherwise normal hosts may fail to react if exposed to overwhelming quantities of a microorganism. Stimuli effective for normal individuals may be insufficient in individuals with congenital or acquired immunodeficiency. The following discussion of developing immunity presupposes immunocompetence in the host and exposure to adequate but not lethal doses of a pathogen.

INTRAUTERINE EXPOSURE

The normal fetus inhabits a sterile environment. Although organisms may enter the amniotic sac under pathologic conditions, most maternal infections do not affect the fetus; additionally, some pathogens do not stimulate immune activity because their presence induces fetal death or premature delivery. Immune response is most likely to occur when a moderate dose of pathogen enters the fetal bloodstream weeks or months before delivery. Direct infection of amniotic fluid rarely elicits a response because the process is usually acute, terminating either in fetal death or accelerated delivery. When infecting agents cross the placenta, long-term contact between fetus and microorganism is established; intrauterine infections that develop shortly before full-term birth may have inadequate opportunity to exert immune effect.

Consequences for the Fetus

Exposure to microbial antigens stimulates precocious development of the fetal immune system. The presence of IgM antibody in fetal or cord blood indicates that there has been intrauterine infection to which the fetus has responded, because IgM of maternal origin does not cross the placenta. IgM antibodies of fetal origin are diagnostic for intrauterine infection but are not protective; despite circulating antibody, fetal tissues contain viable microorganisms, which often persist indefinitely in postnatal life.

Intrauterine infections are more often viral than bacterial. Notorious examples are rubella virus and cytomegalovirus, which cause asymptomatic or trivial infection in the mother but may cause severe developmental anomalies in the fetus who survives transplacental infection. Premature delivery and persisting congenital infection are characteristic of many rubella or cytomegalovirus syndromes. Transplacental infection with syphilis spirochetes (*Treponema pallidum*) causes a variety of congenital anomalies. Other organisms that may provoke immune response in the fetus include species of *Mycobacterium*, *Toxoplasma gondii* and malarial organisms.

SUBCLINICAL INFECTION

An individual with no history of overt disease may nonetheless exhibit immunity to a pathogen because many environmental agents can multiply within the body without causing discernible illness. There are several ways in which the host may become aware that immunity exists. If the individual remains well when others exposed to a known pathogen develop illness, prior immunity can be inferred; so many uncontrolled variables affect clinical disease, however, that this hardly constitutes a reliable test for established immunity. Specific tests are available (see chapters 15 to 18) to demonstrate antibodies, but demonstrating cell-mediated immunity is more difficult. For generations, skin testing for delayed hypersensitivity was the only way to document the presence of cellular immunity to particular antigens or organisms; the skin-test procedure is called the **tuberculin test** when mycobacterial antigens are used. Comparable skin tests are performed with antigens from certain fungi and from other pathogens that characteristically elicit a cell-mediated response. It is now possible to examine cultured cells for reactivity to specific microbial antigens, but these tests are demanding and expensive.

Significance of Antibodies

After known exposure to a pathogen, an individual may want to learn whether he or she has immunity, for example, a man exposed to mumps or a pregnant woman to rubella. Knowledge of prior immune state is sometimes helpful in deciding whether to administer vaccines that are in scarce supply or cause unpleasant or dangerous side effects. The question of immune state is easily answered if serum is examined immediately after exposure; absence of antibody indicates susceptibility to disease, and presence of antibody indicates immunity. In many cases, however, the time of exposure is uncertain, or the realization of exposure comes some time after the fact. When serum is examined well after exposure, absence of antibody still indicates susceptibility, but presence of antibody is harder to interpret. The antibody could have been present for years, indicating prior immunity, or it could have arisen as a prompt reaction to the recent immunizing event. Under these circumstances, it can be very useful to determine immunoglobulin class. Predominance of IgM suggests recent primary immunization, whereas antibodies that are wholly or predominantly IgG indicate previously established immunity.

Significance of Skin Test

Skin tests for cell-mediated immunity are used for epidemiologic studies and to make therapeutic decisions. A healthy individual who fails to react against tuberculin or comparable other antigens is considered free of present or previous infection. Some adults in the United States and most adults in many economically or hygienically deprived areas have a positive tuberculin test; this indicates past experience with the organism, even if there is no history of present or past clinical illness. If an individual known to have had a negative test becomes positive on a subsequent test, this documents recent infective exposure and is an indication to institute treatment. When one person is found to have infective tuberculosis, it is customary to skin test the patient's close contacts. A positive skin test in a child or young person is assumed to reflect recent infection from the original patient, and antituberculosis therapy is given even without signs of illness. Older contacts found to have a positive skin test may or may

---

TABLE 9—4. Significance of the Tuberculin Test

Test Result	Associated Circumstances	Interpretation
Negative test	1. In healthy child or adult 2. In serious illness suggestive of tbc*	1. No present or previous disease 2. Depression of cell-mediated immunity (anergy)
Positive test, no previous results known	1. In seemingly healthy young child 2. In seemingly healthy adult 3. In adult with illness suggestive of tbc	1. Active infection; treatment indicated 2. Exposure to tbc in the past 3. Makes diagnosis of tbc considerably more probable, but is not proof
Positive test, previous test(s) known to have been negative	1. In seemingly healthy adult or child 2. In adult or child with illness suggestive of tbc	1. Recent infective exposure; treatment indicated 2. Strengthens likelihood of diagnosis, but proof by culture still desirable
Negative test, previous test(s) known to have been positive	1. In seemingly healthy adult 2. In adult with serious illness suggestive of tbc 3. In adult with illness not suggestive of tbc	1. May indicate either complete eradication of organism *or* unsuspected presence of illness that depressed cell-mediated immunity 2. Illness may or may not be tbc, but it has depressed cell-mediated immunity 3. Look for malignant or immune disease as cause of depressed cell-mediated immunity

*tbc: abbreviation for tuberculosis

not be considered recently infected, depending upon past circumstances and the results of previous tests if these are known. Table 9–4 outlines some of the ways that tuberculin testing affects clinical judgments.

CHILDHOOD DISEASES

Many diseases with a distinctive clinical course confer long-lasting protection after a single episode of illness; this immunity will be periodically reinforced by subsequent encounters if the organism is widely distributed. Infections with other organisms provoke less individualized clinical manifestations; a number of respiratory and gastrointestinal organisms, for example, produce clinical syndromes that so closely resemble one another that it is impossible, without extensive microbiologic investigation, to assign a specific organism to each episode. In those circumstances, immunity against individual organisms has little practical importance, inasmuch as repeated episodes of very similar illness occur on successive encounters with different organisms.

The diseases sometimes called the **usual childhood diseases** are characterized by distinctive clinical syndromes, by a high level of interpersonal contagion, and by subsequent establishment of lifelong immunity. Before immunization for these conditions was widely prevalent, measles, mumps, chickenpox, whooping cough, and scarlet fever affected large numbers of young children, a population in which close interpersonal contacts occur among individuals with little established immunity. In such circumstances, children encounter the pathogen, suffer and recover from the characteristic illness, and do not again suffer from that disease. Widespread vaccination has made these diseases infrequent in economically developed countries, but in developing parts of the world, distinctive contagious diseases continue to afflict most children.

Age at Exposure

Pathogens highly prevalent in an environment are more likely to cause disease in children than in adults. After maternal antibodies wane, the child is vulnerable to every newly encountered microorganism. With each successive infection, the child expands the list of organisms to which he or she is immune and reduces the number of pathogens capable of causing illness. As long as the pool of pathogenic agents remains constant, symptomatic infections become less and less frequent as age and microbial exposure increase. A change in the pool of organisms or in the state of individual immunity restores susceptibility. Children exposed to the altered social environment of a new school, for example, commonly bring home organisms sufficiently different from those of the parents' previous exposures that the entire household experiences a surge in infections.

Some endemic organisms cause illness that is trivial in children but far more significant when older persons are infected. Hepatitis A virus and the Epstein-Barr virus (EBV) are examples. They cause subclinical infection in infants and children, who thereafter possess permanent immunity; persons who escape childhood exposure and acquire infection only as adolescents or adults often become significantly ill. In unimmunized populations where polio virus is common, most children acquire immunity through subclinical gastrointestinal infection early in life; but if primary infection occurs in later childhood or adulthood, severe or fatal neurologic involvement may result.

FAILURE OF PROTECTION

So-called lifelong immunity is not absolute; levels of protection tend to diminish with time. The immunity that follows clinical illness tends to persist at higher levels than protection induced by artificial immunization. If an infecting dose is large and the level of immunity is low, disease may develop before the anamnestic response can become effective. At any level of immunity, a sufficiently large dose can overcome the protective effect; this is especially likely if other circumstances have compromised innate defense mechanisms. Severe debility, malnutrition, the presence of burns or inflammatory disorders, and the effects of many medications all increase susceptibility to infection, even in persons with previously normal immune function. The disease may be less severe, however, than it would have been in a comparably impaired patient without prior immunity.

Some systemic conditions make infections more frequent and more severe, regardless of prior immune status. Notable in this regard are diabetes mellitus, alcoholism, and widespread malignant neoplasms. Adrenal corticosteroids, given as therapy for a wide range of conditions, suppress non-specific inflammatory defense mechanisms, depress previous levels of immunity, and increase predisposition to infection. Many cytotoxic drugs have a comparable effect. Malignant conditions, diseases of autoimmune etiology, chronic infections, and malnutrition are other common events that make infections more numerous and more severe. Acquired immune defects are discussed in greater detail in chapter 10.

Some examples of seemingly failed protection result from mistaken identity, when several different organisms cause indistinguishable clinical illnesses. For example, otherwise healthy individuals rarely suffer twice from the distinctive illnesses of measles or whooping cough, but widespread skin rashes or epiglottitis can occur several times in the same person, caused by several antigenically distinct organisms.

——————————— **IMMUNITY AT SURFACES** ———————————

Three forms of acquired immunity augment the defensive effect of intact epithelium in protecting surfaces. The most conspicuous is the **presence of antibodies,** largely IgA, in secretions. **Cell-mediated events** and the actions of **IgE** also help protect body surfaces from pathogenic microorganisms.

ANTIBODIES IN SECRETIONS

The IgA present in secretions originates in plasma cells of the mucosa-associated lymphoid tissue; plasma antibodies do not seep into the secretions. Specialized epithelial cells regulate the passage of antigens across the mucosa of bowel and bronchi. Inhaled or ingested antigens stimulate systemic responses as well as surface immune activity. Antigen presentation occurs either in the mucosa-associated lymphoid tissue or in regional lymph nodes that drain the epithelium. Injected antigens rarely stimulate secretory antibodies; most secreted IgA reflects antigens that stimulate the mucosa directly. Antigen presented at a single mucosal site may, however, induce antibody at additional surface locations.

IgA is the only antibody class significantly present in normal secretions; persons with congenital IgA deficiency may, however, have IgM in their secretions. The transport system by which antibodies enter and traverse epithelial cells reacts only with polymerized immunoglobulin. Its affinity for dimeric or trimeric IgA is much higher than for IgM, but if IgA is absent, IgM pentamers engage the receptors and are transported across the epithelium.

Effects of IgA

Secretory IgA prevents antigenic or pathogenic material from penetrating the epithelium and entering the body. The antibody complexes with soluble antigens to reduce absorption of potentially immunizing material. Several antibodies neutralize intraluminal toxins and metabolites, thus preventing damage to epithelial cells. It is probable that whatever toxins and antigens manage to enter the bloodstream are further inactivated by the monomeric IgA present in plasma, but this role for circulating IgA has not been proven.

IgA antibodies against bacteria and viruses prevent these pathogens from adhering to epithelial cells. Possible mechanisms for this effect include reducing motility of the potential invader; blocking receptor sites for epithelial attachment; altering the solubility and the surface electrical charge of the organisms; and enveloping the invaders in a macromolecular complex of antibody, mucus, and antigen. IgA antibodies do not agglutinate organisms but may attach to the surface and exert an opsonic effect, rendering potential pathogens attractive to phagocytic cells that possess receptors for the alpha chain. Inflammatory cells with alpha-Fc receptors are relatively rare in internal tissues but are more numerous in epithelium. Although IgA does not activate complement by the classical pathway, protein aggregates that contain IgA can initiate the alternative pathway and generate the chemotactic and opsonic effects that occur after C3 is cleaved.

IgE-MEDIATED MECHANISMS

The skin and the epithelial surfaces of gut and respiratory tracts contain numerous tissue basophils, called **mast cells,** that bind IgE to their membrane through high-affinity receptors. Encounter with antigen stimulates mucosal T cells to elaborate lymphokines that enhance local production of IgE and increase the number of mast cells. After IgE binds to cells and the cell-bound IgE interacts with antigen, the underlying mast cells release products that induce inflammation, promote smooth muscle contraction, and increase vascular and epithelial permeability. These mechanisms appear to provide a major defense against intestinal parasites, especially helminths like *Schistosoma* species and *Trichinella spiralis*. The inflammatory response allows proteins from the bloodstream to enter the tissue fluid, thus exposing the worms and their larvae to antibodies of all classes. Inflammatory mediators attract macrophages and granulocytes, especially eosinophils, into the antibody-rich area. IgG is opsonic for phagocytic effector cells and serves as the target for antibody-dependent cell-mediated cytotoxicity (ADCC, see chapter 7).

Possible Antihelminthic Effect

IgE molecules that are not bound to mast cells have special actions against helminths; antigen-specific IgE can bind to macrophages and stimulate them to attack specific target organisms, and eosinophils exert a lethal effect on certain parasites that become coated with IgE. Eosinophils also release toxic enzymes and activating factors that bring platelets and macrophages into the battle. Products released from mast cells promote smooth muscle contraction and secretion of mucus, and this assists in expulsion of parasites already damaged by the mechanisms described above. Humoral antiparasitic protection is, however, far from totally effective; individuals with high levels of IgE antibodies against helminth parasites may, at the same time, be heavily infested with the organisms.

CELL-MEDIATED IMMUNITY AT SURFACES

Mucosal surfaces are abundantly supplied with helper T cells and also with cells that have many features of large granular lymphocytes.

Antigen-stimulated T cells elaborate lymphokines that not only enhance antibody production and mucus secretion but also promote accumulation of macrophages, neutrophils, eosinophils, and mast cells. Antigenic material and viable organisms that penetrate the epithelial surface promptly encounter cytotoxic cells and activated macrophages. This cytotoxic activity appears to be less potent against the native organisms than against the host's own cells altered by invading organisms or by contact with their products. These events are poorly understood. If cell-mediated immunity is supposed to prevent multiplication and accumulation of host cells with abnormal properties, the mechanism does not seem to work very well; bowel epithelium and bronchial mucosa are two of the commonest sites at which cancers develop.

EFFECTS OF ANTIBODIES

Antibodies are the major immune defense against bacterial infection, acting to prevent bacterial invasion, to eliminate those organisms that manage to enter and to multiply, and to inactivate many bacterial products. Against viruses, antibodies serve more to prevent infection than to eradicate established intracellular organisms. Many fungal and parasitic infections provoke antibodies, but it is not clear whether the antibodies act to eliminate these pathogens. Organisms that have a significant extracellular phase characteristically elicit a humoral response, whereas a cell-mediated response follows intracellular multiplication of most viruses and of many fungi and protozoa and of certain bacteria.

SPECIFIC EFFECTS ON BACTERIA

Antibodies against cell-wall substances inhibit the movement and multiplication of bacteria and their attachment to target cells. During infection, bacteria synthesize an enormous range of structural, metabolic, and secreted materials that mediate motility, cellular adhesion, evasion of phagocytosis, and incorporation of nutrients. Antibodies against these materials reduce the efficiency with which the organisms cause infection. The organisms may not be killed directly, but if antibody-mediated actions reduce their numbers and viability, they are more vulnerable to non-specific defense mechanisms.

IgM antibodies produce many *in vitro* effects, but it is unclear how many are physiologically significant in the living host. It is doubtful whether agglutination occurs commonly, although it may serve to clear pathogens from the bloodstream. Complement-mediated lysis of bacteria and some viruses is known to occur, but this mechanism seems to have significant antimicrobial effects only against *Neisseria meningitidis* and *Hemophilus influenzae*.

IgM, Complement, and Inflammation

Complement activation is, however, crucially important in promoting opsonization and initiating the anaphylatoxic effects that magnify inflammation. Only a few IgM molecules need combine with antigen to initiate the classical pathway, which generates large amounts of C3a and C5a; these attract inflammatory cells and promote localized accumulation of blood-borne proteins like antibodies, fibrinogen, complement proteins, fibronectin, and kinin precursors. Combination of antibody with surface antigen causes numerous C3b molecules to attach to the cell surface; macrophages and neutrophils, which have C3b receptors, are attracted to the site by the anaphylatoxic effects of complement, and their phagocytic actions are enhanced by the opsonic effects of complement.

IgG antibodies develop late in the primary response and predominate in anamnestic reactions to organisms previously encountered. Large numbers of IgG molecules must complex with an organism to activate complement. IgG coating by itself has significant opsonic effect, because numerous phagocytic cells have high-affinity receptors for the Fc portion of gamma chains; microorganisms coated with both IgG and C3b are even more attractive to macrophages and granulocytes than those coated with either protein alone. Antibody-coated organisms are also susceptible to ADCC.

ANTIBODIES TO METABOLITES

The metabolites of multiplying bacteria often exert independent pathogenic effects, such as inhibition of coagulation, lysis of tissue proteins, repulsion of inflammatory cells, or inhibition of essential physiologic interactions. Antibodies that neutralize these products reduce the competitive advantage that their unmodified action gives to the infecting bacteria. In some diseases, the major clinical effects result from the actions of bacterial toxins rather than from the multiplication of the organisms. Examples are enterotoxic diarrhea in cholera, the systemic events in staphylococcal toxic shock syndrome, neurotoxic effects in tetanus and botulism, and damage to cardiac and neurologic functions in diphtheria. Antibodies against these toxins are therapeutically more useful than those directed against bacterial cell-body antigens.

Some bacterial diseases should not, strictly speaking, even be called infections because no bacteria multiply in the host. Staphylococcal food poisoning is a relatively innocuous example and botulism a potentially fatal example of problems that follow ingestion of preformed bacterial toxins. Treatment for botulism is not antibiotic medication but administration of antibody to the type of toxin identified.

ANTIVIRAL ANTIBODIES

Viruses are obligate intracellular parasites; they replicate only within living cells, where it is difficult for immune mechanisms to penetrate. The virus must, however, enter the body, arrive at the target organ, and then invade individual cells. Antiviral antibodies have several opportunities to interrupt this sequence, but once the virus is inside the cell, cell-mediated immunity is the major defense. Antibodies do better in preventing than in curing viral diseases.

Antibodies may counteract the effects of viral proteins, prevent penetration of the target cell, or directly lyse the intact virus. IgA antibodies in epithelial secretions protect susceptible cells against many respiratory or gastrointestinal viruses; antibodies in the bloodstream attack organisms traveling from their site of entry to distant target organs. The complement cascade may produce direct lysis or may interfere with mechanisms for attachment and penetration. Cells infected by virus often express virus-derived surface antigens; these can combine with complement-activating antibodies that initiate lysis of the infected cell. This is beneficial only if antibody in the surrounding tissue fluid destroys organisms released by lysis of the initially infected cell. When viruses spread directly from one cell to another, antibodies must intervene before additional cell-to-cell spread occurs.

Nonprotective Marker Antibodies

Most viruses have both surface and interior epitopes. Because protective antibodies are, in general, those that react with surface antigens, immunization procedures are intended to evoke these antibodies. Antigens inside the virus activate the immune system only if viral multiplication occurs within the host's cells. Antibodies to surface antigens can result from artificial immunization, but the presence of antibodies to interior viral antigens indicates ongoing or past infection; they constitute useful diagnostic markers but provide little protection. Antibodies against enzymes of the viral coat or interior similarly indicate present or past viral multiplication. Fluid-borne antibodies to these enzymes do not protect against infection because the processes mediated by these enzymes occur inside the invaded cells.

Immunosuppressive Viruses

Some viruses acquire an unfair advantage by depressing immune mechanisms of the infected host. The most notorious example is HIV-1, the retrovirus that causes acquired immune deficiency syndrome

(AIDS). It uses the CD4 antigen to invade T cells, destroying the infected helper cells and profoundly diminishing immune reactivity. Other viruses, notably cytomegalovirus and EBV, exert significant but less dramatic and less permanent immunosuppressive effects on lymphocyte populations.

CELL-MEDIATED IMMUNE EVENTS

Complement-mediated membrane damage is a direct consequence of humoral immunity, but most other immune defenses involve cellular activity, either alone or associated with antibody actions. Antibodies augment cellular defenses through opsonization, ADCC, and enhancement of acute inflammatory events. The cell-mediated arm of immune defense comprises, as we have seen in chapter 7, a variety of phagocytic and non-phagocytic events that may help protect against microbial invasion.

THE EFFECTS OF LYMPHOKINES

In the form of cell-mediated immunity described as delayed-type hypersensitivity (DTH), a small number of antigenically specific T cells influence activity of numerous non-specific lymphocytes, granulocytes, and phagocytic cells. Immune reactivity of this type is effective against many organisms that resist antibody defenses either because their intracellular location prevents contact with antibody or because their surfaces fail to evoke protective antibodies. The classical example is the mycobacterium, the etiologic agent for tuberculosis and leprosy, which remains infective and metabolically active inside macrophages. Comparable effects are seen with various fungi and with *Listeria*, another intracellular bacterium.

Effects on Tissue

In DTH, antigen-activated T cells produce lymphokines, which promote the effector actions of macrophages. When there is established immunity, T cells respond to the presence of the microorganism by secreting lymphokines that attract macrophages and markedly increase their antimicrobial effectiveness. The actions of lymphokines include enhancing phagocytosis and intracellular bacterial killing; inducing increased surface receptors for complement and immunoglobulin; increasing the generation of reactive oxygen species; and stimulating secretion of many proteins, including transport mechanisms, coagulation factors, and enzymes that cleave proteins, fats, and carbohydrates. Also enhanced is production of leukotrienes and

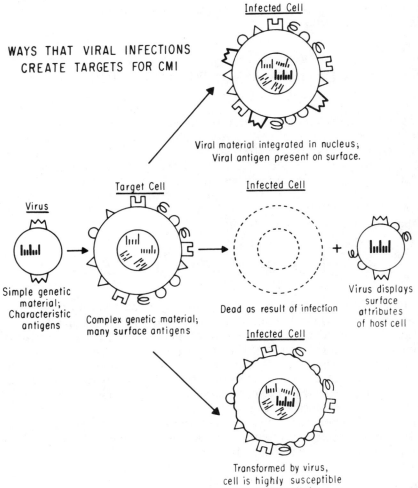

WAYS THAT VIRAL INFECTIONS
CREATE TARGETS FOR CMI

Infected Cell

Viral material integrated in nucleus;
Viral antigen present on surface.

Virus

Simple genetic
material;
Characteristic
antigens

Target Cell

Complex genetic material;
many surface antigens

Infected Cell

Dead as result of infection

+

Virus displays
surface
attributes
of host cell

Infected Cell

Transformed by virus,
cell is highly susceptible
to NK attack

FIGURE 9–3. The two figures on the left show virus, with distinctive genetic material and surface antigens, infecting a host cell with many intrinsic genetic and surface attributes. Infection modifies the host cell in ways that elicit cell-mediated immunity. The top figure shows that an infected cell may express on its membrane viral antigens that the immune system will perceive as foreign. The middle figures show that virus, released into body fluids after infecting and rupturing a host cell, may manifest host-cell antigens that render the virus a target for MHC-restricted recognition. At the bottom, viral infection has transformed the host cell in a way that exposes it to attack by NK cells.

prostaglandins, and of interleukin 1 (IL-1) with all its systemic effects (see chapter 7).

The good news about this cellular stimulation is increased capacity to engulf and to destroy organisms that otherwise evade inflammatory and humoral defenses. The bad news is that these events damage the host tissue at the infected site, causing tissue loss and scarring. (See pages 260–261 for further discussion.)

OTHER CELLULAR EVENTS

Cell-mediated immunity exerts significant effects on cellular antigens and intervenes in infectious events in two additional ways. Certain viruses—notably measles, cytomegalovirus, and some herpes viruses—acquire surface proteins from the cells in which they have multiplied. Viruses with these acquired antigens stimulate T lymphocytes to DTH actions that the unmodified virus might not otherwise elicit. Conversely, viruses contribute antigens to the membrane of host cells. Infected cells characteristically develop surface properties that arise from viral genetic material incorporated in the cell nucleus. Because cells expressing these viral antigens continue to express their own major histocompatibility complex (MHC-I) antigens, they become targets for cytotoxic CD8 cells that recognize foreign antigens in the context of autologous class I antigens. Infected host cells also become more attractive to natural killer (NK) cells, which do not recognize specific antigens but characteristically interact more effectively with infected cells than with normal cells of the same tissue type. These antiviral mechanisms are illustrated in Figure 9–3.

Interferons constitute another avenue of antimicrobial defense. Production of alpha and beta interferons does not require antigen-specific recognition. Secreted by macrophages, fibroblasts, and other cells, these products promote cellular resistance to viral invasion and enhance the actions of macrophages and of antigen-specific lymphocytes. Gamma interferon is an immune product secreted only by T cells that have recognized specific antigen; viral infection may constitute the immune stimulus, but many other antigens are also effective. Many complex cellular antigens elicit gamma interferon, but bacteria characteristically do not. Gamma interferon intensifies non-specific cellular defense events by enhancing the actions of macrophages and of NK cells.

───────── SUGGESTIONS FOR ─────────
FURTHER READING

Borysiewicz LK, Sissons JGP: Immune response to virus-infected cells. Clin Immunol Allergy 1986; 6:159–88

Drutz DJ, Mills J: Immunity and infection. In: Stites DP, Stobo JD, Wells JV, eds. Basic and Clinical Immunology, 6th ed. Norwalk CT: Appleton and Lange, 1987:167–85

Ivanyi J: Pathogenic and protective interactions in mycobacterial infections. Clin Immunol Allergy 1986; 6:127–57

Jawetz E, Melnick JL, Adelberg EA: Review of Medical Microbiology, 17th ed. Norwalk CT: Appleton and Lange, 1987:160–69 (Host-parasite relationships)

Kubens BS, Opferkuch W: Defense against bacterial infections. In: Rother K, Till GO, eds: The Complement System. New York:Springer-Verlag, 1988:469–87

Schoenfeld Y, Isenberg DA: Mycobacteria and autoimmunity. Immunol Today 1988; 9:178–82

Sills RH: Splenic function: physiology and splenic hypofunction. CRC Crit Rev Onc Hematol 1987; 7:1–36

Underdown BJ, Schiff JM: Immunoglobulin A: strategic defense initiative at the mucosal surface. Adv Immunol 1986; 4:389–417

CHAPTER 10

Immunodeficiency Conditions

The complexity of the immune system provides innumerable opportunities for deficiency and malfunction. Defects can be classified into the following categories: B cells and immunoglobulin levels; T cells and cell-mediated events; combined B- and T-cell relationships;

complement factors and regulators; and functions of phagocytic cells. Primary defects in one area frequently affect other functions as well, but this overall classification is useful in organizing a complex subject. Table 10–1 outlines the ways in which different deficits cause

---

TABLE 10–1. Site of Defects in Acquired or Congenital Immunodeficiency States

Element Affected	Pathologic Event
Marrow Stem Cells	Reticular dysgenesis
	Severe combined immunodeficiency syndrome
	Immunosuppressive drugs; x-ray exposure
T Lymphocytes	
Thymus	DiGeorge syndrome
Numbers of mature cells	Corticosteroids
	Malignant disorders
	Some viral infections
	Thermal burns
Function of mature cells	Chronic mucocutaneous candidiasis
	Acquired metabolic disorders (e.g., diabetes, alcoholism, uremia)
	Autoimmune disorders
B Lymphocytes	
Pre-B cells	Infantile hypogammaglobulinemia (X-linked)
Numbers of mature cells	Corticosteroids; malignant disorders
Immunoglobulin synthesis	Selective Ig class deficiencies
	? Common variable immunodeficiency
	Malignant disorders
	Malnutrition
Immunoglobulin levels	Hypercatabolism
	Protein-losing diseases
Phagocytic Cells	
Marrow production	Autoimmune disorders
	Many drugs, viral infections
Motility and chemotactic recognition	Complement disorders
	Acquired metabolic disorders (e.g., diabetes, steroids, alcohol, aspirin)
Phagocytosis	Splenectomy
	Hyperhemolysis (e.g., sickle cell disease, malaria)
	Complement disorders
Enzyme release and intracellular bacterial killing	Chronic granulomatous disease
	Chediak-Higashi syndrome
	Inborn enzyme deficiencies
	Thermal burns

disease. It is also important to divide immunodeficiency conditions into inborn constitutional defects and conditions determined by developmental or environmental events.

MANIFESTATIONS OF IMMUNODEFICIENCY

Defective immunity predisposes to infection. In immunodeficient individuals, there is an increase in number, severity, range of etiologic organisms, and clinical complications of infectious conditions. With inborn immunodeficiencies, these infections begin early in life, and untreated patients may not survive long enough to manifest later complications. Therapeutic strategies in current use, however, now permit many individuals to survive years of immunodeficiency, only to experience autoimmune problems and/or malignant lymphoreticular neoplasms in later life.

TIME SEQUENCE

Infants born to an immunologically intact mother begin life with an impressive array of IgG antibodies; regardless of later immune status, bacterial infections are relatively rare in the newborn period. Viral infections are more numerous than bacterial infections in normal infants, especially those due to viruses that elicit antibodies with no protective effects. Inasmuch as maternal cells do not cross the placenta, the mother's cell-mediated immunity does not pass to the infant. Intracellular bacteria, many fungi, and the more polymorphic viruses can and do cause infections in the normal newborn, but most infants manage to eliminate most invaders.

Childhood Exposures

After maternal antibodies disappear and before active immunity develops, normal infants experience an interval of pronounced susceptibility to environmental agents. Infections that occur reflect the opportunities for exposure. An infant with intimate exposure to only a few adults in a few locations will have fewer infections than one who interacts with persons of varying age in varying surroundings. With advancing age and an expanding social sphere, previously protected infants eventually encounter most of the common environmental pathogens. Entering daycare or school nearly always increases the episodes of infection, regardless of previous social contacts.

The immunodeficient child reacts abnormally to these normal environmental encounters. If cell-mediated immunity is defective, fun-

TABLE 10–2. Manifestations of Primary Immune Deficiency

Characteristic Time that Signs Occur	Immunologic Defect
Earliest infancy	Reticular dysgenesis Severe combined immunodeficiency syndrome DiGeorge syndrome
2–6 months	Infantile hypogammaglobulinemia Mucocutaneous candidiasis
6 months to 2 years	Transient hypogammaglobulinemia of infancy Chronic granulomatous disease Wiscott-Aldrich syndrome (bleeding may occur earlier)
Childhood	Ataxia-telangiectasia (ataxia may occur earlier) IgA deficiency (if symptomatic)
Adolescence or adulthood	Deficiency of C1 esterase inhibitor Deficiencies of C5-C8 Common variable immunodeficiency

gal or viral infections begin in the first few weeks and persist despite what would otherwise be effective therapy; defects of humoral immunity characteristically remain undetected until passive immunity dissipates at several months of age. Limited defects may not emerge until later in childhood, when infectious exposure is more extensive and subtle departures from the normal become more apparent. The age of onset for many inborn immunodeficiencies is given in Table 10–2.

RANGE OF ORGANISMS

Antibody protection works best against extracellular bacterial pathogens and viruses that must travel through the bloodstream to reach their target organs. Patients with antibody deficiencies are conspicuously susceptible to septicemia and to infections of upper and lower respiratory tracts and of the central nervous system. Commonly identified pathogens are the gram-positive and gram-negative cocci, enteroviruses, and agents that cause infectious diarrheas, notably rotavirus, giardia, and salmonella.

The pyogenic infections characteristic of antibody deficiency are more easily treated than the infectious consequences of defective cell-mediated immunity, in which lifelong vulnerability becomes apparent through persistent fungal infections and repeated viral infections of skin, mucosal surfaces, and respiratory tract. Other organisms common in patients with defective cell-mediated immunity include intracellular bacteria, like mycobacteria and listeria; the protozoa *Pneumocystis carinii,* cryptosporidium, and toxoplasma; many viruses, especially those of the herpes, adenovirus and enterovirus groups; and environmental fungi of all sorts.

Defects of Accessory Systems

Phagocytic defects become apparent either very early or somewhat later in childhood. Patients with defective phagocytosis have particular problems with staphylococci and gram-negative bacteria, which characteristically cause repeated and persistent infections rather than sudden or overwhelming sepsis. Fungal infections are also frequent.

Patients deficient in the late components of complement have unexplained susceptibility to neisserial infections. Disseminated gonococcal infection and meningococcal infections of the central nervous system and/or the bloodstream are strikingly frequent; this may not become apparent until late childhood or adolescence when neisserial exposure becomes more common. Other infections tend to be somewhat more frequent and more troublesome in these patients than in normals. Organisms that characteristically complicate immunodeficiency conditions are listed in Table 10–3.

───────── ACQUIRED CONDITIONS OF ───────── DEPRESSED IMMUNITY

Discussions of immunologic disorders often overbalance toward constitutional abnormalities. Individuals with genetically determined defects of clearly defined immune functions are rare, but many insights into immune mechanisms have come from researchers investigating these patients and working backward from clinical observations to basic cellular and molecular understanding. The conceptual importance of constitutional deficiencies should not, however, distort our view of clinical reality; the vast preponderance of individuals are born normal. The overwhelming majority of immune abnormalities result from age, environment, and intercurrent diseases. Acquired immune deficiencies often present with complex manifestations that defy single-cause explanations. Immunodeficiency occurs incomparably more often through environmental or secondary events than through inborn defects of immune activities. In an unselected patient population, there will be many whose immune

TABLE 10–3. Common Pathogens in Immunocompromised Conditions

Defective Element	Common Microorganisms	
T-Cell Deficiencies	Bacteria:	Intracellular: *M. tuberculosis, Listeria monocytogenes* Extracellular: salmonella, legionella, nocardia
	Fungi:	Candida, histoplasma, cryptococcus, aspergillus
	Viruses:	Cytomegalovirus, herpes simplex, herpes zoster
	Protozoa:	Pneumocystis, toxoplasma, cryptosporidium
B-Cell Dysfunction		
Hypogammaglobulinemia	Pyogenic extracellular bacteria	
IgA deficiency	Bacteria infecting sinuses, lungs; *Giardia lamblia;* hepatitis viruses	
Splenectomy	*Streptococcus pneumoniae*, salmonella	
Phagocytic/Bactericidal Deficiency	Many staphylococci and streptococci, *Hemophilus influenzae*, candida	
Complement Deficiencies		
C3	*Streptococcus pneumoniae*	
C5-C9	Neisseria species	

reactivity is abnormal, but very few with constitutional immunodeficiency states. Table 10–4 outlines some of the causes for acquired problems in immune function.

SYSTEMIC CONDITIONS AFFECTING IMMUNITY

Anything that impairs bodily economy can affect immune function. Vulnerable activities include cell division and multiplication; protein synthesis and secretion; metabolic interrelationships; and the ways in which cells and soluble molecules react with one another. Certain metabolic abnormalities and diseases are especially likely to depress immunity.

Generalized Changes

Overall nutritional state and the metabolism of oxygen, carbon dioxide, and simple nutrients significantly affect immune efficiency.

TABLE 10—4. Conditions That Suppress Immune Function

Cause	Induced Defects
Disease States*	
Diabetes mellitus	Depressed chemotaxis and phagocytosis
	Depressed T-cell functions
Alcoholism	Depressed delayed hypersensitivity (mild)
	Increased immunoglobulins, especially IgA
	Depressed neutrophil chemotaxis
Widespread tuberculosis	Anergy (i.e., severely depressed delayed hypersensitivity)
Uremia	Depressed macrophage functions
	Depressed T-cell functions
	Depressed neutrophil chemotaxis
Malnutrition	Depressed cellular multiplication and antibody production
	Depressed phagocytosis
	Depressed T-cell functions
Protein-losing GI or renal conditions	Hypogammaglobulinemia
Thermal burns	Disruption of epithelial barrier
	Loss of serum proteins
	Accelerated degradation of serum proteins
	Depressed T-cell function
	Depressed phagocytosis and chemotaxis
Prolonged hemolysis (e.g., sickle cell disease, malaria)	Exhaustion of macrophage activity
External Events	
Splenectomy	Depressed antibodies to capsular polysaccharides
Adrenal corticosteroids	Depressed number and function of T and B cells
	Depressed neutrophil chemotaxis
	Depressed macrophage numbers, chemotaxis, phagocytosis
	Depressed synthesis of interferons
Cytotoxic drugs	Epithelial damage, leading to reduced barrier function
	Depressed numbers of all marrow-derived cells
	Depressed multiplication of T and B cells
	Activation of latent CMV or EBV infections (sometimes), leading to depressed T-cell functions
General anesthetics	Depressed T-cell functions
X-irradiation	Depressed number and function of lymphocytes, neutrophils
	Depressed macrophage function
	Damage to epithelial surfaces (sometimes)

*For effects of autoimmune and malignant diseases, see chapters 11 and 12.

States of malnutrition or protein deficiency depress cell multiplication and antibody production. When nutrition is poor, previously established protection diminishes and new exposures fail to evoke immunity. Any medical or surgical condition that impairs nutrition subjects the patient to the additional burden of depressed antimicrobial defense; in areas where nutrition is poor because of severe economic deprivation, entire populations experience increased risk of infection.

Another cause of immune deterioration is advancing age, but individuals differ enormously in levels of deficiency. The physiology of aging is poorly understood, and immune changes are no exception. In general, antibody levels decline in and beyond the eighth decade; cellular responsiveness, which is much more difficult to quantify, diminishes to an indeterminable degree. Older persons also exhibit increasing frequency of immune dysfunction and autoimmune conditions.

Specific Conditions

Certain diseases exert an immunosuppressive effect disproportionate to measurable metabolic effects. **Diabetes mellitus,** both insulin-dependent and non-insulin-dependent, impairs T-cell functions and also depresses activities of neutrophils and macrophages. In severe **liver disease,** serum protein synthesis is depressed and complement levels fall. **Cirrhosis,** which alters hepatic circulation and distorts processing and presentation of many antigens, often provokes increased production of immunoglobulins that have no identifiable specificities, and the patient manifests decreased resistance to infection. **Alcohol abuse** impairs many cell functions, especially the chemotactic and phagocytic aspects of inflammation and probably also T-cell activities. **Uremia** distorts many cellular activities, including those of T cells and possibly also of phagocytic cells.

Anesthetic agents depress T-cell activity for days or weeks after the acute exposure and may also affect B-cell responsiveness. The mechanism of depression is not known, but depressed immunity and increased susceptibility to infection almost invariably follow general anesthesia.

PROTEIN LOSS

Antibody levels decline if there is increased loss or destruction of serum proteins; the resulting **hypogammaglobulinemia,** if severe, may depress bacterial immunity. This is most conspicuous in **protein-losing enteropathies** (some of which probably have an immune etiology) and the renal and metabolic condition described as the **nephrotic syndrome**. Passive administration of immune serum globulin is ineffective because the injected proteins are lost along with autologous immunoglobulins.

Thermal burns create special vulnerability to infection. Large-scale damage to skin removes the physical barrier to microbial entry and leaves an exposed surface that is excessively permeable to fluid and protein. Huge quantities of serum protein are lost across the warm, moist, weeping surfaces, which also provide excellent conditions for bacterial multiplication. Although antibody synthesis is unimpaired, the increased metabolism that follows extensive burns causes accelerated degradation of all plasma proteins, in addition to the physical loss across burned surfaces. Further complicating the clinical picture is depression of cellular function, which affects both T cells and the chemotactic and phagocytic actions of inflammatory cells. Infection is the most common cause of death after severe burns.

IMMUNOSUPPRESSIVE DRUGS

Many drugs depress immune functions. Drugs are often given expressly to diminish activity in dysfunctional immune states (see chapter 11); in many other conditions, agents given for specific indications cause unwanted immunosuppression as an unavoidable consequence. Immunosuppressive therapy, often lifelong, is given after organ transplants, and autoimmune or allergic diseases are often treated with immunosuppressives. Adrenal corticosteroids are probably the most commonly used agents. Given for a broad range of clinical problems, they inhibit proliferation and function of lymphocytes and interfere with many inflammatory interactions. Adrenal steroid regimens are monitored to employ the smallest effective dose in an attempt to reduce the immunosuppressive and other side effects of these potent agents.

Malignant diseases are treated with agents that suppress cellular multiplication at many different sites and phases. Cytotoxic drugs and radiation reduce proliferation of malignant cells but also suppress the normally multiplying cells of the immune system and bone marrow. Depressed immune and inflammatory functions and severe risk of infection are inevitable consequences of cytotoxic therapy.

INFECTIONS

Infectious organisms may cause immunosuppression in addition to local tissue damage. The most notorious example is the human immunodeficiency virus (HIV-1), which causes the acquired immunodeficiency syndrome (AIDS). This retrovirus enters helper T cells through the CD4 molecule, profoundly depressing their number and function. Without helper T cells, cell-mediated immunity fails and production and regulation of antibodies are severely distorted. Not only are normal immune responses depressed, but failure of immune regulation leaves AIDS patients particularly susceptible to developing certain malignant diseases that accompany acquired or inborn immune deficiency.

Other viruses cause less permanent alteration of immune function. Cytomegalovirus multiplies in T cells and depresses cellular reactivity; Epstein-Barr virus infects B cells, but response to the B-cell infection causes an increase in the number and function of suppressor T cells; rubella and rubeola (measles) viruses transiently depress T cells. Prolonged or repeated infection with many other common viruses may affect T-cell number and/or function.

Infections with mycobacteria (tuberculosis and leprosy) and many fungi characteristically activate cell-mediated specific and non-specific defenses; massive infection with these same agents may overwhelm cellular responses, leading to the non-responsive state called **anergy**.

THE LYMPHORETICULAR SYSTEM

Neoplasms of lymphoreticular tissue inevitably depress or alter immune function. Neoplastic diseases frequently arise in the bone marrow, the lymph nodes, and the non-nodal reticuloendothelial tissues. Malignant disease originating in the bone marrow is called **leukemia;** when solid organs are the primary focus, the term **lymphoma** is used. Special categories of lymphoreticular malignancies include multiple myeloma and macroglobulinemia. Chapter 11 discusses these conditions in more detail. Besides depressing immune defenses, these diseases induce dysfunctional and autoimmune activity. Many systemic and multiorgan neoplasms of immune origin depress normal immune activities and also induce pathologic activities. Immune energy seems to be deflected from the appropriate goal of antimicrobial defense toward inappropriate targets in the host's own system.

Individuals whose spleen has been removed or inactivated have increased susceptibility to blood-borne bacterial infections. Although *Streptococcus pneumoniae* (pneumococcus) is the most notorious agent, many other bacteria may produce sudden and overwhelming sepsis in asplenic individuals.

———— PRIMARY CONDITIONS AFFECTING ———— BOTH T AND B CELLS

Common hematopoietic precursor cells generate divergent mature populations, so disorders of cellular development often affect several populations simultaneously. There are no inborn disorders that globally suppress the marrow, inasmuch as total hematopoietic failure would be incompatible with intrauterine survival.

RETICULAR DYSGENESIS

Developmental arrest at the earliest detectable stage causes a combined defect of lymphocytes and granulocytes called **reticular dysgenesis**. Growth occurs normally in the uterus, where inflammatory and immune capability are not needed, but postuterine life is severely abbreviated. The usual form of this rare condition affects only lymphocytes and granulocytes, but variant forms with additional erythroid and megakaryocyte abnormalities have been reported. The patients exhibit severe lymphopenia and hypogammaglobulinemia, and the lymphoid organs are rudimentary; the thymus is severely maldeveloped; and lymph nodes, tonsils, and mucosa-associated lymphoid tissue are virtually absent. The clinical picture is one of early, intractable fungal infection of mucosal surfaces, followed by diarrhea, pneumonias, viral infections, and death in the first few months.

SEVERE COMBINED IMMUNODEFICIENCY SYNDROME

Severe combined immunodeficiency syndrome (SCIDS) is a descriptive term encompassing any of the immunodevelopmental failures that affect both T and B cells. Both autosomal and sex-linked forms exist; in some, enzymes or metabolites essential for cell multiplication can be identified as deficient, but most remain unexplained. Approximately 15 percent of SCIDS involve enzymes associated with purine metabolism. All cells require these enzymes, but the resulting abnormalities produce more pronounced consequences in lymphocytes than in other cells. In enzyme-associated SCIDS, the defects in immune function may range in severity from total to relatively moderate; in other forms of SCIDS, immunodeficiency is uniform and profound.

Autosomal recessive SCIDS is sometimes called **Swiss-type agammaglobulinemia;** other forms have no distinctive name. The earliest manifestation of SCIDS is persistent candidal infection of mucosal surfaces, beginning in the first month of life. Candida, cytomegalovirus, and pneumocystis continue as particularly common pathogens; patients may suffer widespread systemic infection if exposed to attentuated viruses used in many vaccines. The thymus and other lymphoid tissues are hypoplastic; lymphocytes and plasma cells are absent from blood and bone marrow, except for a subgroup of cases that exhibit increased numbers of B cells. Repeated infections elicit no antibodies, and cell-mediated immunity is absent.

Bone marrow transplanted from an HLA-identical sibling can completely reconstitute the defect in SCIDS; if no suitable sibling exists, haploidentical marrow from a parent has sometimes been effective. These immunodeficient recipients are at severe risk, however, from graft-versus-host disease (GVHD, see chapters 12 and 13), not only after bone marrow transplantation but even after blood transfusions that contain viable lymphocytes. Immunosuppression given after bone marrow transplantation in these patients is intended to prevent GVHD, not to prevent graft rejection.

WISKOTT-ALDRICH SYNDROME

Wiskott-Aldrich syndrome is characterized by X-linked transmission of immunodeficiency associated with thrombocytopenia and eczema. No single defect can be invoked to explain all the findings. Although the first few months of life may be free of immune abnormalities, early manifestations are bleeding from the thrombocytopenia and persistent and progressive eczematous rash. The most common infecting agents are bacteria—of the sort associated with defective humoral immunity—but herpes viruses, cytomegalovirus, and pneumocystis infections frequently complicate the first years of life.

The major immunologic abnormality identified thus far is excessive degradation of immunoglobulins. There are low levels of IgM antibodies, including near absence of ABO blood group antibodies; IgG antibodies are quantitatively normal but seem to provide subnormal protective effect; serum levels of IgA and IgE are increased. T lymphocytes are present and react normally on *in vitro* testing, but cell-mediated protection is clinically deficient.

Although survival is longer with Wiskott-Aldrich syndrome than with untreated SCIDS, patients with this poorly understood condition have a downhill course. Bleeding is a continuous threat, and repeated bacterial and viral infections take a progressive toll. Immunoglobulin-producing cells are in a continuous hypermetabolic state; dysproteinemias are common and, as patients approach adolescence, lymphoreticular malignancies frequently develop. Bone marrow transplantation has shown some promise as definitive therapy.

ATAXIA-TELANGIECTASIA

Another inherited condition with no identifiable unifying defect is **ataxia-telangiectasia,** an autosomal recessive syndrome. This is a relatively common inherited immunologic defect; heterozygous possession of the gene is estimated at 1 percent. Although heterozygotes do not manifest the syndrome, they do experience increased liability to cancers of solid organs. Patients and family members have been shown to have an abnormality of the long arm of chromosome 14 and to have defects in repair of damaged DNA.

Ataxia is disturbance of gait and posture related to cerebellar dysfunction; this begins early and tends to progress. **Telangiectases** are superficial abnormalities of blood vessels which, in this condition, become apparent after age 2. The most conspicuous immunologic abnormality is deficiency of secretory and serum IgA. Serum IgM tends to be high and IgE to be low. Although IgG is quantitatively normal, antibody responses to specific immunogens are depressed, and chronic respiratory tract infections occur frequently. Most patients survive into adulthood, but the neurologic problems tend to worsen, and repeated infections cause pulmonary damage. Lymphoreticular malignancies are frequent in older patients.

PRIMARY DISORDERS OF T CELLS

DiGEORGE SYNDROME

Congenital **thymic hypoplasia,** also called DiGeorge syndrome or third/fourth pharyngeal pouch dysgenesis, is not genetically transmitted; it is a developmental defect that occurs sporadically in equal numbers of male and female infants. Structures in the anterior portion of the embryo develop abnormally, causing absence of the thymus and parathyroid glands, characteristic facial anomalies, and often malformations of the heart and blood vessels. The parathyroid deficiency causes symptomatic hypocalcemia in the first few hours of life; this, along with the facial deformities, provokes diagnostic evaluation that uncovers absence of the thymus.

Defective immunity becomes apparent through superficial fungal infections, frequent diarrhea, susceptibility to pneumonia, and failure to thrive. T lymphocytes are severely reduced in number and function. B lymphocytes are present, and antibodies to T-independent antigens are normal, but, because T-cell help is needed for most antibodies, there is increased susceptibility to a wide range of infections. Implantation of fetal thymus can restore T-cell activity, but the cardiovascular deformities and hypoparathyroidism remain independent problems.

CHRONIC MUCOCUTANEOUS CANDIDIASIS

Chronic mucocutaneous candidiasis is a highly selective T-cell defect that affects both males and females. T cells respond inadequately to antigens of *Candida albicans,* leading to severe infection of skin and mucosal surfaces but not, ordinarily, of deeper tissues. T cells respond normally to antigens other than candida, and B-cell function is unaffected. Abnormalities of IgA levels or of phagocytic activities have been noted in some patients, and other abnormalities occur frequently but unpredictably. The parathyroids, the adrenals, or the ovaries may be hypoactive; antigland autoantibodies may accompany or even precede the endocrine deficiency. Other sporadic problems include chronic hepatitis, diabetes mellitus, iron deficiency, and vitamin B_{12} deficiency. Neither the cause nor a cure for the immune defect has been found. Treatment is directed against the severe and often disfiguring skin infections and the glandular deficiencies.

PRIMARY DISORDERS OF B CELLS

B-cell abnormalities cause immunoglobulin deficiencies, but the reasons for most defective B-cell activity are by no means understood. The organ of instruction for B cells cannot easily be located or shown to be abnormal and, although much is known about immunoglobulin synthesis, the pathways responsible for specific dysfunctions remain unclear.

X-LINKED HYPOGAMMAGLOBULINEMIA

The best-known constitutional immunodeficiency is the X-linked condition first described by Bruton in 1952. **X-linked hypogammaglobulinemia,** also called Bruton's agammaglobulinemia, is easily diagnosed by demonstrating uniformly low levels of immunoglobulins and, often, a family history of infectious problems in male infants. These children appear normal as long as passively acquired maternal antibodies persist; after several months, pneumococcus, streptococcus, hemophilus, and other pyogenic bacteria cause recurrent infections that affect especially the respiratory tract, the skin, and sometimes the central nervous system. Viral and fungal infections are uncommon, except for hepatitis and enteroviruses. Frequent and persistent infections of lung or central nervous system often cause progressive tissue damage; rheumatoid arthritis is common in those who survive past puberty.

Clinical Observations

The entire B-cell population seems to be absent; blood and tissues lack cells with any of the B-lymphocyte markers. T cells are normal or increased in number and exhibit normal functions. Phagocytic cells are functionally normal, but absence of IgM and IgG antibodies reduces opsonic activity, and the bactericidal actions of neutrophils are sharply reduced. Tissue sites normally rich in B lymphocytes are hypoplastic, but the thymus is normal.

Serum in this condition contains less than 250 mg/dl total immunoglobulin, of which most is IgG; secretions contain virtually no IgA. Treatment is prophylactic administration of an immunoglobulin preparation (ISG) containing a wide range of antibody specificities (see chapter 9); episodes of infection are treated promptly with appropriate antimicrobials. Antibiotics are, however, less effective in these patients than in persons with normal antibodies and opsonic activity. Passive immunotherapy cannot correct antibody levels in epithelial secretions, and upper respiratory tract infections, dental caries, and diarrhea remain troublesome. Optimal treatment allows survival into adulthood, but life expectancy is reduced. Patients often suffer from allergic and autoimmune phenomena, and leukemia and lymphomas are frequent late complications. Overwhelming infections with fungi, pneumocystis, pseudomonas, and proteus may prove fatal despite seemingly optimal therapy.

Hypogammaglobulinemia in Females

Hypogammaglobulinemia indistinguishable from the Bruton type sometimes occurs in young girls. It is possible that these female infants carry two abnormal X chromosomes, or there may be other defects not yet identified.

OTHER HYPOGAMMAGLOBULINEMIAS

Some few infants fail, in the second half of their first year, to develop normal immunoglobulin levels. Some come to medical attention because of repeated infections, but others are found only incidentally during study of families with known immunodeficiency. Continued observation often demonstrates eventual but belated antibody production and normal responses to most bacterial challenges, although a few cases have persistently depressed IgA production. This condition has been called **transient hypogammaglobulinemia of infancy**. It appears to be self-limited; passive administration of immunoglobulins is contraindicated, because that may actually suppress antibody formation.

A poorly understood and possibly heterogeneous condition exists in which IgG and IgA are depressed and IgM levels are normal or elevated. These patients suffer repeated respiratory infections, which begin later than those occurring in Bruton's agammaglobulinemia. The volume of lymphoid tissue is normal or increased, but the cell population produces only IgM. Malignant proliferation of IgM-producing cells may occur later in life. Red cells and neutrophils frequently exhibit autoimmune impairment; neutrophil defects probably contribute to the increased susceptibility to pseudomonas and pneumocystis that persists despite passive immunotherapy.

COMMON VARIABLE IMMUNODEFICIENCY

Also known as acquired hypogammaglobulinemia or idiopathic late-onset immunodeficiency, **common variable immunodeficiency** becomes apparent only after one or several decades of normal immune activity. Normal numbers of B cells persist, but immunoglobulin concentration and antigen-specific responses decline. On experimental stimulation, cultured B cells fail to multiply or to differentiate, a defect thought to be constitutional even though normal immune activity occurs in the first years of life. Some patients who initially exhibit the hyper-IgM condition described in the preceding paragraph gradually lose all Ig-producing capacity. Infections tend to be less severe than in Bruton's agammaglobulinemia, but the frequency of autoimmune phenomena and malignant disease is even higher. Intestinal malabsorption syndromes and protein-losing enteropathy are common, as is chronic lung disease. Some patients eventually develop deficiencies of T-cell function as well, much expanding the spectrum of infections to which they are susceptible. Family members have a high incidence of immunoglobulin abnormalities and autoimmune diseases.

SELECTIVE IgA DEFICIENCY

The most prevalent constitutional immune defect in the general population is **selective absence of IgA**. Frequency estimates range from 1 in 320 to 1 in 800 in white populations surveyed; in patients with allergic or autoimmune disorders, prevalence is even higher. The diagnosis is made from depression of serum IgA concentration, which is usually below 5 mg/dl, but the pathologic manifestations result from deficiency of IgA in secretions. The cause of the defect is unknown. Many different abnormalities have been observed: increased suppressor activity directed against IgA-producing cells; inability of IgA-producing plasma cells to release Ig; abnormal distribution of isotypes on cells destined to produce IgA; and abnormal reactivity to chemical agents. In a single kindred, some members may have selective IgA deficiency, and others may have common variable immunodeficiency.

Selective IgA deficiency produces diverse clinical effects. Some patients experience sinopulmonary infections or chronic diarrhea as a result of inadequate surface defenses. Allergic manifestations against ubiquitous environmental antigens, especially cow's milk, are unduly frequent in persons with deficient serum and secretory IgA. Another frequent concomitant condition is autoimmune disease of the collagen-vascular type (see chapter 12). Some affected individuals have no symptoms at all and are identified only through population surveys.

Antibodies against IgA

IgA-deficient patients often have antibodies against all immuno-globulins of the IgA class. Severe anaphylactic reactions have occurred in a very few IgA-deficient persons transfused with IgA-containing blood components. Although circulating anti-IgA antibodies are found relatively frequently, anaphylactic transfusion reactions are very rare. Cell-bound IgE, not circulating antibody, mediates anaphylactic transfusion reactions, but the presence of anti-IgA in serum should prompt caution in undertaking transfusion.

In patients with selective IgA deficiency, infections are treated only as they occur, and allergic or autoimmune manifestations are treated as needed. Passive administration of IgA is contraindicated, because injections do not restore antibody levels in secretions and could possibly provoke class-specific antibodies.

DEFICIENCIES OF OTHER ISOTYPES

Aside from IgA, selective isotypic deficiencies are rare. Some patients who lack IgA also lack IgG2; when added to IgA deficiency, IgG2 deficiency seems to cause no incremental clinical consequences. Some patients with ataxia-telangiectasia have subclass-specific depression of IgG2.

Selective IgM deficiency has been observed, but very rarely. These patients have experienced meningococcal septicemia, pyogenic infections of the upper and lower respiratory tracts, staphylococcal skin infections, and tuberculosis. Other immunoglobulin classes were normal in the few cases studied.

An isolated disturbance of kappa chain production has been reported; lambda chain production was increased in compensation and immunoglobulin status was functionally normal.

DEFICIENCIES IN THE COMPLEMENT SYSTEM

Deficiency of virtually any of the components, factors, and regulators of complement can occur. As of 1984, 242 complement-deficient individuals had been described and classified. C2 deficiency was most common, affecting 77 persons, with equal sex distribution. The gene for absence of C2 has been estimated to occur in 1.2 percent of the white population, giving an expected homozygote frequency of 1 in 28,000. The HLA haplotype A10,B12 has strong linkage disequilibrium with the C2-null gene. Deficiencies of early components in the classical pathway have been reported only in whites; blacks with complement deficiencies have lacked components 5 through 8, which are activated in both classical and alternative pathways. The site for properdin synthesis is on the X chromosome, but all the other complement proteins are determined by autosomal genes. Of 14 persons found to be C3 deficient, all but 2 were males; other defects show no gender bias.

CLINICAL CONSEQUENCES

Given the importance of complement in inflammation and opsonization, it is not surprising that complement deficiencies cause increased susceptibility to bacterial infection. Less readily explained is the striking prevalence of autoimmune diseases in patients lacking the early components of the classical pathway. Late-sequence deficiencies cause susceptibility to neisserial infection, both *N. meningitidis* (meningococcus) and *N. gonorrheae* (gonococcus). Nearly a quarter of individuals lacking C5 through C9 have no clinical abnormalities, and 16 percent of persons deficient in C1, C2, or C4 report no associated problems. Patients who lack C3, the pivotal protein in both the classical and the alternative pathways, are susceptible both to infections and to autoimmune diseases.

The autoimmune diseases seen most often in patients with complement deficiency are systemic lupus erythematosus, discoid lupus, glomerulonephritis, and vasculitis. These affect 85 to 90 percent of patients with defects of C1, C2, or C4 and about 65 percent of C3-deficient patients. About a third of patients with C3 deficiency have increased susceptibility to pneumococcal infection as their only problem. In patients with late-phase deficiencies, abnormalities other than neisserial susceptibility have been seen only with C5 defects, which show an association with glomerulonephritis.

Deficient Control Protein

Hereditary angioedema, which results from deficiency of the control protein **C1 esterase inhibitor** (C1 inhibitor, C1INH), is an inherited deficiency that does not cause immune dysfunction. This alpha-2 globulin prevents generation of the C1qrs esterase by attaching to the C1q molecule in a fashion that causes C1r and C1s to dissociate (see Chapter 8). C1INH is a normal constituent of plasma. It prevents ongoing activation not only of C1 but also of the plasminogen system, which cleaves fibrin and fibrinogen, and of the kinin system, which generates proteins that mediate increased vascular permeability.

All these proteins have interrelated roles in the coagulation and inflammatory systems, and normal physiologic function depends upon precise adjustment of activation and inhibition. In persons who lack C1INH activity, uncontrolled activation of C1qrs leads to excessive cleavage of C4 and C2, generating powerful kinin-related proteins that cause increased vascular permeability. There are no signs of complement deficiency, presumably because the alternative pathway can generate sufficient C3 convertase to compensate for defective classical-pathway activation. Problems arise, however, from the inappropriate excess of vascular permeability. Patients suffer recurrent episodes of localized edema affecting the gastrointestinal tract, the upper respiratory tract, and the skin. The skin problems are the most visible but least dangerous. Gastrointestinal involvement causes episodic abdominal pain and/or diarrhea, and angioedema of the larynx may cause death by asphyxiation.

The deficiency derives from an autosomal dominant gene, of which there are two varieties. The more common variety causes absence of the protein, whereas the less common (15 percent) form codes for a protein that has no physiologic activity. Diagnosis rests upon demonstrating absent or very low C1INH and, during acute episodes, marked depletion of C4 and C2.

——— ABNORMALITIES OF PHAGOCYTOSIS ———

Antibody and complement deficiencies severely impair phagocytic defenses, but an additional category of defects specifically affects phagocytic cells. These cause problems primarily with bacterial defenses; defenses against viruses and protozoa depend so heavily on lymphocytes that granulocyte/macrophage disorders affect them relatively little. Very severe depression of phagocytosis predisposes to fungal infections, but these occur much less commonly than recurrent or persistent bacterial infections.

CHRONIC GRANULOMATOUS DISEASE

Patients with **chronic granulomatous disease** (CGD) suffer frequent infections with organisms that have low virulence in normal persons, notably *Staphylococcus epidermidis* and species of serratia and aspergillus. Characteristic problems are chronically enlarged and draining lymph nodes, persistent mucosal infections, osteomyelitis, and chronic intestinal symptoms. Treatment requires high doses of powerful bactericidal agents.

Chronic granulomatous disease reflects defects in the intracellular processes that kill ingested organisms. Phagocytosis occurs normally, but the cells fail to generate the toxic oxygen species that kill the phagocytized organisms. Several different patterns of genetic transmission exist; the clinical picture is essentially the same for all. In the X-linked form, the missing protein is a component of the neu-

TABLE 10–5. Major Inborn Defects of Immune Function

Defective Element	Name of Syndrome	Inheritance Pattern
Precursor cell for lymphocytes, macrophages, granulocytes	Reticular dysgenesis	Autosomal recessive
B and T lymphocytes	SCIDS, common type*	Autosomal recessive or X-linked
	SCIDS with enzyme defects*	Autosomal recessive
	Wiskott-Aldrich syndrome	X-linked
	Ataxia-telangiectasia	Autosomal recessive
Primarily T lymphocytes	DiGeorge's syndrome	Developmental defect, probably not genetic
	Chronic mucocutaneous candidiasis	Autosomal recessive
Primarily B lymphocytes	Infantile hypogammaglobulinemia	
	Bruton's type	X-linked
	Affecting females	Unknown
	Transient hypogammaglobulinemia of infancy	Familial; more frequent in families with SCIDS syndromes
	Common variable immunodeficiency†	Familial, but transmission pattern not understood
	Selective IgA deficiency	Various: both autosomal recessive and dominant patterns; sometimes familial association with common variable immunodeficiency
Complement proteins		
C1INH	Hereditary angioedema	Autosomal dominant
C1 through 9	Complement deficiency	Probably autosomal recessive
Phagocytic functions	Chronic granulomatous disease	Most common form is X-linked
	Chediak-Higashi syndrome	Autosomal recessive
	Glucose-6-phosphate dehydrogenase deficiency	X-linked
	Defective leukocyte chemotaxis	Various; some associated with carbohydrate storage diseases

*SCIDS: Severe combined immunodeficiency syndrome
†Some element of T-cell dysfunction accompanies many cases of common variable immunodeficiency

---

TABLE 10—6. Evaluation of Immune Competence

Screening
    History: frequent or unusual infections; eczema; growth retardation, or developmental defects; affected family members
    Complete blood count with differential white count
    Test for antibody to HIV-1
    Skin tests for delayed hypersensitivity to commonly encountered antigens
    Serum protein evaluation: protein electrophoresis; levels of anti-A, and anti-B; levels of IgM, IgG, IgA
    Nitroblue tetrazolium (NBT) test for neutrophil function
    Hemolytic complement evaluation (CH50)

T-Cell Evaluation
    Chest x-ray for thymus in infants, thymic tumors in adults
    Quantify peripheral lymphocytes with antibodies to CD3 (all T cells), CD4, and CD8
    Lymph node biopsy to identify number, distribution, and morphology of T cells
    In vitro tests of functional competence: Blast transformation to mitogens
                                                    Stimulation by allogeneic cells
                                                    Lymphokine production after challenge

Evaluation of Humoral Immunity
    Antibody titers before and after specific immunization
    Quantity and distribution of IgG subclasses
    Enumerate peripheral lymphocytes that express mIg or receptors for Fc and EBV
    Bone marrow evaluation for pre-B cells, plasma cells
    Lymph node biopsy, for number, distribution of cells with B-related differentiation markers
    In vitro test of functional competence: Blast transformation to mitogens

Phagocytes and Complement
    Quantify C3, C4; other components if necessary
    Tests for chemotaxis: Skin window, *in vivo;* Boyden chamber, *in vitro*
    Specific intracellular enzymes
    Quantitative tests of bacterial killing, opsonic response

---

trophil system known as the **cytochrome b complex**. An intriguing association exists between the white-cell problems in X-linked CGD and a pattern of abnormalities in red blood cells and striated muscle called **McLeod syndrome,** in which abnormal membrane proteins are associated with unusual blood group characteristics on red cells and progressive damage to neuromuscular elements.

OTHER ENZYMES

Deficiencies in many different enzyme systems can impair granulocyte and macrophage function. Depressed levels of **myeloperoxidase** and **alkaline phosphatase** affect cells throughout the body, but only cells of the granulocyte/macrophage lineage express significant functional deficiency. Patients with severe **glucose-6-phosphate dehydrogenase** deficiency may have depressed intracellular bactericidal function comparable to that of CGD. Two other conditions in which defective phagocytosis is part of a clinical constellation are **Chediak-Higashi syndrome** and the condition known as **Job's syndrome;** both are multiorgan diseases with familial distribution but unknown molecular basis.

Table 10–5 summarizes the major forms of primary immune dysfunction—those owing to constitutional defects.

Table 10–6 lists some of the tests employed to identify and to diagnose immunodeficiencies, either constitutional or acquired.

────────── **SUGGESTIONS FOR** ──────────
FURTHER READING

Davis AE, III: C1 inhibitor and hereditary angioneurotic edema. Ann Rev Immunol 1988; 6:595–628

Dwyer JM: Intravenous therapy with gamma globulin. Adv Int Med 1987; 32:111–36

Ochs HD, Wedgwood RJ: IgG subclass deficiencies. Ann Rev Med 1987; 38:325–40

Pinching AJ: Laboratory investigation of secondary immunodeficiency. Clin Immunol Allergy 1985; 5:469–90

Root RK: The compromised host. In: Wyngaarden JB, Smith LH, Jr, eds: Cecil Textbook of Medicine, 18th ed. Philadelphia: WB Saunders, 1988:1529–38

Schur PH: Inherited complement component abnormalities. Ann Rev Med 1986; 37:333–46

Webster ADB: Laboratory investigation of primary deficiency of the lymphoid system. Clin Immunol Allergy 1985; 5:447–468

CHAPTER 11

Neoplasms of the Immune System

Without cellular multiplication, immune responses could not occur. With this propensity to divide, however, it is not surprising that cells of the lymphoreticular system often exhibit neoplastic proliferation. Malignancies of the lymphoreticular system can best be classified by the nature and maturational state of the cell of origin.

197

CLASSIFICATION OF NEOPLASMS

A **neoplasm** is an accumulation of cells derived from a single progenitor, a clone that proliferates autonomously, unconstrained by physiologic stimuli or external events. Many processes that lead to overaccumulation of cells involve cells of several different genetic compositions; these processes usually reflect normally constituted cells responding in an excessive or abnormal fashion to an external stimulus. A monoclonal proliferation reflects derangement of the internal events that regulate cell division and growth. Neoplastic cells with a single clonal origin can differ in their appearance and function, depending upon level of maturation, exposure to mediators, adequacy of blood supply, and other variables.

BENIGN VERSUS MALIGNANT

Not all neoplasms are malignant. Benign neoplasms are more likely than their malignant counterparts to stop growing spontaneously, to remain distinct from the surrounding tissues, and to maintain a high level of differentiated appearance and function. Malignant neoplasms characteristically infiltrate surrounding tissue, establish new sites of multiplication at distant locations **(metastases),** express immature and undifferentiated cellular characteristics, and recur after attack by surgical removal or cytotoxic agents.

Leukemia versus Lymphoma

Cells of certain types can experience either benign or malignant neoplastic proliferation, but neoplasms of the lymphoreticular system are, almost without exception, malignant. Non-malignant lymphocytes or mononuclear phagocytes may accumulate to an excessive extent, but this represents polyclonal reaction to one or more stimuli. Malignant proliferation that involves primarily circulating cells of blood and/or bone marrow is designated **leukemia;** processes that originate in the solid tissues of the immune system are called **lymphomas**. Malignant leukemic cells may infiltrate solid tissues, and lymphoma cells may be found in the bloodstream; but the diagnostic distinction—admittedly imperfect—is useful both clinically and theoretically.

CELLS OF ORIGIN

Malignant proliferations arise from defects in regulation of the genetic processes that control replication. Cells at any stage of the differentiation process may escape from normal control; all the clonal offspring will express the same dysregulation and will be at the same differentiational stage as the parent cell. In classifying malignancies of the lymphoreticular system, the tools used to identify normal populations can be applied to neoplastic cells. Unchecked multiplication, however, often distorts protein synthesis and intracellular organization, so the malignant population may bear little immediate resemblance to normal cells of the same lineage. Characterization of cells that have lost their normal appearance and function can best be done with monoclonal antibodies to surface molecules and by genetic analysis of deoxyribonucleic acid (DNA) sequences.

Lymphoreticular neoplasms may arise from B cells, T cells, or mononuclear phagocytes, and the proliferating clone may reflect any stage of differentiation. Different entities exhibit different patterns of age distribution, clinical course, and response to treatment. Table 11–1 outlines the developmental origins of most lymphoreticular neoplasms.

TABLE 11–1. Malignancies of the Lymphoreticular System

Cell of Origin	Usual Clinical Condition
Lymphoblast, no other distinguishing features	"Null cell" acute lymphoblastic leukemia (ALL)
Pre-pre-B or pre-B cell	ALL positive for the common-ALL antigen (CALLA, CD 10)
Stage I thymocyte	T-cell ALL
Stage I/II thymocyte	T-cell lymphoblastic lymphoma
Mature or partially differentiated B cell	Chronic lymphocytic leukemia (CLL) Burkitt's lymphoma Various non-Hodgkin's lymphomas Hairy cell leukemia
Immunoglobulin-secreting B cell	Multiple myeloma Waldenström's macroglobulinemia Heavy-chain disease Mediterranean lymphoma
Mature T cell	Adult T-cell leukemia/lymphoma T-cell chronic lymphocytic leukemia (TCLL) Sezary syndrome Mycosis fungoides Various non-Hodgkin's lymphomas
Monocyte/macrophage lineage	Hodgkin's disease (probably) True histiocytic lymphoma Histiocytosis X Monocytic or monoblastic leukemia

EXPLORING THE NUCLEUS

Nuclear events determine the fate of all cells, normal and abnormal. Techniques that have been especially useful in examining chromosomes and individual gene sequences are **cytogenetic analysis** and DNA probing by **restriction fragment length polymorphisms** (RFLP; see page 68). Cytogenetic techniques reveal the morphology of chromosomes captured during mitosis. Histochemical, immunologic, and photographic techniques are used to characterize the size and shape of individual chromosomes and to identify abnormalities of appearance, number, and location of chromosomal segments. With RFLP techniques, the DNA sequence of specific segments can be mapped and compared with segments of known characteristics.

In diagnosing lymphoreticular malignancies, genetic rearrangements are used to assign cells to B or T classifications and to discriminate proliferating neoplastic clones from other cells with which they are admixed. If specific cytogenetic abnormalities are frequently associated with certain neoplasms, it suggests that individual gene sequences influence development of specific kinds of neoplastic multiplication. Mapping procedures have revealed the presence and location of DNA segments, called **oncogenes,** that are present in normal cells but that, after activation by various known or unknown stimuli, seem to mediate unregulated cell multiplication.

MALIGNANCIES OF LYMPHOID PRECURSORS

Neoplastic proliferation of minimally differentiated lymphoid cells is called **acute lymphoblastic leukemia** (ALL). Although cytogenetic and immunologic techniques can assign these prefunctional cells to individual lineages, the untreated clinical course of all such neoplasms is relatively uniform.

CLINICAL LEUKEMIA SYNDROMES

Acute leukemia reflects a block very early in differentiation. Extremely immature cells overrun sites at which lymphocytes normally multiply, especially the bone marrow, where they suppress the division and maturation of red cells, platelets, and granulocytes. Problems arise not only from unchecked multiplication of neoplastic cells but also from absence of normal lymphocyte-mediated activities. The clinical picture usually includes anemia, with consequent weakness and impaired tissue function; thrombocytopenia, with bleeding from mucosal surfaces and into the skin; and granulocytopenia, leading to problems with infection. Impaired humoral and cell-mediated immunity exacerbates the susceptibility to infection.

Predisposition and Prognosis

Any cell of bone marrow origin can exhibit leukemic proliferation; lymphocytes and granulocytes are most commonly involved. In general, acute lymphoblastic leukemia affects children, whereas acute leukemia of granulocyte precursors (myeloblastic leukemia) begins after puberty; children do, sometimes, suffer from acute myeloblastic leukemia and rare adults may have acute lymphoblastic leukemia. Occasional leukemic patients have had exposure to ionizing radiation or mutagenic chemicals, but for the vast majority of cases, no predisposing event is apparent. There have been many attempts to implicate viral infection as causing leukemia, but interpretation of these observations remains controversial. Spontaneous or induced immunodeficiency conditions and certain congenital chromosomal abnormalities impose an excess risk of developing leukemia.

COMMON ALL

When sheep-cell rosetting was the only way to identify T cells, and the presence of membrane immunoglobulin was the only feature that identified B cells, most acute lymphoblastic leukemias could not be classified. The neoplastic cells lacked features that could assign them to T or B lineage but did possess a membrane molecule that came to be called the **common acute lymphoblastic leukemia antigen** (CALLA). This surface marker, now designated CD10, is not specific for leukemia; it is present on the earliest lymphoid precursor cell (see page 78) and is a marker for cellular immaturity. In normal marrow at all ages, approximately 1 percent of cells express CALLA. Nonhematopoietic cells that are CD10 positive include renal epithelium in adults and fetuses, fetal intestinal cells, and myoepithelial cells of the adult breast. In about 80 percent of patients with ALL, the malignant cells are CALLA positive; occasionally CALLA may be seen on the malignant blasts seen in the terminal stage of chronic granulocytic leukemia.

Other Markers

Leukemic cells that express CALLA frequently are positive for the Ia surface antigen (see page 70) and the enzyme terminal deoxynucleotidyl transferase (TdT). Although sometimes considered a marker for immature T cells, TdT remains in the nucleus of B-lineage cells through the rearrangement of chromosome 14. When the DNA of CALLA-positive cells is examined, it usually shows the rearrangement of chromosome 14 characteristic of B-cell commitment; most cases of "common" ALL can more properly be considered leukemias of the pre-pre-B cell. In about 10 percent of lymphoblastic leukemias, neither CALLA nor Ia nor chromosomal rearrangements are found; the nucleus of these "null" cells is usually positive for TdT.

MORE DIFFERENTIATED PRECURSORS

Of patients with childhood ALL, 10 to 15 percent have cells that form sheep-cell rosettes and react with antibodies against T9 and T10 antigens. T-cell ALL carries a worse clinical prognosis than null-cell or CALLA-positive lymphoblastic leukemia. In all types of childhood ALL, predictors of an unfavorable clinical course include male sex, high white-cell numbers at presentation, and older age at onset; precisely these features are common in T-cell ALL. Patients with T-ALL also tend to have malignant cells in solid organs, particularly those sites where normal T cells pass from the circulation into solid tissue.

Cells that have mu heavy chains in the cytoplasm are considered pre-B cells; 15 to 20 percent of ALL involves pre-B cells, which are also positive for CALLA and for TdT. They lack immunoglobulin monomers on the membrane, the hallmark of the mature B cell, but do have CD21, the receptor for Epstein-Barr virus (EBV) recognition (see Table 5–4). Rarely, ALL involves mature B cells, which express membane Ig, Fc receptors, and the Ia antigen and lack CALLA and TdT. Only 2 to 5 percent of ALL cases fall into this category; these patients respond very poorly to therapy and rarely survive more than 4 to 6 months.

As a patient's disease worsens, markers on the neoplastic cells may change. CALLA may disappear if initially present or develop if initially absent. Features that distinguish T from B cells, however, do not exchange. T-cell forms do not acquire B-cell characteristics or vice versa, and null cells do not later assume distinguishing features.

LYMPHOMAS

Lymphomas are solid tumors of the lymphoreticular system. Many clinical syndromes and morphologic entities exist; attempts to classify and to systematize the lymphomas are fraught with confusion and controversy. Most lymphomas involve cells in middle or late stages of differentiation. The small proportion that embody early evolutionary phases are often described as **lymphoblastic lymphomas** and have a very poor prognosis despite aggressive therapy.

About 85 percent of lymphoblastic lymphomas are of T-cell origin; the cells tend to be slightly more mature than those of acute leukemia. As with T-cell ALL, males outnumber females. Mediastinal mass is a common initial event, but involvement of bone marrow and peripheral blood frequently follows. Null-cell and pre-B lymphoblastic lymphomas occur less often and are less likely to present with a mediastinal mass, but they, too, rapidly progress to widespread dissemination and poor prognosis.

NEOPLASMS OF MATURE B LYMPHOCYTES

The mature B cell displays membrane immunoglobulin (mIg) and other markers described in chapter 5 but has not differentiated into an Ig-producing plasma cell. Neoplasms of mature B lymphocytes include both solid-tissue malignancies (lymphomas) and primary bone marrow conditions (leukemias).

CHRONIC LYMPHOCYTIC LEUKEMIA

In **chronic lymphocytic leukemia,** the bone marrow is heavily populated by partially mature B lymphocytes that do not secrete immunoglobulin, but adequate production of normal hematopoietic elements continues in the early phases of the disease. The neoplastic cells of chronic lymphocytic leukemia multiply much less rapidly than those of lymphoblastic leukemia. The leukemic cells have an abnormally prolonged life span and, eventually, enormous numbers of cells accumulate. The disease usually remains indolent until, in the late stages, there is loss of normal marrow function and infiltration of lymph nodes, spleen, and other tissues by leukemic cells. Terminally, the previously mature neoplastic cells may undergo irreversible transformation to immature blast configuration; even if blast crisis does not occur, previously normal-looking cells become larger and more atypical as the disease progresses.

Serum immunoglobulin concentration may be quantitatively normal, but functional immunity is often impaired. Along with reduced normal immune response goes increased likelihood of dysfunctional immune activity. Autoantibodies to red cells occur fairly frequently, sometimes causing significant hemolysis. Autoantibodies to platelets occur less commonly but may cause symptomatic thrombocytopenia. As in many other immunodeficiency and dysfunctional states, patients with chronic lymphocytic leukemia have increased likelihood of developing other malignant neoplasms.

HAIRY CELL LEUKEMIA

The name **hairy cell leukemia** derives from the peculiar filamentous projections of cytoplasm characteristic of these neoplastic cells

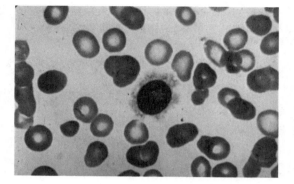

FIGURE 11–1. This "hairy cell" takes its name from the irregular cytoplasmic filaments seen in this Wright-stained preparation. On scanning electron microscopy, these cells have a densely ruffled contour.

(Fig. 11–1). Features characteristic of B cells include rearrangement of heavy-chain and light-chain genes, the presence of membrane immunoglobulin, and existence of receptors for gamma-chain Fc, although not, usually, for C3. Unlike normal B cells, hairy cells are capable of limited phagocytosis, and they exhibit some reactivity with antibody against one of the monocyte-macrophage antigens. Another distinctive feature is strong expression of CD25, the receptor for interleukin 2 (IL-2). An early name for this molecule was **Tac,** denoting a marker for **T**-cell **ac**tivation; IL-2 is now known to stimulate B as well as T cells, so presence of its receptor need not identify the underlying cell as a T cell. Hairy cells seem most plausibly to be B lymphocytes in the phase of activation that precedes evolution into Ig-secreting plasma cells.

The clinical course of hairy cell leukemia is less aggressive than that of acute lymphoblastic leukemia but somewhat more aggressive than most chronic lymphocytic leukemias. Middle-aged males are most frequently affected; splenomegaly and leukopenia are characteristic findings on presentation. Splenectomy has long been the treatment of choice, but alpha-interferon therapy has recently given excellent results in this type of leukemia. The most common and severe complications result from infections, but many patients also manifest autoimmune problems of various kinds.

LYMPHOMAS

B-cell lymphomas, which range from indolent to aggressive, may embody any stage of cellular maturation. Different classification systems place varying emphasis on cellular appearance, on the putative origin of the cells, on the overall tissue patterns, and on the clinical course. A reasonable summary is that lymphomas in which small, fairly uniform-looking cells grow in a non-destructive pattern have a less aggressive clinical course and embody a later stage of maturation than conditions with large and/or pleomorphic cells and a growth pattern that effaces normal architectural features.

Other than Burkitt's lymphoma (see below), frequency of B-cell lymphomas increases with age. As lymphomas become more aggressive, normal B-cell activity diminishes and predisposition to autoimmune abnormalities increases. Bone marrow involvement occurs late or not at all, so abnormalities of red cells, granulocytes, and platelets are rarer in the lymphomas than in the leukemias; anemia of chronic disease, weight loss, and other dysfunctions characteristic of systemic malignancies occur in advanced phases.

BURKITT'S LYMPHOMA

This neoplasm of small lymphocytes was first described in Africa, where it predominantly affects children. Cells are TdT negative, and the membranes nearly always display CALLA, membrane Ig, and the Ia antigen. In affected tissues, diffusely proliferating lymphocytes are interspersed with large, pale phagocytic cells to give an appearance described as "starry sky."

Untreated Burkitt's lymphoma is highly aggressive, growing and destroying the bone or other site of origin and spreading rapidly to other tissues. Prompt and intensive chemotherapy often induces a rapid, dramatic, and long-lasting response; although recurrence sometimes follows successful therapy, many patients have lifelong remission. In certain areas of Africa the tumor occurs so frequently that it is described as endemic; sporadic cases of Burkitt's lymphoma occur in other parts of the world. Bones of the jaw are the commonest primary site for African tumors, followed by sites in the abdomen; lymph nodes, the mucosa of the upper respiratory tract, and the bone marrow are seldom involved. In non-African cases, the nervous system, kidneys, gonads, retroperitoneal tissue, liver, and spleen are primary sites. In African but not sporadic cases, Epstein-Barr virus (EBV) is closely associated with the lymphoma. The chromatin of tumor cells contains genetic elements of EBV, and virus can be recovered from cultures.

Translocation and Oncogene

Burkitt's lymphoma provides an exciting illustration of consistent chromosomal abnormality and the association of oncogene with neoplasia. The neoplastic cells of Burkitt's lymphoma characteristically express a translocation in which material from the long arm of chromosome 8 becomes attached to another chromosome, usually the long arm of chromosome 14 but sometimes the short arm of chromosome 2 or the long arm of 22. (Fig. 11–2). The displaced fragment of chromosome 8 carries the oncogene called *c-myc;* the acceptor sites are those that control the manufacture of the immunoglobulin heavy chain, the kappa light chain, and the lambda light chain, respectively. The physiologic significance of this translocation is not entirely clear, inasmuch as the neoplasm is not associated with immunoglobulin abnormalities, and specific manifestations of *c-myc* activity cannot often be identified. As the activities of oncogenes are more fully understood, the significance of an oncogene associating with a functionally distinctive chromosomal site will doubtless be illuminated.

Significance of EBV

Yet another oddity of Burkitt's lymphoma is the association of EBV and restricted geographic areas with tumor occurrence. Epstein-Barr virus is known to modify cell growth and multiplication. Inser-

Translocation (8;14) in Burkitt's Lymphoma

8

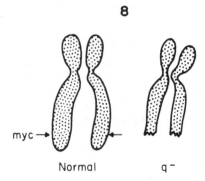

myc →   Normal   q⁻

14

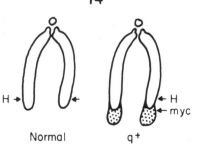

H →   Normal   q⁺   ← H
                                            ← myc

FIGURE 11–2. Normal examples of chromosome 8 *(top)* and 14 *(below)* are on the left. The *myc* site is near the end of the long arm of chromosome 8. The site that directs manufacture of immunoglobulin heavy chains (designated H) is near the end of chromosome 14. In 8;14 translocation, shown in the two figures at right, chromosome 8 loses a fragment that breaks at the *myc* site and chromosome 14 acquires the additional material, bringing *myc* and the H-chain site into proximity.

tion of DNA from EBV into the genome of cultured cells causes the recipient cells to become "transformed"; they express growth and metabolic properties characteristic of cultured neoplastic cells, and they continue dividing indefinitely as long as culture conditions are favorable. *In vivo*, EBV infects B lymphocytes through the CD21 antigen, which serves as a virus receptor. Infection of B cells affects T-cell behavior, inducing enhanced numbers and activity of suppressor T cells and altered helper-cell control.

Epstein-Barr virus infection is widespread throughout Africa, but only in certain areas is Burkitt's lymphoma endemic. These are areas characterized by intensely prevalent malarial infection. Malaria is known to distort T-cell function. It is plausible to assume that abnormal immune regulation might occur in children whose immune systems mature in an environment of repeated malarial infections. The normal response of suppressor T cells to EBV infection is to suppress *in vivo* proliferation of B cells, but T-cell abnormalities induced by malaria could well interrupt this regulatory function. Because translocational events are more likely to occur during exuberant cell division, unchecked multiplication of EBV-infected cells could provoke damage to chromosome 8 and transposition of the oncogene. Adding plausibility to this hypothesis is the increased occurrence of Burkitt's lymphoma in patients with acquired immunodeficiency syndrome (AIDS), who are known to have aberrant T-cell function and in whom EBV infection is extremely common. Quite possibly the numerous non-African cases of Burkitt's lymphoma reflect other types of prolonged or repeated immune dysregulation. Such a scenario does not, however, explain why the crucial chromosomal sites are selectively involved, nor does it explain the unique sensitivity of the lymphoma to cytotoxic chemotherapy.

MALIGNANCIES OF DIFFERENTIATED B CELLS

Fully differentiated immunoglobulin-secreting cells may undergo malignant proliferation. Monoclonal protein derived from the multiplying cells can often be found in the serum, but the fundamental event is cellular multiplication, not accumulation of protein.

Neoplasms of immunoglobulin-producing cells usually cause serum protein abnormalities. Either a normal molecule is present in abnormal quantities or a protein accumulates that is not normally present in blood or body fluids. The presence of any serum protein abnormality can be called **dysproteinemia;** the term **paraproteinemia** usually refers to protein that is qualitatively abnormal. Most dysproteinemias reflect excess production of structurally normal immunoglobulins or their constituent chains, but in some proliferative disorders, structurally variant proteins accumulate in serum or tissues.

MONOCLONAL GAMMOPATHY

Monoclonal gammopathy denotes accumulation of protein that originates from a single proliferating clone. The traditional way to demonstrate monoclonal origin has been electrophoretic analysis of the protein, but newer analytic techniques permit direct demonstration of uniform molecular properties in the proliferating protein-producing cells.

Migration of a protein in an electric field is determined by molecular size, shape, and charge, which reflect the amino acid sequence and associated side chains. Molecules of different structures express different migration patterns on an electrophoretic strip; densitometer analysis of the strip gives a tracing that depicts the migration rate and relative concentration of the separated proteins. When several different molecules migrate close to one another, the group of incompletely separated proteins appears as a diffuse, irregularly shaped elevation on the densitometer tracing. A single protein at high concentration produces intense staining at the sharply focused site where that molecule accumulates; on the densitometer tracing, this appears as a narrow, sharply defined peak with height proportional to the concentration of monoclonal protein (Fig. 11–3). Such a peak is called an **M spike;** M stands for monoclonal or myeloma (the most frequent cause for this diagnostic finding)—not for mu chain or immunoglobulin M class.

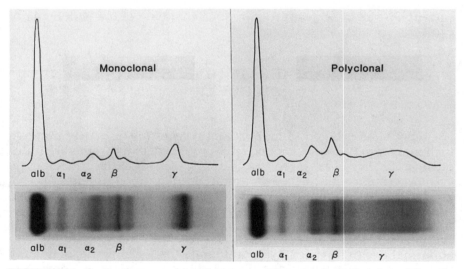

FIGURE 11–3. In the monoclonal gammopathy at left, molecules of the abnormally increased globulin have migrated on the gel strip as a dense, homogeneous band in the gamma region. The densitometer tracing depicts a clearly defined peak. In the polyclonal increase shown at right, the entire gamma region is diffusely dark and the densitometer tracing shows an irregular hump.

MULTIPLE MYELOMA

Multiple myeloma, a malignant neoplasm of plasma cells, largely affects older adults. It is characterized by masses of neoplastic cells in bone and marrow at various sites; "myelo" denotes marrow, and "-oma" means mass. Early in the process, the plasma cells have nearly normal appearance and function, but as neoplastic multiplication progresses, the cells lose differentiation of function and appearance.

Clinical Events

Where neoplastic cells accumulate, the bone is usually painful and may be so weakened that fractures occur spontaneously. Although monoclonal protein is conspicuous in serum, overall levels of immunoglobulin decline, and susceptibility to infection increases. Anemia is common, reflecting depression of erythropoiesis rather than marrow infiltration by neoplastic plasma cells. Serum calcium is usually high, and this, along with abnormalities of urine protein levels, often impairs renal function. Therapy usually induces a favorable response, and survival is characteristically measured in years. Common causes of death are infection, hematologic complications, or renal failure.

The most striking diagnostic feature in multiple myeloma is accumulation of monoclonal protein, its nature determined by the phenotype of the proliferating plasma cell. The monoclonal protein is IgG in 50 percent of cases, IgA in 25 percent of cases, IgM in 15 to 20 percent, and IgD or IgE much less commonly. These frequencies parallel the proportions in which immunoglobulin classes are normally produced, suggesting that neoplastic proliferation affects plasma cells at random and does not reflect a specific activating event or intrinsic susceptibility.

Bence-Jones Protein

Besides production of complete immunoglobulin molecules, the neoplastic cells secrete excessive light chains, either kappa or lambda, that are not paired with heavy chains. Light-chain monomers, much smaller than the four-chain immunoglobulin molecule, rapidly pass from blood into urine and rarely accumulate in the serum. For more than a century, their presence in urine has been used as a diagnostic feature for multiple myeloma. Light chains in urine are called **Bence-Jones protein**. These unpaired light chains do not react with many chemical indicators for protein and will not be detected with most urine dip sticks. The unique property of Bence-Jones protein is that it redissolves at temperatures near the boiling point after precipitating when heated to about 55°C; most proteins are irreversibly denatured by heat, and the cloudy precipitate that forms on heating remains despite further heating or cooling (Fig. 11−4).

BENCE-JONES PROTEIN VS. OTHER URINARY PROTEINS

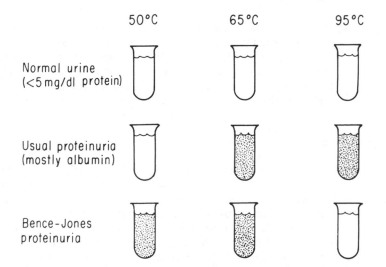

FIGURE 11—4. Heating precipitates most proteins. Heating normal urine, shown in the top panel, causes no precipitation because little or no protein is present. In most pathologic states, urine protein is largely albumin, shown in the middle panel, which precipitates irreversibly at about 65°C. Bence-Jones protein, shown in the bottom panel, precipitates at a lower temperature than albumin but redissolves when the temperature approaches the boiling point.

The heat test is a dramatic but insensitive way to demonstrate Bence-Jones proteinuria. Electrophoresis of concentrated urinary proteins, a more sensitive technique, demonstrates Bence-Jones protein in urine of 50 to 70 percent of patients with multiple myeloma. About 20 percent of myeloma patients have Bence-Jones proteinuria as the only indication of dysproteinemia. Highly concentrated light chains in the urine damage renal epithelium; in myeloma patients, the development of renal failure parallels the magnitude and duration of Bence-Jones proteinuria. Patients with isolated Bence-Jones proteinuria without an M spike in serum more often suffer from amyloidosis (see later section) and generally have a poorer prognosis than those whose neoplasms secrete intact immunoglobulin molecules.

Other Problems

Clinical problems in multiple myeloma include hyperviscosity of blood and elevation of serum calcium. Although hyperviscosity occurs more consistently and dramatically with other paraproteinemias, it can be significnt in multiple myeloma. Hypercalcemia is thought to result both from bone destruction by the proliferating malignant cells and from abnormalities of renal and bone metabolism.

WALDENSTRÖM'S MACROGLOBULINEMIA

Conceptually similar to multiple myeloma but clinically distinct is **Waldenström's macroglobulinemia,** in which the paraprotein is IgM, usually the pentamer but sometimes also in the monomeric form. The neoplastic cells are not plasma cells but lymphocytes of abnormal appearance. The usual site of cellular proliferation is the solid tissue of the lymphoreticular system, rather than bone marrow. Patients are, on average, somewhat older than those with multiple myeloma, and the clinical course ranges from relatively indolent to fairly aggressive. Common presenting complaints are anemia and symptoms caused by abnormal serum proteins.

Accumulating IgM exerts many harmful effects. It causes a bleeding tendency by interfering with platelet function and with the finely regulated interaction of coagulation proteins. Large numbers of individual and aggregated IgM molecules make the blood flow sluggishly, especially in the peripheral portions of the circulation where red cells may stick to each other and interact abnormally with the cells that line blood vessels. The resulting defects of flow often cause clinical symptoms in the brain, the eyes, and the fingers and toes. Kidney damage is common in Waldenström's macroglobulinemia; contributing factors include deposition of protein, accumulation of aggregated cells in vessels and interstitium, and immune activity against soluble or structural proteins.

Antibodies to Red Cells

Occasional examples of monoclonal IgM express specificity for antigens on the patient's red cells. If the antibody reacts at physiologic temperatures, the result may be the syndrome called **cold agglutinin disease**. Circulating blood achieves somewhat lower temperatures in peripheral areas like fingers, toes, and the tips of the ears than in more central locations. IgM autoantibodies, which react better at cooler temperatures than at 37°C, may agglutinate red cells and obstruct small vessels in cooler peripheral sites, or they may activate the complement cascade. The affected cells may either succumb within the vessels to the membrane attack phase of the complement cascade, or they may return to the central circulation and be damaged by splenic macrophages that express C3 receptors, a phenomenon called **extravascular** hemolysis.

HEAVY-CHAIN DYSPROTEINEMIAS

Unpaired overproduction occurs less commonly for heavy chains than for light chains. In heavy-chain dysproteinemias, abnormally rearranged genetic material often causes production of structurally abnormal chains. Patients characteristically experience depressed levels of normal immunoglobulins, predisposition to infection, and generalized marrow depression. Dysproteinemias have been reported that involve any heavy-chain isotype except epsilon, but only alpha-chain disease occurs with any frequency.

Clinical Syndromes

In **alpha heavy-chain disease,** also called Mediterranean lymphoma, the lymphoid tissue of the gut is massively infiltrated by lymphocytes and plasma cells of appearance ranging from relatively normal to highly bizarre. Diarrhea, malabsorption, and abnormal muscular activity accompany the mucosal changes. This condition occurs in geographic areas where the population suffers frequent and recurrent intestinal infections with numerous bacteria, viruses, and parasites. A similar mucosal abnormality affecting only the respiratory tract occurs sporadically in Europe and the United States. In some patients with intestinal manifestations, antimicrobial therapy has induced complete remission. Antilymphoma therapy has been successful in other patients, but many patients have a progressively fatal course despite all therapy. No evidence links infection with the much rarer conditions of gamma (50 cases), mu (15 cases), or delta (1 reported case) heavy-chain disease.

AMYLOIDOSIS

Amyloid is a fibrillar protein that accumulates in many different tissues under various clinical circumstances. When amyloidosis occurs in patients with the chronic immune stimulation of persistent infection or with disorders of plasma cells, the condition is called **secondary amyloidosis**. Other forms are **primary,** in which there is no other associated abnormality; a **familial** form; and a **degenerative** form, in which increasing age is associated with increasing deposition of protein in heart and brain.

Similarities to Ig Chains

Amyloid, which looks featureless and homogeneous on light microscopy, has proven on analysis to include several different kinds of fibrillar material, which are listed in Table 11–2. The protein seen in primary amyloidosis and in patients with plasma cell disorders shares structural characteristics with the immunoglobulin light chain, more often lambda than kappa. All amyloid of this type includes the V portion of the light chain; some examples also express part or all of the C domain. Molecular weight varies between 5 and 25 kD. It is not clear why these proteins accumulate or whether the deposited material reflects degradation of previously intact chains.

TABLE 11–2. Proteins Associated with B-Cell Neoplasms

Protein	Disease	Structure	Clinical Features
Monoclonal Ig*	Multiple myeloma	Normal four-chain immunoglobulin	Hyperviscosity may occur Frequency of involved isotypes parallels normal Ig proportions
Bence-Jones protein	Multiple myeloma	Normal kappa or lambda light chain	Present in urine but not serum Precipitates at 55°C, redissolves at 95°C
Macroglobulin	Waldenström's macroglobulinemia	Normal IgM, sometimes as monomer	Hyperviscosity is common Autoantibody to red cells may cause hemolysis or vascular occlusion
Alpha heavy chain	Mediterranean lymphoma	Alpha heavy chain, often of abnormal structure	Masses of cells infiltrate gut, cause GI tract symptoms
Amyloid† AL form	Primary amyloidosis	V portion of light chain; also C?	Present in tongue, gut, muscle, skin, etc.
AL form	Plasma cell disorders	V portion of light chain; also C?	Present in liver, spleen, kidneys, etc.
AA form	Chronic infections	Unique configuration	May accumulate anywhere
AS form	Senile degeneration	Resembles prealbumin	Present in heart, brain

*Ig: abbreviation for immunoglobulin
†Terminology from Third International Symposium on Amyloidosis

TABLE 11–3. Selected Neoplasms of B Lymphocytes

Disease	Presumed Cell of Origin	Predominant Population Affected	Significant Clinical Events	Prognosis (With Appropriate Treatment)
Acute lymphoblastic leukemia (ALL)	Pre-pre-B or pre-B	Prepubertal children	Leukemic cells replace normal marrow Infections, bleeding common	Up to 70% long-term survival, when onset between age 2 and 10
Chronic lymphocytic leukemia (CLL)	Partially-to-fully mature B cell	Older adults	Peripheral-blood lymphocytosis Autoimmune problems Second tumors common	Prolonged course (3–20 yrs) but no cures
Hairy cell leukemia	B cells, possibly in activated state	Middle-aged men	Splenomegaly Pronounced marrow infiltration Neutropenia and infections	Usual course 3–5 years
Burkitt's lymphoma	Mature B cells	Children and adolescents M:F = 2:1	Rapidly enlarging extranodal tumors Translocation of chromosome 8 Association with EBV in African type	Up to 50% long-term survival after prompt, intensive treatment
Non-Hodgkin's lymphomas (approx. 65%)	Various phases	Older adults	Painless lymphadenopathy Extranodal tumors	Moderate to poor
Multiple myeloma	Plasma cells	Middle-aged and elderly	Monoclonal gammopathy Bence-Jones protein Bone lesions and hypercalcemia	Survival 3–6 years
Waldenström's macroglobulinemia	Ig-secreting lymphocytes	Elderly	Hyperviscosity Cold-agglutinin syndrome	Plasma exchange ameliorates symptoms Survival approx. 3 years
Mediterranean lymphoma	IgA-secreting plasma cells	Young adults	Mucosal tumors of small intestine	Variable; some cures, some rapid progression

Other Forms

Some forms of amyloidosis are protein abnormalities associated with immune system dysfunction, but many are not. The structure of the amyloid that accompanies chronic infections and other chronic illnesses has a unique structure unrelated to any other known protein. The form that accumulates in senile heart and brain is chemically related to prealbumin. No specific therapy exists for any of these conditions. For amyloidosis of chronic infection or plasma-cell disorders, treating the primary disease prevents further progression, but the material already deposited does not regress.

BENIGN MONOCLONAL GAMMOPATHY

Electrophoresis of serum proteins from some seemingly normal older individuals reveals an M spike. Of otherwise normal persons above age 70, 5 to 8 percent have this abnormality, but its significance is controversial. Some patients subsequently develop malignant monoclonal proliferative conditions; in others, the monoclonal protein remains stable for many years and lymphoreticular abnormalities never develop. The term **benign monoclonal gammopathy** is used when an M spike is found as the only abnormality in an otherwise healthy person. If cellular proliferation develops, the diagnosis becomes that of the evolving disorder. If the serum protein abnormality remains stable and asymptomatic, the diagnosis of benign monoclonal gammopathy stands. Because this condition affects older people and because plasma cell disorders take many years to become apparent, it is probable that many "benign" monoclonal conditions never reveal their malignant aspect because the patient dies of unrelated causes.

Table 11–3 summarizes significant neoplasms of B-cell origin.

—————— MALIGNANCIES OF MATURE —————— T LYMPHOCYTES

Despite the fact that T cells constitute about 70 percent of peripheral-blood lymphocytes, proliferative disorders of T cells involve solid tissues more often than bone marrow or circulating blood. Of the chronic lymphocytic leukemias, only 2 to 5 percent involve T cells; although morphologically indistinguishable from cells in B-cell chronic lymphocytic leukemia, the leukemic cells show genetic rearrangement of the T-receptor sites and express the pan-T antigen CD2, the sheep-cell rosette receptor. In most T-cell chronic leukemias, the cells have cytoplasmic granules and high enzyme levels, suggesting possible kinship with large granular lymphocytes or with T cells at the prolymphocyte stage of maturation.

ADULT T-CELL LEUKEMIA/LYMPHOMA

A disease of enormous recent interest is a T-cell leukemia most commonly found in certain parts of Japan and the Caribbean basin. Called **adult T-cell leukemia/lymphoma,** this aggressive process involves the skin in addition to blood and the solid lymphoreticular tissues. The leukemic cells display markers of mature T cells, including CD4 and the IL-2 receptor. Functionally active, they exert a suppressor effect on other lymphocytes, and they secrete a lymphokine that leads to bone damage and hypercalcemia. Uniquely significant is the association of this disease with infection by the retrovirus called human T-lymphotropic virus type I (HTLV-I) or human T-cell leukemia virus. Viruses have long been implicated in animal and avian leukemias, but this is the first virus proven to cause human leukemia.

CUTANEOUS T-CELL LYMPHOMA

CD4-positive lymphocytes infiltrate the skin in a group of conditions known as **mycosis fungoides** and **Sezary syndrome**. In Sezary syndrome, neoplastic cells of uniform appearance are present both in skin and in circulating blood; in mycosis fungoides there is greater diversity of cells in the skin, but circulatory involvement is rare. Both pursue an indolent course, but, in long-standing cases, the neoplastic cells eventually infiltrate lymph nodes, spleen, and liver. Hypergammaglobulinemia and elevation of serum IgE and IgA are frequent, but cell-mediated immunity remains active until the advanced phases; liability to infection is rarely a problem.

SYSTEMIC LYMPHOMAS

Relatively few lymphomas have T-cell phenotypes, but, as a group, they are marked by an aggressive course and comparatively poor prognosis. The neoplastic cells vary in size and shape, and the diffuse growth pattern effaces preexisting architectural features. Inflammatory cells frequently accompany the neoplastic cells, possibly in response to chemotactic lymphokines. These diffuse mixed-cell lymphomas express CD4 more often than CD8. A category of large-celled, highly aggressive lymphomas called **immunoblastic sarcoma** usually derives from B cells, but 5 to 15 percent are of T-cell origin. These tumors, which respond poorly to therapy, often occur in patients with preexisting immune dysfunction.

TABLE 11–4. Selected Neoplasms of T Lymphocytes

Disease	Presumed Cell of Origin	Predominant Group Affected	Predominant Clinical Events	Post treatment Prognosis
Acute lymphoblastic leukemia (ALL)	Immature T cell	Children >5 years M>F	Leukemic cells replace normal marrow Infections, bleeding common	Less favorable than B-cell types
Lymphoblastic lymphoma	Partially differentiated thymocyte	Older children and young adults; Elderly	Mediastinal mass Dissemination to meninges, marrow	Generally poor
Adult T cell leukemia/ lymphoma	Mature T cell expressing CD4	Adults, especially blacks	Association with HTLV-1 Bone lesions and hypercalcemia Solid-tissue infiltration	Very poor
Cutaneous lymphomas	CD4-positive T cells	Adults	Localized skin lesions Blood, other organs involved later	Local therapy helps skin lesions Survival worsens when disease disseminates

Mature T cells and their lymphokines are implicated in a condition variously called **angiocentric immunoproliferative lesion,** atypical lymphocytic vasculitis, and polymorphic reticulosis. Lymphocytes and inflammatory cells infiltrate and progressively destroy blood or lymphatic vessels. The lymphokine-stimulated cells display conspicuous phagocytosis of blood cells, especially erythrocytes.

Table 11–4 summarizes significant neoplasms of T-cell origin.

HODGKIN'S DISEASE

Hodgkin's disease is a lymphoreticular neoplasm with a pronounced inflammatory component; its cell of origin has not been unequivocally characterized. The lymphocytes, plasma cells, granulocytes, and fibroblasts that constitute the mass of the lesions are thought to be reactive, not neoplastic, and to represent a polyclonal response to neoplastic cells that are present in relatively small numbers. The pathognomonic cell of Hodgkin's disease is the **Reed-Sternberg cell,** a large cell with abundant cytoplasm and, classically, two or more nuclei with prominent nucleoli. These cells are thought to originate from the monocyte/macrophage lineage, but room for equivocation persists. Although it does not appear to be a primary T-cell neoplasm, Hodgkin's disease causes depressed T-cell activity even in its early phases.

CLASSIFICATION

Different cases of Hodgkin's disease present different histologic appearances and clinical syndromes; these have been systematized into several classifications used to predict prognosis and, to a certain extent, to plan therapy (Table 11–5). Age distribution is bimodal. One peak occurs in young adults, and then few cases occur until gradually increasing numbers of cases develop after age 50. The forms that occur in young adults respond much better to therapy than those of older patients. Many young adults have been aggressively treated and are alive and healthy many years later, but older patients rarely have an outcome that favorable.

In the most favorable form, called **lymphocyte predominance,** Reed-Sternberg cells are few, small lymphocytes are numerous and uniform, and there is little inflammatory-cell admixture. Another pattern with an excellent prognosis occurs primarily in young women. Called **nodular sclerosis,** it is characterized by abundant fibrous tissue which encircles nodules of reactive and neoplastic cells in varying proportions. The form called **mixed cellularity** is common in older patients; it has numerous and sometimes atypical Reed-Sternberg cells and a reactive cell population that includes variable proportions of

TABLE 11–5. Features of Hodgkin's Disease*

Cells Involved
Reed-Sternberg cell: ? monocytoid, ? interdigitating cell
Reactive cells: lymphocytes, plasma cells, granulocytes, fibroblasts

Patterns of Lymph Node Change (Rye Classification)
Lymphocyte predominance: 5–15% of cases; often asymptomatic; excellent prognosis
Nodular sclerosis: 40–75% of cases; multiple nodes involved; often in young women; good prognosis
Mixed cellularity: 20–40% of cases; usually symptomatic; patients are middle-aged; fair prognosis
Lymphocyte depletion: 5–15% of cases; presents at advanced stage; poor prognosis

Clinical Staging (Ann Arbor Classification)
(A) denotes absence, (B) denotes presence of fever, night sweats, weight loss of >10% of body weight
  I: Single node region or localized, single extralymphatic site
  II: Two or more node regions or one node region and one localized extralymphatic site on same side of diaphragm
  III: Node regions on both sides of diaphragm, with or without involvement of spleen and/or localized involvement of extralymphatic site
  IV: Multiple or disseminated extralymphatic sites, with or without lymph nodes

Therapeutic Approaches, with 5-year Disease-free Survival Rates
Localized radiation therapy, for stages I and II, A or B: 70–90%
Total irradiation, with or without chemotherapy, for some stage IIIA: 70–80%
Combined chemotherapy, with or without irradiation, for some stage IIIA: 65–75%
Combination chemotherapy, for stage IIIB: 60%
Combination chemotherapy, for stage IV, A or B: 50%

*Adapted from Glick JH: Hodgkin's Disease. *In* Wyngaarden JB, Smith LH, Jr, eds: Cecil Textbook of Medicine. 18th ed. Philadelphia: WB Saunders, 1988:1014–1022

lymphocytes, plasma cells, neutrophils, eosinophils, histiocytes, and fibroblasts. The form with the worst prognosis is called **lymphocyte depletion;** it has numerous, often strikingly pleomorphic, neoplastic cells and very few reactive cells.

CLINICAL FINDINGS

Hodgkin's disease, although a primary neoplasm of lymph nodes, may involve any part of the lymphoreticular system and virtually any organ of the body. The primary complaint is usually enlarged lymph nodes, but sometimes investigation is precipitated by fever, anemia, or unexplained laboratory findings. Some cases come to medical attention only because enlarged lymph nodes are found on chest or abdominal x-rays taken for some other reason.

It is important to know how far the disease has progressed before beginning and subsequently evaluating therapy. Disease at presentation is classified into stages I through IV, according to the number and location of involved lymph nodes and the presence of disease in spleen or non-lymphoid organs. These are described in Table 11–5. Within each stage of extent, the letters A and B are used to connote the absence or presence, respectively, of such symptoms as weight loss, fever, night sweats, or bone pain.

NEOPLASMS OF MONOCYTE/ MACROPHAGES

Before solid tumors could be accurately phenotyped, many non-Hodgkin's lymphomas were described as "histiocytic" or "reticulum cell" tumors. With better diagnostic techniques, the neoplastic cells in most of these can now be identified as lymphocytes at varying stages of differentiation and maturation. Only a few lymphomas—perhaps 5 to 10 percent—derive from monocyte/macrophage lines. In these, the malignant cells possess receptors for Fc and complement and frequently manifest phagocytic capability. This group of non-Hodgkin's lymphomas is called **true histiocytic lymphoma** and carries a poor prognosis.

MONOCYTIC LEUKEMIA

Pure monocytic or monoblastic leukemia is malignant proliferation of bone marrow cells derived from myelocyte/monocyte precursors. It is a relatively uncommon subcategory of leukemia and is more a hematologic than a lymphoreticular neoplasm.

HISTIOCYTOSIS X

This category includes several diverse clinical syndromes of unknown etiology. The most prominent conditions are **eosinophilic granuloma, Hand-Schüller-Christian disease,** and **Letterer-Siwe disease**. In all, there is systemic immunodeficiency and proliferation of non-phagocytic mononuclear cells that are probably related to the Langerhans cell normally found in the skin. Bone and lung are the most common sites for the localized conditions, but destructive changes may affect virtually any organ when there is systemic involvement. These conditions usually occur in early childhood.

───────────── **SUGGESTIONS FOR** ─────────────
FURTHER READING

Beckstead JH: An approach to practical problems in the diagnosis of lymphoproliferative disorders using cytochemistry and immunocytochemistry. Clin Lab Med 1988; 8:211–22

Brodeur GM: The involvement of oncogenes and suppressor genes in human neoplasia. Adv Pediatr 1987; 34:1–44

Harris NL: Lymphoma 1987: an interim approach to diagnosis and classification. Pathol Annual 1987; 22:1–67

Paoletti M, Bitter MA, Vardiman JW: Hairy-cell leukemia: morphologic, cytochemical and immunologic features. Clin Lab Med 1988; 8:179–95

Sobol RE, Bloomfield CD, Royston I: Immunophenotyping in the diagnosis and classification of acute lymphoblastic leukemia. Clin Lab Med 1988; 8:151–62

CHAPTER 12

Immune-Mediated Disease

The immune system performs vital protective functions, as described in chapter 9, and dire consequences follow absence of immune activity, as described in chapter 10. Besides protecting against disease, however, immune events can also cause disease. Unregulated or misdirected immune processes provoke or exacerbate many pathologic conditions. The past several decades of clinical and experimental literature testify abundantly to these adverse effects, and increasing understanding of immune mechanisms reveals increasing numbers of disease states in which immune influences are significant. Overall, however, the protective consequences of immune activities far outweigh the problems they cause.

CONSIDERATIONS OF TERMINOLOGY

The vocabulary that describes immune influences on disease is important for precise communication but potentially confusing. Table 12–1 summarizes some of these terms, which are discussed in the section that follows.

GOOD NEWS AND BAD NEWS

The term **immunity** has always had beneficial connotations; many terms have been applied to harmful manifestations of immune activity. In 1906, the term **allergy** was introduced to describe how second or subsequent exposure to an agent changes the nature of physiologic responses, including both beneficial and undesirable consequences. In current usage, these changes are called **immune reactivity;** the agent that induces such alterations is termed an **antigen**. The harmful effects of immune reactivity are called **hypersensitivity** or **allergy**.

Detrimental Effects

Allergy is a particularly confusing term. Some writers include under "allergy" any and all untoward events mediated by the immune system. Others use "allergy" only for specific events that follow activation of IgE. Everyone agrees that allergy is an unwanted immune event, but the term is difficult to use precisely. The term "hypersensitivity" implies a wide range of immune mechanisms and manifestations that confer no benefit to the host.

Induction of protective immunity is called **immunization;** induction of immune events with harmful effects can be described as **sensitization**. One must remember, however, that many physiologic events are beneficial in some ways and harmful in others. Protective processes often damage tissue, and mechanisms with pathologic outcomes may be physiologically indistinguishable from beneficial interactions.

Anaphylactic versus Anaphylactoid

In 1902, Richet and Portier used the term **anaphylaxis** to describe a sequence of shock, collapse, and death in animals experiencing, for a second time, certain materials that had initially exerted no

---

TABLE 12–1. Terms Used to Describe Immune Events

Beneficial to the Host

Immunity: Protection against specific environmental agents; from Latin for "exempt"

Immunization: Acquisition of protection by contact with antigenic material

Harmful or Unpleasant to the Host

Hypersensitivity: Any pathologic effect of immune reactivity; from Greek for "above, higher" and Latin denoting "perception" or "response"

Allergy: Detrimental effects of immunity; connotes especially local events mediated by cell-bound antibodies; from Greek term that means "other"

Anaphylaxis: Systemic effects of mediators released after cell-bound antibodies react with antigen; from Greek, meaning "the reverse of protection"

Atopy: Predisposition to allergies against common agents in the environment; from Greek for "out of place"

Experimentally Induced Phenomena

Arthus phenomenon: Immune complex reaction at injection site where antigen combines with circulating antibodies

Prausnitz-Küstner reaction: Transfer of immediate-type hypersensitivity by introducing antibody into an intact skin site, where it binds to basophils

Schultz-Dale reaction: Transfer of immediate-type hypersensitivity by introducing antibody into an isolated tissue preparation that contains basophils

Schwartzman phenomenon: Inflammatory and vascular response occurring locally or systemically after a second injection of bacterial endotoxin

---

visible effect. In current usage, anaphylaxis denotes systemic events that follow activation of cell-bound IgE, causing problems ranging from discomfort to death. Some workers distinguish between "anaphylactic" and "anaphylactoid" reactions, the former meaning release of mediators after activation of IgE and the latter referring to other mechanisms that cause mediator release. This distinction is seldom significant and is often difficult to make under clinical circumstances. We will use the term "anaphylactic" for all these events.

THE GELL AND COOMBS
CLASSIFICATION

The years between 1906 and the 1960s brought enormous illumination of both helpful and harmful immune activities. Humoral immunity and complement were more extensively understood than cell-mediated immunity. In their 1962 book, *Clinical Aspects of Immunology*, the British immunologists PGH Gell and RRA Coombs devised a classification for "the kinds of allergic reaction . . . [that] may do damage of some kind, whether or not the effect in the long run may be beneficial." Gell and Coombs defined four different ways in which immune activity mediates tissue damage, a classification that has remained extremely useful. Most modern writers modify the system somewhat, and many include ideas or mechanisms that the original authors did not, in 1962, propose.

Original Formulation

Gell and Coombs attributed immune-mediated damage to four different mechanisms, categorized according to type. **Type I** events occur when reaction between antigen and a cell-bound antibody stimulates release from the underlying cell of physiologically active substances. Tissue events reflect the actions of cell-derived mediators; the role of the antigen-antibody reaction is to stimulate their release. In **type II** events, free antibody molecules react directly with antigen, either an intrinsic constituent of a membrane or molecules adhering to its surface. Reaction of antibody with cell-surface antigen damages or destroys the cell; complement is often involved. **Type III** reactions occur when antibody reacts with free or fluid-borne antigen to generate complexes that precipitate in tissue and induce inflammation. Gell and Coombs gave only two examples—serum sickness and the Arthus phenomenon (discussed below)—but many pathologic conditions are now known to result from immune-complex effects. **Type IV** reactions embody delayed or "tuberculin-type" sensitivity. Gell and Coombs gave, as examples, the tuberculin reaction, contact dermatitis, some infectious and autoallergic diseases, and, they surmised, the rejection of homografts. They considered the mechanisms to be "the reaction of specifically modified mononuclear cells containing a substance or mechanism capable of responding specifically to allergen deposited at a local site." The type IV category now includes an ever-expanding list of cell-mediated reactions in which antibody and complement play no part.

Modified Categories

In the material that follows, we will slightly modify the above categories. Type I reactions are events initiated when cell-bound antibody reacts with specific antigen to cause release of various mediator and effector substances from the underlying cell. Type II reactions are the events that follow direct combination of antibody with antigen on a cell surface or tissue membrane. Type III reactions are those initiated when soluble antigen and soluble antibody form an insoluble complex that precipitates in tissue or on cells and initiates localized tissue effects. Type IV includes all the tissue-damaging effects of T-cell and macrophage activity—a large and highly diverse category. Table 12–2 summarizes these categories, which are discussed in detail later in the chapter.

NATURE OF THE ANTIGEN

Anything that the immune system perceives as foreign can elicit an immune response. These materials may arise from outside or inside the body and may be animal, vegetable, or mineral. Material originating outside the host can be described as **exogenous;** elements native to the host are **endogenous**. Exogenous stimuli originating from non-human sources are called **heterologous** or **xenogeneic;** material of human origin introduced into a different human individual is described as **homologous** or **allogeneic**. Self constituents that elicit immune reactivity are called **autologous** antigens or **autoantigens**.

SOME HISTORIC TERMS

Some historical experiments and observations continue to be useful in illustrating theoretical concepts, even though the experimental conditions are not currently employed. The student should be familiar with the concepts embodied in these historic terms.

The **Arthus phenomenon** denotes localized damage that follows immune-complex deposition provoked when antigen is injected at a single site in a subject with circulating antibodies. As fluid-borne antibody combines with localized antigen, complexes deposit on the walls of blood vessels in the area and elicit necrotizing inflammation (Fig. 12–1). If antigen enters the circulation to unite with circulating antibody, the resulting immune complexes deposit in many different tissues to produce systemic effects. The Arthus phenomenon is a type III reaction; it requires circulation of preexisting antibody, which recognizes and reacts with antigen injected at a single site.

Clinically similar but less well understood is the **Schwartzman phenomenon,** which occurs when bacterial endotoxin is introduced a second time one or several days after a first dose. Intradermal injection causes a localized reaction; intravenous injection precipitates systemic consequences. The tissues undergo intravascular coagulation, necrosis, and inflammation suggestive of intense complement

TABLE 12–2. An Outline of Immune-Mediated Disease

Gell and Coombs Classification	Descriptive Term	Immune Mechanism	Mechanism of Injury	Antigens Often Involved
I	Immediate hypersensitivity	Reaction between antigen and cell-bound ab* stimulates cell to release mediators	Vascular and cellular changes provoked by mediators released from granulocytes	Hetero†: Inhaled, ingested or injected plant or animal proteins Allo‡: Very rare Auto§: Extremely rare
II	Antibody-mediated	Attachment of ab to antigen-bearing surface exerts direct effects	Inflammatory or lytic effects of complement, if activated Actions on inflammatory or immune cells with Fc receptors Inactivation of cell or molecule expressing antigen	Hetero: Rare: some drugs that attach to cell surfaces Allo: Surface antigens on transfused or transplanted cells Auto: Surface antigens of blood, endocrine, epithelial cells; basement membranes; receptor molecules on cell membranes
III	Immune complex	Combination of complement-activating ab with soluble antigen	Inflammatory effects of complement	Hetero: Drugs, microbial antigens, inhaled plant or animal proteins Allo: Rare, to transfused proteins Auto: Nuclear and cytoplasmic cell constituents; serum globulins
IV	Cell-mediated	Mediators produced by activated T cells Direct cytotoxic action of T cells	Inflammatory actions of macrophages, lymphocytes Enzymes, other proteins secreted by activated macrophages Enhanced NK cell actions	Hetero: Microbial antigens, plant oils, organic or inorganic haptens, drugs Allo: MHC products on transplanted cells; graft-versus-host disease Auto: Functional cells of nearly any organ, especially liver, pancreas, CNS

*ab: antibody
†Hetero: Antigens from any source other than humans
‡Allo: Antigens from human individuals genetically different from host
§Auto: Antigens native to host, but usually not unique to host

227

THE ARTHUS PHENOMENON

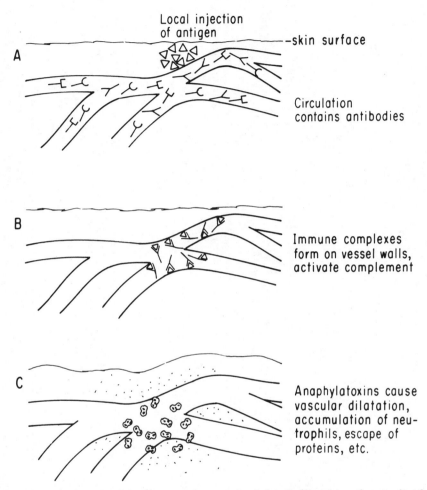

FIGURE 12–1. Panel A shows antigen injected into the skin of an individual with circulating antibody of that specificity. Immune complexes deposit on the walls of blood vessels, shown in panel B, and activate complement. Anaphylatoxic cleavage fragments cause dilatation and increased permeability of blood vessels, edema and swelling of the skin, and accumulation of neutrophils, as shown in panel C.

activation. Specific antigen and antibody recognition need not be present; it is possible that the Schwartzman phenomenon reflects alternative-pathway activation of complement.

The **Prausnitz-Küstner** reaction illustrates *in vivo* transfer of immediate (type I) hypersensitivity from one individual to another (Fig. 12–2). Küstner was allergic to fish. His serum was injected into the

PASSIVE TRANSFER OF
IMMEDIATE HYPERSENSITIVITY

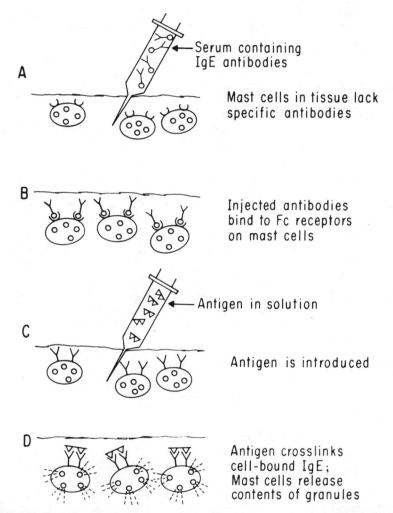

A — Serum containing IgE antibodies

Mast cells in tissue lack specific antibodies

B Injected antibodies bind to Fc receptors on mast cells

C — Antigen in solution

Antigen is introduced

D Antigen crosslinks cell-bound IgE; Mast cells release contents of granules

FIGURE 12–2. Immediate hypersensitivity can be transferred from one individual to another by injecting highly concentrated specific IgE into a site (usually skin) where mast cells are abundant. Panel A shows the injection, and panel B shows antibody bound to Fc receptors on the mast cells. Introduction of antigen at that site, shown in C, allows the passively acquired antibody to be crosslinked by antigen, as shown in D. Crosslinking the membrane-bound antibody signals the granules to release their contents, causing detectable tissue consequences.

skin of Prausnitz, who was non-allergic; subsequent introduction of fish extract at the injection site elicited inflammation and edema. The antifish antibodies present in Küstner's serum attached to mast cells in the skin at the injection site, where they could combine with locally injected fish antigen to provoke release of inflammatory mediators.

The **Schultz-Dale** reaction demonstrates the same events without requiring an intact recipient. The indicator is an isolated strip of smooth muscle in which release of cellular mediators induces contractions that can be measured. If the muscle strip comes from an animal already sensitive to a specific antigen, topical application of that antigen provokes contraction. If the original animal was unsensitized, serum from an animal with circulating IgE antibodies can be applied to the muscle strip and the passively transferred antibody will bind to mast cells in the muscle. The passively transferred antibody, now bound to cells in the muscle strip, reacts with locally applied antigen, provoking release of cell contents that cause contraction.

TYPE I IMMUNOPATHOLOGY

Type I conditions are called **immediate hypersensitivity reactions** because manifestations begin seconds or minutes after contact with the antigen. The mediators that induce these events are already present in the cells and need only to be released to begin immediate activity (Fig. 12–3). The reaction may continue for prolonged periods, however, as new mediators evolve and the early changes elicit later chemical and cellular events.

MEDIATORS OF IMMEDIATE HYPERSENSITIVITY

Type I reactions occur predominantly in the skin, the respiratory tract, and the gastrointestinal tract; the major changes are vasodilatation, increased vascular permeability and consequent edema, contraction of smooth muscle, and increased secretion by stimulated epithelial cells. The first mediator discovered to cause type I reactions was **histamine;** it is the first mediator released after cell-bound antibody combines with antigen. Cells that possess histamine receptors undergo changes that begin within seconds of exposure and end in 10 to 30 minutes.

Two types of histamine receptors exist, H_1 and H_2; cells with H_1 receptors are more significant in hypersensitivity reactions. Engagement of H_1 receptors causes smooth muscle contraction in bronchioles and upper respiratory tract; increased permeability of venules in mucosal surfaces; constriction of pulmonary blood vessels; and increased epithelial secretion in the upper respiratory tract. Activation

TYPE I: IMMEDIATE HYPERSENSITIVITY

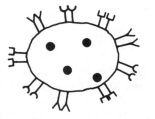

Basophil binds IgE
antibodies to membrane

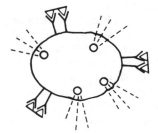

Antigen crosslinks antibody,
stimulates granules to
release contents

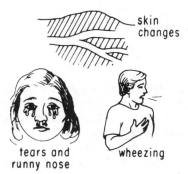

Mediators cause vascular changes,
smooth muscle contraction,
secretions from epithelium

FIGURE 12–3. Immediate hypersensitivity requires that specific IgE antibodies bind to the membrane of a basophilic granulocyte, shown in the top figure. The immunologic reaction consists of crosslinking by the corresponding antigen, as shown in the middle figure. This stimulates the cell to release previously synthesized materials stored in the granules. These materials cause the physiologic events perceived as hypersensitivity symptoms, shown at the bottom.

of H_2 receptors causes widespread increased permeability of venules and capillaries, increased mucus production, and secretion of acid by cells that line the stomach. Histamine attracts eosinophilic granulocytes, which release materials that promote bronchoconstriction and elaborate proteolytic substances that may damage many parasitic worms. Eosinophil-derived materials also neutralize histamine actions. Tissue undergoing a type I reaction characteristically contains many eosinophils.

Other Secreted Materials

Several other materials released from granules prolong and modify events initiated by histamine. The **eosinophil chemotactic factor of anaphylaxis** (ECF-A) attracts eosinophils to the area, and a closely related substance has a comparable effect for neutrophils. Eosinophil chemotactic factor of anaphylaxis stimulates eosinophils to release material harmful to helminths; it stimulates the antihistamine and anti-immune-complex actions of eosinophils but also exerts effects on eosinophils that neutralize their activity. Several **kinin-generating activators** interact with precursor and activator substances in plasma and tissue fluid to generate bradykinin and to activate Hageman factor and the contact portion of the coagulation cascade. Materials released from mast cell granules evolve into **kallikrein,** which cleaves a serum precursor to activate **bradykinin**. Bradykinin induces moderately prolonged smooth muscle contraction, increased vascular permeability, and increased secretory activity and is thought to be involved in stimulation or perception of pain and itching. **Heparin** and **serotonin** are released from basophil granules and are known to be involved in animal models of anaphylaxis, but their functions in immediate-type hypersensitivity in humans are not clear.

Late-developing Mediators

The prolonged consequences of type I reactions result from mediators generated in response to the initial events. Some are synthesized by granulocytes, some by endothelial cells in the involved blood vessels, and some by macrophages. **Platelet activating factor** (PAF) is generated by basophils and macrophages. As its name implies, it causes platelets to aggregate and to release materials that promote coagulation and inflammation. It also acts directly on tissues, causing pronounced bronchoconstriction and alterations of vascular function that, locally, cause skin reactions and, if introduced systemically, cause hypotension and cardiovascular collapse.

A constellation of late effects was formerly attributed to an agent called **slow-reacting substance of anaphylaxis** (SRS-A), but SRS-A has never been isolated as a specific material. The effects arise from the cumulative actions of metabolites generated from arachidonic acid precursors through the **lipoxygenase** pathway. The resulting **leukotrienes,** designated LTB4, LTC4, and LTD4, are powerful stimulants to vasodilatation, smooth muscle spasm, and increased vascular permeability. Another pathway of arachidonic acid metabolism, the **cyclooxygenase** pathway, generates **prostaglandins, prostacyclins,**

TABLE 12—3. Some Mediators Involved in Immediate Hypersensitivity

Name	Functions
Preformed, released from granules after antigen-antibody reaction	
Histamine	Through H_1 receptors: Increases vascular permeability Stimulates smooth muscle of bronchioles, GI tract Stimulates mucus production in upper respiratory tract Attracts eosinophils Promotes synthesis of prostaglandins Through H_2 receptors: Stimulates secretion of gastric acid Increases vascular permeability Stimulates mucus production in lower respiratory tract
Eosinophil chemotactic factor of anaphylaxis (ECF-A)	Attracts eosinophils and neutrophils Increases expression of complement receptors on eosinophils Deactivates eosinophils and neutrophils
Heparin	Prevents coagulation Inhibits complement Binds to histamine
Activators for prekallikrein, Hageman factor	Activates coagulation and contact cascades
Kallikrein	Generates kinins
Generated as secondary part of response	
Platelet activating factor	Aggregates platelets, also neutrophils and monocytes Promotes release of platelet factors affecting vasculature, coagulation, inflammation Promotes bronchoconstriction
Lipoxygenase pathway products (leukotrienes)	Attract neutrophils, eosinophils Induce sustained smooth-muscle constriction Increase vascular permeability and dilatation
Cyclooxygenase pathway products (prostaglandins and thromboxanes)	Induce sustained increase in vascular permeability Induce smooth-muscle constriction and bronchoconstriction

and **thromboxanes,** which also affect smooth muscle, vascular function, and platelet activation. These cyclooxygenase metabolites variously promote or suppress inflammation and coagulation, depending upon the changing microenvironmental conditions that regulate their concentrations.

Other Effects

A poorly understood aspect of immediate hypersensitivity, called **late-phase reactions,** includes cutaneous and respiratory events that occur hours after initial stimulation. Eosinophils and mononuclear cells that accumulate during earlier events are thought to be responsible, but specific mediators have not been characterized.

Table 12–3 lists the major mediators involved in immediate-type hypersensitivity.

CLINICAL EVENTS

Most of the clinical events in type I reactions can be attributed to the mediators described above. Skin reactions begin with localized pallor followed by flushing, itching, and accumulation of fluid in swellings called **wheals** or **hives**. Vasoactive mediators promote the increased blood flow that causes flushing and the increased permeability that causes edema. The itching has been variously attributed to bradykinin, to direct effects of histamine, or to unknown interactions.

The most conspicuous upper respiratory change is **increased secretion** by mucous and tear glands, leading to the weeping eyes and runny nose all too familiar to allergy sufferers. The consequences of **edema** are nasal stuffiness, swelling around the eyes, and, most dangerous of all when it occurs, laryngeal edema. In the lower respiratory tract, increased production of mucus and constriction of smooth muscle cause narrowing of small bronchi and bronchioles; this leads to **wheezing** that is more noticeable on expiration than inspiration. Smooth muscle contraction in the gastrointestinal tract causes **diarrhea** and/or **vomiting**. Gastric hyperacidity and profuse watery secretions in small and large intestines occur when epithelial secretion is stimulated.

Dangerous Systemic Changes

In systemic type I reactions, there are profound changes in vascular permeability and vessel tone throughout the body. As vessels dilate and vascular permeability increases, blood flow slows and fluid accumulates in the interstitium. This leads to decreased peripheral resistance, falling arterial blood pressure, and reduction in the volume of blood in the circulatory system and returning to the heart. These hemodynamic changes cause **hypotension,** which may progress to irreversible **shock,** especially if laryngeal edema and/or bronchospasm cause **respiratory difficulties** that compromise oxygenation. Air reaches the lungs only after passage through the larynx, the narrowest part of the upper respiratory tract; rapidly developing **laryngeal edema** can asphyxiate the victim within minutes.

ATOPY

Hay fever, some food sensitivities, many cases of asthma, and some skin rashes are type I reactions against antigens commonly encountered in the environment. The descriptive term for this group of conditions is **atopy** or, sometimes, the unmodified term "allergy." Predisposition to the atopic form of type I reactions is familial. Atopic conditions occur in an estimated 10 percent of the population. The child of two atopic parents has a 75 percent chance of being affected; if one parent is atopic, the chance is 50 percent.

Entry of Antigens

The heritable abnormality that causes the atopic state has not been characterized. The offending antigens (allergens) are usually of moderate size (10 to 70 kD) and characteristically enter the body through the respiratory or gastrointestinal tract. Atopic manifestations in the skin usually reflect antigens that have been inhaled or ingested; skin problems arising from materials that directly penetrate the skin are called **contact dermatitis** and are usually cell mediated (see later section). Pollens, feathers, dust mites, animal danders, and airborne fungal spores are common inhaled allergens; proteins from fish, milk, eggs, nuts, and legumes are the foodstuffs most often incriminated. Affected patients seem more likely than normal persons to absorb these substances in antigenically active form.

The constitutional defect has been attributed to some or all of the following: reduced barrier function of mucosal surfaces; increased production of IgE; alteration in antigen processing or presentation; or some peculiarity of a poorly defined aspect of the major histocompatibility complex called "immune response genes." Persons congenitally deficient in IgA are especially prone to atopic conditions. This suggests that secretions on mucosal surfaces normally exert protective action against exogenous materials.

Local Symptoms

Hay fever, asthma, atopic dermatitis, and allergic gastroenteritis are site-specific manifestations of mediators released locally. Basophils in individual tissue locations bind, through their membrane receptors, antibodies against environmental antigens; where antigen reaches the tissue in significant quantity, mediators are released at levels proportional to the degree of immune reactivity. As the atopic patient grows older, the intensity of reactions and the number of allergens that elicit them often decline. Allergic asthma occurs more often and more severely in small children than in adults, partly because of age-related differences in sensitivity and partly because the child's small bronchi suffer proportionately greater narrowing from smooth-muscle constriction than the larger bronchi of adults. Atopic manifestations often change with age; the child who suffered from rashes or asthma may develop hay fever as an adult, or a person with gastrointestinal intolerance to eggs may later exhibit a rash after eating fish.

ANAPHYLAXIS

In contrast with localized, often unpleasant but rarely dangerous, atopic reactions, **anaphylaxis** is a generalized condition that can be fatal within a relatively short time if severe and if inadequately treated. Relatively little genetic predisposition has been demonstrated, and atopic individuals are not excessively liable to anaphylactic hypersensitivity. Antigenic material that enters the circulation, sometimes in minute quantities, causes system-wide release of mediator substances. The most familiar triggering agents are **venoms** of stinging insects (the Hymenopterae family), **penicillin,** and local **anesthetic agents** such as procaine. Many protein and non-protein drugs have been incriminated with varying frequency, and such foods as seafood, legumes, or egg albumin cause anaphylaxis in a few individuals.

Laryngeal edema, intractable shock, and cardiac dysrhythmias are the most dangerous manifestations. Not life-threatening but unpleasant are severe wheezing; edema of the face or extremities; cramping pain of the intestines or uterus; diarrhea and/or vomiting; and urinary or fecal incontinence. Some anaphylactic reactions strike with full force in just a few minutes, but more often, symptoms crescendo, with superficial edema, respiratory distress, cramping, or hypotension providing sentinel events that indicate the need for prompt therapy.

Table 12–4 summarizes clinical considerations in atopy and anaphylaxis.

IMMUNE MECHANISMS

Most cell-bound antibodies are IgE, although IgG is occasionally implicated. It is not clear why some antigens provoke IgE antibodies or why some people exposed to such antigens develop these antibod-

TABLE 12—4. Atopy versus Anaphylaxis

	Atopic Conditions	Anaphylactic Reactions
Immune mechanism	Type I hypersensitivity	Type I hypersensitivity
Nature of reaction	Localized	Systemic
Sites frequently involved	Upper respiratory tract Lower respiratory tract GI tract Skin	Soft tissue of face and neck Larynx Small vessels of systemic circulation Respiratory bronchioles GI tract
Familial tendency	Pronounced	Minimal
Nature of antigen	Ubiquitous environmental proteins, often multiple	Specific agent, often insect venom or drug
Usual treatment	Antihistamines; sometimes subcutaneous adrenal steroids, bronchodilators	Epinephrine; sometimes massive adrenal steroids, bronchodilators, agents to elevate blood pressure

ies. It is known that some clones of helper T cells promote production of specific immunoglobulin classes, and some antigens stimulate suppressor cells more effectively than others. Such observations suggest mechanisms whereby selectivity could occur, but they do not explain differences between individuals. Affected individuals usually have elevated total serum IgE; sometimes reactivity to specific antigens can be demonstrated but serum IgE circulates in nanogram concentrations, making this kind of investigation difficult to perform.

Clinical Considerations

Diagnosing type I hypersensitivity reactions requires two steps: (1) establishing that IgE-mediated immune reactivity is, in fact, the cause of the clinical problems; and (2) detecting what antigens are responsible. A careful clinical and family history is crucial for the first determination, because these conditions produce virtually no specific test findings. Eosinophilia in the blood or mucosal secretions may confirm a suspicion, but negative results do not rule out the diagnosis. With severe atopic conditions, some patients have elevated levels of total serum IgE, but here, too, affected patients may have normal findings. It is important to rule out other possible causes for respiratory, skin, or gastrointestinal symptoms, especially infections and immunodeficiency conditions.

Skin testing remains the most effective way to identify specific allergens. Even if manifestations are most prominent in the gastrointestinal tract or the respiratory tract, introducing the responsible antigen into the skin reliably elicits local signs. Antigen-antibody combination induces acutely increased vascular dilatation and permeability within 15 to 20 minutes, generating the skin changes described as **wheal and flare**. The problem is to decide which potential allergens to test and to obtain pure, potent preparations suitable for skin challenge. Suitable controls are important, in order to rule out hyperreactivity of the skin to every form of stimulation.

In Vitro Testing

A laboratory test to detect elevation of IgE with antigenic specificity is intellectually appealing but, in most cases, offers no greater sensitivity or specificity than skin testing. The procedure is called **radioallergosorbent testing** (RAST) (Fig. 12–4). The suspected allergen is adsorbed to some solid phase like a disk, well, or microtiter plate. When serum is incubated with the solid-phase antigen, all antibody molecules that recognize that antigen will attach; this includes antibodies of the IgG class, which are likely to be present in much higher concentration than IgE. The presence and quantity of bound IgE is determined by adding radiolabeled antiglobulin serum specific for IgE. (An enzyme label, as described in chapter 18, can be used instead.)

Radioallergosorbent testing procedures present both technical and clinical problems. The test is only as good as the antigen used. Preparing pure and potent antigen is just as demanding for RAST as for skin testing, and selecting antigens for trial requires the same diagnostic decisions. Even when massively elevated, serum levels of IgE are several orders of magnitude lower than those of IgG, so the antiglobulin reagent must be rigorously specific for IgE. There is no satisfactory way to obtain absolute nanogram concentration from the level of radioactivity generated. Results are expressed relative to a known positive control serum, but it can be difficult to extrapolate this relative reactivity to the clinical events seen in a specific patient. Many allergists believe that *in vitro* testing is more advantageous than skin testing only if there are widespread skin lesions that make such testing impossible, if the patient is on medications that will suppress reactivity, or if the patient's skin is so hyperreactive that needle prick alone can elicit a wheal and flare.

RADIOALLERGOSORBENT TEST
RAST

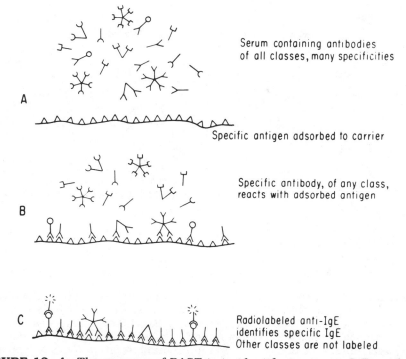

A

Serum containing antibodies
of all classes, many specificities

Specific antigen adsorbed to carrier

B

Specific antibody, of any class,
reacts with adsorbed antigen

C

Radiolabeled anti-IgE
identifies specific IgE
Other classes are not labeled

FIGURE 12—4. The purpose of RAST is to identify, in serum, IgE antibody of a single specificity. The selected antigen is adsorbed to a solid phase, as shown in A, and allowed to interact with serum. Antibodies of any class that are specific for that antigen will bind to the surface, as shown in B. Panel C shows that many antigen sites attract antibodies of IgG and other classes. The relatively few IgE molecules that bind are detected and quantified by a radiolabeled antiglobulin serum specific for the epsilon chain of IgE.

BLOCKING ANTIBODIES

Antigens that elicit IgE antibodies often elicit IgG antibodies as well. When soluble IgG antibody and cell-bound IgE of a single specificity compete for a limited amount of antigen, IgG usually prevails. This preferential reaction with IgG is exploited in the immunologic treatment of atopic and anaphylactic conditions. Very small doses of the incriminated antigen can be introduced in a repetitive schedule that elicits maximum anamnestic production of IgG. The presence in tissue fluid of so-called **blocking** IgG antibodies often prevents antigen from reaching and reacting with cell-bound IgE (Fig. 12–5). For

BLOCKING ANTIBODIES

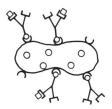

Cell-bound IgE has modest
avidity for antigen.

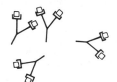

Soluble IgG has high
avidity for antigen.

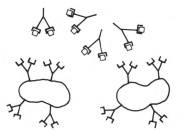

Antigen enters tissue, is rapidly
bound by IgG, does not reach IgE.

A   B

FIGURE 12–5. When the same antigenic specificity resides in antibodies of different classes, soluble IgG characteristically reacts with much greater avidity than cell-bound IgE, as shown in panel A. Panel B depicts tissue that contains both soluble IgG and cell-bound IgE specific for a single atopic allergen. As allergen enters the tissue, it is promptly bound by IgG and has no opportunity to elicit symptoms by crosslinking the cell-bound IgE.

many hay fever victims and those sensitive to Hymenoptera venoms, immunotherapy of this kind can provide quite satisfactory relief. For most drug and food allergens, the best treatment is avoidance.

CELLULAR EVENTS

IgE binds to the cell membrane through its Fc portion, leaving the Fab portions free. Crosslinking the Fab portions signals the underlying cell to release its contents. Under natural conditions, antigen engages contiguous Fab portions to crosslink the molecules; under experimental conditions, antibodies to the IgE isotype can induce a crosslinked configuration. Crosslinking initiates complex and highly modulated intracellular events that affect membrane phospholipids, protein kinases, and calcium channels, eventually signaling granules to release their contents. The intracellular messengers **cy-**

clic **adenosine monophosphate** (cAMP) and **cyclic guanosine monophosphate** (cGMP) have reciprocal effects on granules. Decreased cAMP or increased cGMP promote release, whereas rising cAMP or diminished cGMP inhibit these processes. One hypothesis about constitutional susceptibility is that atopic conditions occur if generation of cAMP and cGMP is improperly regulated.

Therapeutic Applications of Antihistamines

Antihistamines are therapeutically effective only after histamine has been released from granules. Antihistamines interact with histamine receptors, either H1 or H2. Most symptoms of atopic disease involve cells with H1 receptors, so allergies are best treated with this class of antihistamines. Antagonists to H2 receptors suppress gastric acid production and are useful in peptic ulcer disease but have relatively little immunologic application. Antihistamines affect only the clinical events mediated by histamine. They do not ameliorate life-threatening immune manifestations and do not modify the events leading to release of mediators.

Therapy with Hormones

Pronounced and long-lasting changes in vascular permeability, smooth muscle constriction, and disturbances in cardiac rhythm initiate compensatory physiologic responses mediated through the autonomic nervous system. **Epinephrine,** the hormone of the adrenal medulla, causes vasoconstriction and smooth muscle relaxation, thus directly reversing many of the effects we have been discussing. Epinephrine, or pharmacologic agents with selected effects of epinephrine, are used to treat systemic events mediated by IgE.

Another group of drugs useful in immune-mediated conditions are the **steroid hormones** of the adrenal cortex. Corticosteroids exert physiologic actions in many systems; in this context, they are useful in counteracting inflammatory events and altering generation and release of proteins.

Other Agents

Several other agents are useful in treating individual type I conditions, through mechanisms not fully understood. **Theophylline,** a substance related to caffeine, is a bronchodilator useful in treating asthma. **Disodium cromoglycate** (cromolyn) interferes in an unknown fashion with release of mediators from mast cells but does not counteract their tissue effects. Because cromolyn is not absorbed across membranes, its major use is topical application to the eyes, nose, or respiratory tract when exposure to inhaled allergens is likely.

———————— **TYPE II IMMUNOPATHOLOGY** ————————

Gell and Coombs included in type II only cytolysis or cell death resulting directly from antibody attachment. Some later workers place into type II all cytolytic events, including cell-mediated forms of damage; other workers merge type II and type III, because it can be difficult to distinguish whether antibody has bound directly to membrane antigens or is part of an immune complex adsorbed to the cell surface. We will include in type II only reactions to antigens that are an intrinsic constituent of a cell or membrane.

MECHANISMS OF DAMAGE

Effects of Complement

Antibodies that react with surface antigens may initiate several forms of tissue damage. Gell and Coombs originally emphasized the lytic effects of classical-pathway complement activation, and this remains the most dramatic and easily identified form of type II damage. The immune event involves a minimum of one IgM molecule or two closely adjacent IgG molecules. Complement binds directly to the membrane displaying the antigen; in addition, the cleavage products C3a, C4a, and C5a exert anaphylatoxic effects that attract inflammatory cells and promote vasodilatation and increased vascular permeability. Acute inflammation induced in this way will affect whatever tissue displays the antigen recognized by the complement-activating antibody.

Antibody on Cell Membranes

In addition to lysis and anaphylatoxic actions, C3 causes the antigen-bearing cell to become susceptible to prompt and efficient phagocytosis by cells with receptors for C3b. Opsonization can be a type II effect even without activation of complement. Surface-bound antibody enhances phagocytosis because cells with C3b receptors also have receptors for the Fc portion of IgG. In addition, antibody on a cell membrane exposes the coated cell to direct cytotoxic attack. Although large granular lymphocytes are the effectors of antibody-dependent cell-mediated cytotoxicity (ADCC), ADCC can be considered a type II effect because antibody must first unite with surface antigen.

Anti-Receptor Actions

Antibodies against receptor molecules on cell membranes cause damage of a different kind. In most cases, antibodies that react with

---

TABLE 12–5. Mechanisms of Tissue Injury in Type II Reactions

Associated with Complement Activation
　　Cell lysis, through membrane attack unit
　　Opsonization, through surface-bound C3b
　　Acute inflammation, through anaphylatoxic cleavage fragments
Independent of Complement Activity
　　Opsonization, through surface-bound IgG
　　Antibody-dependent cell-mediated cytotoxicity, through surface-
　　　　bound IgG
　　Depression of cell activity, through inactivation of receptor molecules
　　Stimulation of cell activity, through crosslinking of receptor mol-
　　　　ecules

---

receptor molecules inactivate or impair the receptor and depress activity of the underlying cell. Characteristically the receptor-antibody complexes are interiorized, leaving the cell surface unable to interact with stimulatory agents. A dramatic exception is the effect of antibody to the receptor for thyroid-stimulating hormone; when this antibody combines with receptor, it crosslinks the receptor and stimulates the underlying thyroid cell to increased secretion of hormone. Anti-idiotype antibodies may stimulate immunoregulatory cells in a comparable fashion, leading to immune enhancement through a feedback mechanism. Table 12–5 summarizes the mechanisms of type II diseases.

EXOGENOUS ANTIGENS

Antibodies exert their protective effects by interacting with microorganisms in the mechanisms just described. These reactions with surface antigens of exogenous microorganisms are not pathological; they are physiologically essential and are described in chapter 9.

Damaging type II reactions against exogenous antigens are relatively rare; the target is usually a drug. Most drugs are dissolved or suspended in body fluids; reactions with anti-drug antibodies usually lead to insoluble immune complexes that induce type III reactions. If the drug is fixed to a cell membrane, however, antibody that reacts with drug may damage the underlying cell. Penicillin, if present at very high plasma concentrations, may adsorb to red cells; antibodies to penicillin, usually IgG, may react with the surface-bound drug and leave the cell coated with antibody. Through their Fc-gamma receptors, phagocytic cells in spleen, bone marrow, and liver may damage the membrane of the antibody-coated cell, even though the antibody is not directed against cell constituents.

ALLOGENEIC ANTIGENS

Allogeneic antigens derive from humans with genetically determined traits different from those of the host. Under natural conditions, pregnancy and childbirth are the major routes through which one human experiences material from another human; not infrequently, fetal cells enter the mother's circulation at delivery and, to a much lesser extent, during the pregnancy. Twentieth-century medicine, however, has devised other opportunities for allogeneic exposure, notably transfusion, transplantation, and the injection of protein preparations.

Natural Immunization

The major naturally occurring type II reaction against allogeneic antigens is **hemolytic disease of the newborn** (HDN). This can develop if fetal red cells enter the mother's circulation and provoke antibodies against antigens that the fetus acquired from paternal genes. The antibodies do not harm the mother, because her cells lack the antigen. If the fetus of a later pregnancy is positive for the same antigen, however, the IgG antibodies can cross the placenta, bind with antigen on the fetal cells, and cause the cells to undergo accelerated destruction. By far the most common antibody that causes severe HDN is anti-D, which develops in Rh-negative women who have successive Rh-positive infants. Immunoprophylaxis against Rh sensitization, introduced in the late 1960s, has markedly reduced the frequency of symptomatic HDN. In rare cases, alloantibodies to granulocyte or platelet antigens may damage fetal neutrophils or platelets in a comparable manner. Antisperm antibodies, which may impair fertility, are another alloimmune event that can develop after natural exposure.

Iatrogenic Immunization

Transfusion introduces the recipient to numerous allogeneic antigens of red cells, platelets, or white cells; some recipients develop antibodies against these foreign antigens. Such antibodies characteristically cause harm only if the individual later receives another transfusion of cells that express the same antigen. Pretransfusion compatibility testing detects most potentially harmful antibodies against red cells, allowing transfusion of selected cells that lack the implicated antigens. If incompatible cells are transfused, the antibody causes cell damage either from complement-mediated intravascular

TYPE II: ANTIBODY INTERACTS WITH SURFACE ANTIGEN

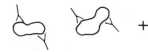

Complement-activating antibody on RBCs	Complement components	Membrane attack unit lyses cells (intravascular hemolysis)

FIGURE 12–6. Complement-binding antibody specific for a red-cell antigen attaches to the cell surface and initiates the complement cascade. At completion, the membrane attack unit lethally damages the membrane, and the circulating cell is hemolyzed. Intravascular hemolysis is almost always caused by IgM antibody.

lysis (Fig. 12–6) or from phagocytosis by sinusoidal lining cells with Fc receptors (Fig. 12–7). It is more difficult to identify antibodies against platelets and white-cell antigens than against red-cell antigens; alloantibodies frequently cause reactions after transfusion of platelets or granulocytes.

Transplantation of solid organs exposes the recipient to foreign antigens that remain immunologically active as long as the graft remains in place. Both humoral and cell-mediated reactions occur against these allogeneic antigens. This is discussed in more detail in chapter 13.

TYPE II: ANTIBODY INTERACTS WITH SURFACE ANTIGEN

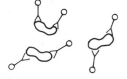 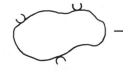 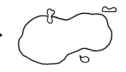

IgG antibody on RBCs	Macrophages with Fc-gamma receptors	Damage to RBCs (extravascular hemolysis)

FIGURE 12–7. IgG antibody specific for a red-cell antigen may remain attached to the cell as it travels through the spleen or other reticuloendothelial site. When they engage the immunoglobulin molecule, macrophages with receptors for Fc-gamma damage the underlying red-cell membrane. These damaged red cells are removed from the circulation and destroyed.

AUTOLOGOUS ANTIGENS

Many autoimmune diseases reflect the action of antibodies directed against antigens of the host's own cells or proteins. Autoreactive antibodies may accompany conditions in which the initial tissue damage derives from some other agent, but often antibodies to self constituents are the primary cause of injury (Table 12–6). Autoimmune diseases are classified as either organ-specific or generalized. Generalized conditions, in which several different organs or cell types are affected, more often have a type III origin and are discussed in the next section. In organ-specific conditions, antibody reactive against a defined tissue constituent provokes disease in the organ that expresses the antigen.

Goodpasture's syndrome is unusual in that autoantibody of a single type produces disease at several sites. The antibody reacts with basement membrane protein; the organ most conspicuously involved is the glomerulus of the kidney. Antibody attaches to the glomerular capillaries and activates complement, provoking inflammation and altered vascular function. The resulting condition, called **antiglomerular basement membrane** (GBM) **glomerulonephritis,** causes rapid deterioration of renal function (Fig. 12–8). The same antibody also recognizes basement membrane antigen in pulmonary capillaries, activating complement to cause lung damage that is primarily hemorrhagic rather than inflammatory. Basement-membrane protein is present in many tissues but is apparently more accessible to the antibody in glomeruli and lung than anywhere else.

Hematologic Conditions

Perhaps the most common type II condition is **autoimmune hemolytic anemia** (AIHA), in which antibody interacts with elements of the red-cell membrane. The antibody may be IgM or IgG; complement activation may or may not contribute to shortened red-cell survival. Sometimes other immune dysfunctions accompany the red-cell autoantibody, but in many patients the autoantibody occurs as an isolated and apparently spontaneous event. Platelet antibodies are also frequent, producing the condition called **immune** (or idiopathic) **thrombocytopenic purpura** (ITP), in which antibody-coated platelets are removed from the circulation more rapidly than the bone marrow can replace them. **Autoimmune neutropenia** occurs much less often than hemolysis or thrombocytopenia, but has the same mechanism.

Endocrine Conditions

Autoantibodies cause depressed secretory function in many glandular tissues. In **pernicious anemia,** antibodies act against gastric lining cells and reduce the manufacture of intrinsic factor, which is needed for absorption of vitamin B_{12}; antibodies may also be directed

TABLE 12—6. Autoantibodies Associated with Type II Reactions

Disease	Antigen	Mechanism
Autoimmune hemolytic anemia (AIHA)	Red-cell membrane	Cells damaged by macrophages with receptors for Fc
Immune thrombocytopenic purpura (ITP)	Platelet membrane	As for AIHA
Autoimmune neutropenia	Neutrophil antigens	Probably as for AIHA
Pernicious anemia	Gastric parietal cells	Genetic predisposition
	Intrinsic factor	Atrophic changes in epithelium; blockage of intrinsic factor activity
Lymphocytic thyroiditis	Thyroglobulin Microsomal antigens	Genetic predisposition ? Interaction of macrophages with colloid ? ADCC* against epithelial cells
Graves' disease (Toxic goiter)	Receptor for thyroid-stimulating hormone	Crosslinking of receptor stimulates hormone production
Addison's disease (Adrenal insufficiency)	Microsomal antigens	Genetic predisposition
	Adrenal epithelial cells	? ADCC against epithelial cells
Pemphigus vulgaris	Desmosomes (protein structures that hold skin cells together)	Complement-mediated blister formation Detachment of skin cells from one another Possible secondary response to damaged tissue
Goodpasture's syndrome (Glomerulonephritis and/or pulmonary hemorrhage)	Basement membrane	Acute inflammation mediated by complement activation
Myasthenia gravis	Acetyl choline receptor	Inactivation of receptor function
Insulin-resistant diabetic states	Insulin receptor	Inactivation of receptor function
Insulin-dependent diabetes mellitus (type I)	Islet cells	Inflammatory damage to insulin-producing cells (cell-mediated immunity also significant)

*ADCC: Antibody-dependent cell-mediated cytotoxicity

TYPE II: ANTIBODY INTERACTS WITH SURFACE ANTIGEN

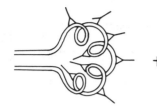

Anti-GBM attaches to glomerular basement membrane

Complement components

Complement provokes acute inflammatory damage to glomerulus

FIGURE 12–8. Circulating antibody to glomerular basement membrane (anti-GBM) adheres to the target tissue and initiates the complement cascade. Anaphylatoxic consequences of the complement cascade predominate, and the resulting cellular and vascular events cause inflammatory renal injury.

against intrinsic factor. Thyroid cells and their products express many antigens, to which several different autoantibodies may develop. These induce functional or inflammatory changes in the gland and may cause enlargement of the gland (goiter) or systemic hypothyroidism or both. Organ-specific antibodies may depress glandular function in the adrenal glands, the ovaries, or the parathyroid glands; often, however, autoantibodies to these tissues exist in the blood without causing endocrine hypofunction. In the insulin-dependent form of **diabetes mellitus** (type I), there may be antibodies against insulin-producing cells, against insulin receptors, or against insulin itself, but cell-mediated mechanisms are probably of greater pathogenic importance.

Anti-Receptor Antibodies

Antibodies against membrane receptors depress cellular functions in **myasthenia gravis** (acetyl choline receptors), in **insulin resistance** (insulin receptors), and in certain abnormalities of the autonomic nervous system (beta-2 adrenergic receptors) (Fig. 12–9). Anti-receptor antibodies have the opposite effect in the form of hyperthyroidism called **Graves' disease,** in which antibody is directed against receptors for the thyroid-stimulating hormone (TSH) secreted by the pituitary. Antibody to the TSH receptor crosslinks the membrane molecule; the underlying cell reacts as though TSH had engaged the receptor and responds by producing thyroid hormone. Production of thyroid hormone normally fluctuates in response to

TYPE Ⅱ: ANTIBODY INTERACTS WITH SURFACE ANTIGEN

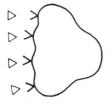 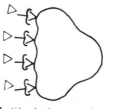 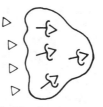

Receptors allow mediator
to stimulate target cell

Antibody to receptor
prevents stimulation

Antibody-receptor
complex is interiorized.
Membrane lacks receptors.

FIGURE 12–9. Stimulation by mediators requires accessible receptors on the target cell. Antibody against the receptor molecules not only blocks the steric interaction between mediator and receptor but often causes the mediators to disappear from the cell membrane.

changing levels of TSH. In Graves' disease, the antibody to TSH receptor remains at a constant high level; because physiologic events are unable to modulate thyroid function, excessive production of thyroid hormone occurs continuously.

——————— TYPE III IMMUNOPATHOLOGY ———————

Type III disease occurs when soluble antibody unites with soluble antigen and the macromolecular complexes precipitate out of solution. Damage results not from the union of antigen and antibody but from the associated activation of complement. Tissue damage occurs at those sites where deposition of the complexes promotes local accumulation of anaphylatoxic cleavage fragments and activated components. Most tissue effects result from anaphylatoxic effects of C3a and C5a; the membrane attack unit (C8 and C9) can lyse circulating red cells, but fixed tissue seldom undergoes lytic damage in type III reactions.

MECHANISMS

Soluble molecules of antigen and antibody combine into complexes whose size depends largely on the relative concentration of each constituent. The size of the reacting molecules does affect the size of the complex, but concentration is more significant. If excess antigen is present, there is saturation of combining sites on the antibody molecules before an effective lattice can accumulate; in antibody excess, free antigen sites may be so sparse that multivalent antibody molecules cannot find multiple attachments to form a lattice. (See discussion of precipitation, pages 309–312.) In blood or body fluids, very small complexes either pass directly into the urine or remain suspended; they do not deposit in tissue. Very large complexes are removed and degraded by the reticuloendothelial system before they cause damage. Immune complexes that form in conditions of mild antigen excess are just the right size to deposit in such sites as glomerular basement membrane, vascular endothelium, joint linings, and pulmonary alveolar membranes.

Complement and Other Mediators

Precipitated complexes activate complement through the classical pathway. The anaphylatoxic effects of C3a and C5a attract neutrophils and promote degranulation of mast cells. C5a also stimulates smooth muscle contraction, increases vascular permeability, and attracts and activates macrophages. Interleukin-1, a product of activated macrophages, probably causes the systemic symptoms of fever and malaise that occur early in an acute episode. Accumulating neutrophils damage tissue by generating oxygen radicals and releasing proteolytic enzymes; damaged tissue elements then exert independent inflammatory effects that perpetuate the process. These events enhance the increased vascular permeability initiated by complement action and promote additional accumulation of proteins, including coagulation proteins that evolve into fibrin. Materials released from mast cells promote platelet activation and further enhance vascular permeability, as described in the section on type I reactions. Generation of leukotrienes and prostaglandins further modulates the inflammatory events. Table 12–7 summarizes the sequence of tissue events.

Subsequent Events

These processes may cease spontaneously if degradation of antigen or depletion of antibody interrupts evolution of immune complexes. If complement activation is intense and explosive, depletion of complement may halt the process. If, however, immune complexes continue to form and to deposit, inflammation persists and produces permanent tissue loss and scarring. Tissue damaged by the acute events sometimes initiates an autoimmune response that further perpetuates the tissue damage. Table 12–8 lists some of the clinical events seen with these types of reactions, and Figure 12–10 illustrates the mechanisms.

TABLE 12–7. Sequence of Tissue-Damaging Mechanisms in Type III Reactions

---

Initiating Events
Immune complex forms and deposits in tissue
Antibody in complex activates complement through classical pathway
Anaphylatoxic cleavage fragments are generated
Complement-mediated Effects
Attraction of neutrophils and macrophages
Activation of macrophages and mast cells
Increase in vascular permeability
Contraction of smooth muscle
Secondary Events

Neutrophils:	Damage to cells and extracellular proteins
Macrophages:	Production of IL-1, other locally and systemically active proteins
Mast cells:	Increased vascular permeability; platelet activation; smooth muscle constriction
Platelets:	Promotion of coagulation events; release of platelet-derived growth factor; stimulation of vascular endothelium
Vascular changes:	Accumulation of immunologically active proteins; formation of fibrin; generation of prostaglandins and leukotrienes

Long-Term Changes
Loss of tissue elements that cannot regenerate
Accumulation of scar tissue
Initiation of autoimmunity against damaged tissue constituents

---

EXOGENOUS ANTIGENS

Serum sickness and the Arthus reaction (see earlier section) were the first forms of immune complex disease to be recognized. Spontaneous **Arthus reactions** occur infrequently. Classical **serum sickness** was common in the era before antibiotics, when passive immunization with animal serum was important in treating infections. The resulting syndrome caused malaise, fever, and generalized symptoms 1 to 2 weeks after injection of the animal serum. Antibodies to the foreign protein developed sufficiently rapidly that substantial amounts of the injected material remained in the system to combine with the evolving antibody. If a patient had had previous experience with the protein and already had antibodies, injection of animal serum provoked more rapid and intense symptoms, sometimes causing systemic cardiovascular catastrophe.

TABLE 12–8. Some Diseases Caused by Type III Reactions

Organ Involved	Initiating Event	Clinical Consequences
Kidney		
Poststreptococcal glomerulonephritis	Infection with "nephritogenic" strain of organism	Usually resolves spontaneously as antigens are eliminated
Glomerulonephritis of systemic lupus erythematosus (SLE)	Immune dysfunction allows formation of anti-DNA	Acute episodes remit with depletion of antibody and complement; recurrence and progressive damage are common
Lungs		
Acute allergic alveolitis	Inhaled antigens combine with circulating antibodies	Acute episode resolves if exposure ceases; repeated episodes may cause scarring
Joint Lining		
Postinfectious arthritis	Infection, often viral, induces circulating antibody	Systemic malaise, other symptoms common; usually resolves with no permanent damage
Drug-sensitivity arthritis	Circulating drug combines with antibody induced by previous exposure	Usually resolves promptly when drug is discontinued; systemic symptoms often present
Rheumatoid arthritis (RA)	Immune dysfunction allows formation of autoantibodies to IgG	Progressive damage follows recurrent episodes; not all patients with RA have demonstrable antibody to IgG
Blood Cells	Immune complexes settle on circulating cells; inciting antigen is usually a drug	Sudden, dramatic destruction of red cells or platelets follows exposure to very small amounts of antigen; complete recovery follows removal of antigen
Blood Vessels		
Serum sickness	Reexposure to animal proteins	Cardiovascular collapse, multiple organ involvement if severe; usually resolves
Henoch-Schoenlein purpura	Unknown; may be drug or microbial antigens	Hemorrhage into skin, joint pain, glomerulonephritis; gastrointestinal problems; usually remits in 7–10 days

TABLE 12—8. *Continued*

Organ Involved	Initiating Event	Clinical Consequences
Drug-induced vasculitis	Reexposure to immunizing drug	Skin, kidneys usual sites of involvement; usually resolves if drug is identified and withdrawn
Polyarteritis nodosa	Usually autoimmune; may occur after hepatitis	Progressive necrotizing inflammation of medium-size arteries
Wegener's granulomatosis	Unknown; possibly hypersensitivity to inhaled antigens, possibly auto-immune	Necrotizing inflammation of small arteries and veins; nearly always involves lungs, upper respiratory tract; T cells and macrophages are also involved

Drug Reactions

The term "serum sickness" is sometimes used for any systemic ill effects arising from immune-complex deposition after exposure to foreign material. Animal serums are so immunogenic that they have little current therapeutic use, but many widely used **drugs** provoke systemic immune-complex syndromes. Sulfonamides, penicillins and other antibiotics, thiazides, thiouracils, and hydantoins have all been implicated in immune-complex reactions characterized by fever and widespread inflammatory or hemorrhagic manifestations in skin, joints, or kidneys.

A rare but dramatic form of **red-cell destruction** occurs with immune complexes involving drugs. Quinine derivatives, some analgesics that are no longer marketed, and several other drug classes may provoke antibodies that unite with circulating drug to form complexes that precipitate on blood cells. The complexes activate the complement cascade, which swiftly generates the membrane attack unit and causes intravascular lysis of the underlying cells, which may be red cells or platelets. This kind of cell damage is sometimes called "innocent bystander" hemolysis.

Organisms and Inhaled Antigens

Infections may cause immune complex-mediated disease if **antigens of microorganisms** remain present long enough to react with

TYPE Ⅲ: IMMUNE COMPLEXES ACTIVATE COMPLEMENT

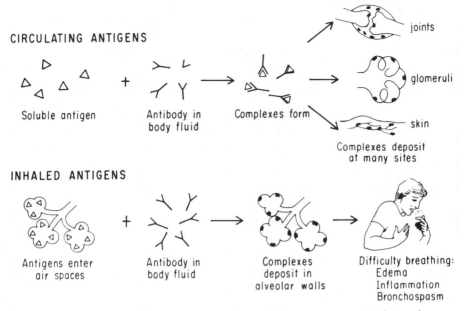

FIGURE 12–10. The consequences of type III hypersensitivity depend upon the site of immune complex deposition. Complexes containing soluble antigen and antibodies from the bloodstream may be deposited on membranes of blood vessels, joints, or kidney. At these sites, the anaphylatoxic effects of activated complement cause acute inflammation. When antigens are inhaled and react with circulating antibodies, complement-activating complexes rapidly deposit in the alveolar walls and cause prompt appearance of symptoms.

antibodies that the infection elicits. The classic example is **immune-complex glomerulonephritis,** which occurs 10 days to 2 weeks after infection with certain strains of streptococcus. Viral hepatitis sometimes causes skin and joint symptoms thought to have the same origin, and other viruses may, less frequently, cause this kind of syndrome.

Several kinds of **hypersensitivity pneumonitis** are due to inhaled antigens, but not all are type III conditions. **Extrinsic allergic alveolitis** is a type III inflammation of air spaces that develops when a person with circulating antibodies inhales antigens. Alveolitis of this sort is usually due to moldy or contaminated hay, but other finely divided plant or animal proteins can induce the syndrome in susceptible individuals. Symptoms develop within a few hours of exposure and disappear when the inhalant is removed. Pulmonary hypersensitivity conditions that develop more slowly and continue more persistently are usually cell mediated and are described in a later section.

ALLOGENEIC ANTIGENS

Human plasma proteins in transfusion components virtually never cause a serum-sickness syndrome. Individuals congenitally deficient in IgA sometimes form allo-anti-IgA if exposed by transfusion to this immunoglobulin class. Usually the antibodies are IgG and cause few or no symptoms after transfusion of IgA-containing components. Rarely, transfusion provokes catastrophe in an immunized IgA-deficient person; the clinical picture is one of anaphylactic, immediate hypersensitivity, presumably resulting from cell-bound IgE antibody and not from circulating IgG antibody.

AUTOLOGOUS ANTIGENS

A large group of systemic, multiorgan diseases involve immune-complex reactions with autologous antigens. Sometimes called **collagen-vascular** or **connective-tissue** diseases, they are characterized by antibodies against such universally present constituents as single- or double-stranded deoxyribonucleic acid (DNA), nucleohistones, IgG proteins, phospholipids, and various cytoplasmic proteins. Clinical characteristics of disease are influenced by the specific disease syndrome, the genetic constitution of the patient, and the environmental events the patient experiences. Frequent clinical findings are intermittent inflammatory episodes involving small or medium blood vessels, membrane surfaces, joints, or glomeruli. Table 12–9 lists some of the antibodies associated with this group of poorly understood conditions.

The classic example is **systemic lupus erythematosus** (SLE), which has a frequency of 15 to 50 per 100,000 population, with a female-to-male ratio of 9:1. The most consistent serologic findings in SLE are antibody to nuclear antigens and to DNA and, during exacerbations, immune complex deposition on glomerular basement membranes. In the kidneys and other sites of acute inflammation are deposited complexes that contain DNA, immunoglobulin, and complement. The pathogenetic defect seems to be dysregulation of B-cell activity, manifested by aberrant antibodies that form immune complexes with essential self constituents.

Another common but poorly understood autoimmune disease is **rheumatoid arthritis,** which has less striking female-to-male preponderance than SLE and tends to occur somewhat later in life. The conspicuous autoantibody in rheumatoid arthritis is called **rheumatoid factor,** which is IgG or IgM with specificity against the IgG immunoglobulin class. Deposits of antibody, IgG, and complement can be found in the membranes of inflamed joints; many of the manifestations of rheumatoid arthritis can be explained by immune complex deposition. Other tissues and organs may experience destructive changes in which antibodies do not seem to be implicated.

TABLE 12–9. Some Autoantibodies Associated with Systemic Diseases

Antibody Specificity	Major Disease Associations	Methods of Detection	Comments
Nuclear Elements			
Native (double-strand) DNA[1]	SLE[3]	IF[4], RIA[5], CIE[6], others	Highly characteristic of SLE
Single- or double-strand DNA	SLE; other connective tissue diseases	IF, RIA, CIE, others	High titers in SLE; lower titers, less consistent occurrence in other diseases
Deoxynucleoprotein	SLE and drug-associated lupus	IF, RIA, latex particle agglutination	Cause of "LE cell" phenomenon
RANA[2]	Rheumatoid arthritis, Sjögren's syndrome	IF, immunodiffusion	Reacts *in vitro* only with cells transformed by EBV
Cytoplasmic Elements			
Mitochrondria	Primary biliary cirrhosis; SLE	IF	Marker antibody, no pathogenetic role identified
Smooth muscle antigens	Chronic active hepatitis	IF	Marker antibody, no pathogenetic role identified
Non-cellular antigens			
IgG	Rheumatoid arthritis; SLE; postviral syndromes; otherwise normal elderly	Latex particle agglutination	Antibodies are called "rheumatoid factors" May be IgG or IgM Found in complement-activating complexes in affected joints
Phospholipids	SLE; many autoimmune and malignant diseases	Prolongation of prothrombin time test	Often called "lupus anticoagulant" Causes thrombotic tendency, not bleeding Common cause of "biologic false-positive" result in non-specific tests for syphilis

1. DNA: deoxyribonucleic acid
2. RANA: rheumatoid arthritis-associated nuclear antigen
3. SLE; systemic lupus erythematosus
4. IF: immunofluorescence
5. RIA: radioimmunoassay
6. CIE: counterimmunoelectrophoresis

Other conditions in this category of connective-tissue disorders include **scleroderma, polymyositis, mixed connective tissue disease, polyarteritis nodosa,** and other forms of arteritis. Demonstration of autoantibodies is useful in diagnosing these conditions, but the pathogenetic mechanisms remain unclear.

TYPE IV HYPERSENSITIVITY DISORDERS

Type IV tissue damage results solely from cellular events. Antibody activity is not a factor, although, in some cases, there may simultaneously be antibodies to the same antigens. In type IV conditions, antigen stimulates idiotype-specific T lymphocytes either to perform direct cytotoxic actions or to secrete factors that incite other cells to destructive activities. When the body defends against microorganisms, it is difficult to separate the beneficial and the harmful results of cellular events because cell-mediated attack on intracellular pathogens almost inevitably does some damage to the host tissues. Reactions to environmental antigens, on the other hand, have obvious harmful effects and few detectable benefits. Cell-mediated autoimmune reactions are clearly destructive, but they often represent physiologically useful activities gone wrong in target or intensity. Table 12–10 lists some of the diseases in which cell-mediated immunity damages tissue.

TISSUE CHANGES

Lymphocytes and macrophages are prominent in tissue undergoing cell-mediated damage. Contact with specific antigen provokes clonal expansion of effector T cells; some of the activated daughter cells secrete lymphokines that induce tissue effects, whereas others perpetuate memory. If the antigen causing primary immunization is one that remains present for long periods, immune reactivity may become apparent days to weeks after initial exposure. For antigens that disappear or are degraded, immunization becomes detectable only with later exposure to the same antigen. Lymphokines secreted by antigen-stimulated T cells promote accumulation of macrophages that do not recognize specific antigens. Interactions between antigen-specific lymphocytes and non-restricted macrophages enhance the activity of both cell types. The accumulating lymphocytes express increased secretory capacities and augmented cytotoxic capabilities.

Macrophages increase in number and state of activation, manifesting altered morphology, enhanced phagocytosis, and increased production of numerous proteins. In addition to proteolytic enzymes, macrophages release materials that enhance coagulation and platelet

---

TABLE 12–10. Examples of Type IV Immune Conditions

Exogenous Antigens
   Contact dermatitis
   Adult-type tuberculosis
   Infections with many intracellular bacteria and fungi
   Lepromatous leprosy
   Tertiary manifestations of syphilis
   Chronic hypersensitivity pneumonitis
   ? Sarcoidosis
Allogeneic Antigens
   Allograft rejection
   Graft-versus-host disease
Autologous Antigens
   Insulin-dependent diabetes mellitus
   Chronic active hepatitis
   Allergic encephalomyelitis
   Multiple sclerosis
   ? Sarcoidosis
   ? Granulomatous colitis
   ? Idiopathic myocarditis

---

activity, stimulate production of fibrous tissue, and cause vasodilatation and increased vascular permeability. Tissue undergoing this type of reaction contains many lymphocytes that do not express antigenic specificity; the role of these cells is not understood.

A Nondestructive Example

The classic example of the cell-mediated immune response is the **tuberculin reaction** (see pages 162–164) in which immunity becomes apparent through tissue effects that begin 12 to 48 hours after introduction of a previously encountered antigen. The involved tissue seldom experiences permanent damage because the vascular and cellular events degrade the small amount of injected material; as the antigen disappears, the reaction dissipates. Individuals with very strong tuberculin reactivity may, however, respond to the small amount of injected antigen with an inflammatory reaction that causes tissue necrosis. Type IV reactions are consistently destructive if the eliciting antigen persists or renews itself and stimulates continuing cytotoxic, vasoactive, and proteolytic activity.

CONTACT SENSITIVITY

The poison ivy reaction is, undoubtedly, the type IV condition with which the largest number of people are familiar. It belongs to the

TYPE IV : CELL-MEDIATED TISSUE DAMAGE
CONTACT SENSITIVITY

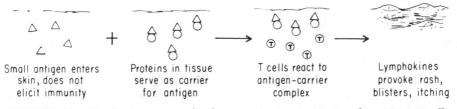

Small antigen enters skin, does not elicit immunity

Proteins in tissue serve as carrier for antigen

T cells react to antigen-carrier complex

Lymphokines provoke rash, blisters, itching

FIGURE 12–11. Antigens involved in contact sensitivity characteristically require combination with host proteins to elicit primary immunization. Once sensitivity is established, exposure to very small quantities of antigen can provoke pronounced cell-mediated symptoms.

large category of **contact dermatitis** reactions, in which antigen penetrates the skin to elicit a local cell-mediated immune response. Contact dermatitis illuminates the roles of **hapten** and **carrier** in the induction and expression of immunity. Characteristically, the allergen is very small (MW less than 1 kD) and incapable of inducing by itself primary immunization. After penetrating the epidermal barrier, the allergen combines with the host's own proteins, which act as carrier to create a fully immunogenic complex. Once primary immunization has occurred, subsequent exposure to hapten provokes cell-mediated reactivity at the site of antigen exposure (Fig. 12–11). The most conspicuous effects are itching, reddening, edema, and blister formation.

Poison Ivy Reactions

Poison ivy, poison oak, and poison sumac, which belong to the **Rhus** genus, elaborate oils capable of penetrating intact skin. The skin reactions occur only after direct contact with the plant oil; contact with fluid from evolving blisters does not spread the rash. Sometimes new areas of rash and blisters appear well after an episode of known exposure or at a skin site that had no contact with the plant. These new lesions do not represent secondary spread from originally involved tissue. The late-reacting area has usually experienced unnoticed contact with a small amount of oil-bearing material; since the provoking dose is so small, the reaction takes longer to develop. The oily allergen can persist for many days on unwashed surfaces, so a person can experience sensitizing contact long after parting company from the plant. The oil can also spread by aerosol; highly sensitive individuals standing downwind of burning foliage may experience severe skin or respiratory effects.

Reactions to Chemicals

Besides the Rhus allergens, common causes of contact dermatitis include nickel compounds, rubber compounds, dichromates, and paraphenylenediamine. Cross-reactivity is common; after a person develops a sensitivity, contact with related substances also elicits symptoms. Nickel is found in alloys used for jewelry and fasteners on clothing; rashes develop where earrings, zippers, watch buckles, and other appliances touch the skin. Persons sensitive to rubber observe lesions on the hands after wearing rubber gloves. Dichromates are used in processing animal skin; this sensitivity affects tannery workers and those who wear or handle leather articles. Paraphenylenediamine sensitivity often becomes apparent as reaction to para-aminobenzoic acid (PABA), a common ingredient in sunscreens. Related compounds like sulfonamides, azo dyes, sulfonylurea, or topical anesthetics of the benzocaine type are likely to cause skin problems in persons sensitive to PABA.

Photoallergic Events

A related form of contact dermatitis is **photoallergic dermatitis,** which requires the additional presence of ultraviolet (UV) radiation to modify or to activate the sensitizing events. Subsequent contact with the allergen produces a reaction only if UV is present at the same time. The lesions of photoallergic dermatitis occur where skin is exposed to the sun—commonly the face, the V of the neckline, and the arms and hands. Chemicals in germicidal soaps and some ingredients of deodorants and cosmetics are common sensitizers.

MICROBIAL ANTIGENS

Cell-mediated immunity is important in protection against such invaders as listeria, salmonella, cryptococcus, and candida. Cell-mediated attack on the infecting organism, however, characteristically damages the tissues where the encounter occurs. This is most conspicuous in infections with *Mycobacterium tuberculosis* and with the fungus *Histoplasma capsulatum.*

In individuals who lack immunity to these organisms, primary infection is often characterized by rapid multiplication and dissemination of the organisms, which may overrun the liver, bone marrow, spleen, and other reticuloendothelial sites. Disseminated *M. tuberculosis* infection occurs most often in young children whose immune system is immature, or in debilitated individuals with depressed cellular immunity.

Tissue Destruction

Cellular immunity to these organisms provokes an inflammatory reaction consisting of lymphocytes and large numbers of highly acti-

TYPE Ⅳ : CELL-MEDIATED TISSUE DAMAGE
MYCOBACTERIA AND SIMILAR ORGANISMS

   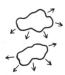

| Macrophages attempt to destroy organisms | T cells respond to organisms by producing lymphokines | Activated macrophages attack organisms more effectively | Activated macrophages secrete products that damage tissue, promote scarring |

FIGURE 12–12. The destructive consequences of cell-mediated attack on microorganisms arise from events intended as protective. Antigen-specific T cells respond to the organisms by secreting lymphokines, which enhance inflammatory mechanisms, especially in macrophages. This increases antimicrobial activity but also generates cellular and enzymic events that destroy tissue elements and engender fibrosis.

vated macrophages. Enzymes from the activated macrophages damage the infected tissue, often by slow but progressive necrosis. Fibrous tissue is abundant, partly from the scarring that follows tissue damage and partly in response to growth-promoting factors derived from the inflammatory cells. After extensive tissue loss, scarring and fibrosis distort what functioning tissue remains. These tissue changes, although initiated by the infection, are largely the consequence of the immune response (Fig. 12–12). Therapy should be directed at halting the destructive process by containing and eliminating the organisms, not at suppressing immune activity. If other illness, malnutrition, drugs, or radiation depress the normal level of immune reactivity, organisms previously confined and inactivated by effective immunity may begin to multiply. In individuals with destructive but localized infection, anything that depresses cellular immunity may permit rapid multiplication and dissemination of the organisms. If medication and macrophages succeed in eradicating the organisms, the destructive process stops, but lost tissue cannot be restored, nor can the effects of scarring be reversed.

OTHER EXOGENOUS ANTIGENS

Inhaled antigens may provoke cell-mediated pulmonary disease. Allergic alveolitis resulting from immune complexes (type III damage) is a brief, intense inflammation of the air spaces, with cough, dyspnea, and fever developing shortly after exposure to known allergens. In the cell-mediated forms of **hypersensitivity pneumonitis** (type IV disease), lymphocytes and macrophages cause problems that develop slowly and persist for long periods after exposure occurs. Cellular immunity to molds, dusts, or animal proteins cause many of the episodic or progressive lung conditions related to environmental or occupational events.

Cell-mediated immunity also underlies the poorly understood disease called **sarcoidosis**. Any organ can be involved, but the lungs are most consistently affected. The characteristic lesion contains CD4 cells and activated macrophages, but decades of intense investigation have failed to identify a specific antigenic stimulus. Sarcoidosis may reflect dysfunctional immune modulation, such that any of numerous different antigenic stimuli elicit excessive and non-selective cell-mediated activity.

ALLOGENEIC ANTIGENS

Cell-mediated immunity is a major cause for **rejection of tissue grafts**. The immune system is attacking non-self constituents, and this is exactly what immunity is supposed to do, but the result is considered harmful because the foreign tissue was intentionally introduced. Overall body health would be better served by allowing the non-self cells or tissue to remain, but the host's immune system has no way of knowing this. Chapter 13 discusses transplantation at greater length.

Graft-versus-host disease (GVHD) is a remarkable cell-mediated condition that occurs when transfused or transplanted T lymphocytes react against antigens of the recipient's tissue. Most recipients of foreign cells or tissue effectively eliminate T cells introduced with the blood or graft. If the recipient is severely immunodeficient, however, the donor's T cells can multiply unopposed and respond to their unfamiliar environment by attacking antigens of the host's tissues.

AUTOLOGOUS ANTIGENS

Cell-mediated reactivity against self constituents can be demonstrated in an ever-increasing number of diseases and abnormalities. Autoreactive cells quite probably cause damage to many target tissues, but it is not safe to conclude that, in every case, autoimmunity has caused the observed disease. The demonstration, in the laboratory, that cells react against autologous antigens does not necessarily prove that comparable events occur in the living body. In some conditions, microbial, chemical, or physical events have damaged cells and altered their antigenic properties to render them "foreign" to immune receptors. Within these etiologic constraints, however, the role of cell-mediated autoimmunity is becoming increasingly apparent in many diseases.

Consequences of Viral Infections

In many instances of T-cell accumulation and progressive tissue damage, an attractive explanation is that viral infection is the initiating event. Viral material enters the genome of the host cell and may induce permanent alteration of its antigenic features even if there is not active viral multiplication. Effector cells activated by antigens of altered autologous cells could be expected to cross-react with cells of the same type that do not harbor infection (Fig. 12–13).

Viral infection followed by autoimmune destruction of insulin-producing cells has been invoked as the cause of **insulin-dependent** (type I) **diabetes mellitus;** alteration of hepatocytes by the viruses of hepatitis B or non-A, non-B may underlie many cases of **chronic active hepatitis**. Bacterial or chlamydial infections have been proposed

TYPE Ⅳ : CELL-MEDIATED TISSUE DAMAGE

AUTOIMMUNE EFFECTS

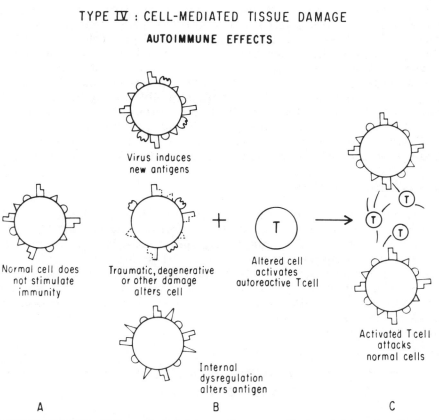

FIGURE 12–13. Cell-mediated immunity may affect autologous cells previously damaged by viral infection, traumatic injury, or growth disturbances. Once a population of activated T cells develops, there may be continuing cross-reactive damage to autologous cells that are not abnormal.

as the initiating event in several kinds of seemingly immune-mediated arthritis, including a syndrome with associated inflammatory changes of skin, eye, and genitalia. Several chronic inflammatory and demyelinating conditions of the central nervous system have been attributed to cellular autoimmunity, although it has been difficult to identify consistent viral invaders. The most promising examples are **multiple sclerosis, acute idiopathic polyneuritis** (Guillain-Barré syndrome), and **acute postviral encephalomyelitis** that sometimes follows viral illnesses or immunizations. Suspicion without conclusive evidence has attached to a wide variety of other conditions, including inflammatory conditions of the large and small intestine, the heart, and various endocrine glands.

Viral Effects on Immunoregulation

A different viral effect on autoimmunity may be disruption of immunoregulation. One explanation offered for normal tolerance of self antigens is that continual contact with autologous antigens maintains continuous activation of antigen-specific suppressor cells that prevent the actions of autoaggressive effector cells. Viral infection is known to influence the function of cells that are not, themselves, harboring organisms. For example, the Epstein-Barr virus infects B lymphocytes but impairs the suppressive actions of CD8-positive T lymphocytes. It is certainly plausible to suggest that viral events could disturb normally effective suppression of anti-self activity. The target of such "escaped" autoimmunity need not be the cells or tissue where the infection occurred, and it would be extremely difficult to detect the time sequence for these hypothetical interactions.

Constitutional Effects

Genetic constitution affects susceptibility to many diseases of immune dysfunction. The clearest association is between HLA-B27 and the spinal arthritis called **ankylosing spondylitis**. Except for that involvement of a B-series antigen, the HLA-DR phenotypes have been the traits most suggestively associated with immune-mediated diseases. The haplotype that determines A1, B8, and DR3 is notably overrepresented in patients with autoimmune diseases. Such associations are by no means consistent, and many other influences can be invoked for most conditions.

─────────────── **SUGGESTIONS FOR** ───────────────
FURTHER READING

Cohen IR: The self, the world and autoimmunity. Sci Am 1988; 258 (issue 4):52–60

Eisenbarth GS: Type I diabetes: clinical implications of autoimmunity. Hosp Pract 1987; 22 (issue 9):167–84

Hamilton RG, Adkinson NF, Jr: Clinical laboratory methods for the assessment and management of human allergic diseases. Clin Lab Med 1986; 6:117–38

Harris EN, Asherson RA, Hughes GRV: Antiphospholipid antibodies—autoantibodies with a difference. Ann Rev Med 1988; 39:261–71

Rabinowe SL, Eisenbarth GS: Polyglandular autoimmunity. Adv Int Med 1986; 31:293–307

Terr AI: In vitro tests for immediate hypersensitivity. Ann Rev Med 1988; 39:135–45

Whaley K: Complement and immune complex diseases. In: Whaley K, ed. Complement in Health and Disease. Norwell, MA: MTP Press, 1987:163–83

CHAPTER 13

Transplantation Immunology

Transplantation introduces tissue from a donor into a recipient in whom it is expected to survive and to function permanently. This contrasts with transfusion, in which cells and proteins are expected to remain functional only for a limited time. Successful transplantation establishes in the recipient a permanent mass of self-renewing tissue derived from another individual. Inasmuch as the express function of immunity is to prevent the establishment of foreign materials, it is no surprise that overcoming immune differences is the major problem in tissue grafting. Problems of blood supply and incoming and outgoing connections are effectively addressed by surgical manipulation, but manipulation of immune events requires complex physiologic and pharmacologic intervention.

266

——— PRINCIPLES OF TRANSPLANTATION ———

Differences among individuals arise from differences in genetic composition. Appearance and function differ among living beings because different genetic endowments code for proteins with highly diverse structures and functions. Immune defenses identify and react against non-self elements; the greater the disparity, the greater the immune response. Success in transplantation results from selection of the least immunogenic material, accompanied by strategies to modify the reactions that almost inevitably develop.

TYPES OF GRAFTS

It is customary to describe grafted tissue according to the relationship between donor and host. Tissue removed from one site and reintroduced into another site in the same individual is an **autograft**. Tissue exchanged between different individuals with identical genetic composition is called a **syngraft**. In humans this occurs only with monozygotic ("identical") twins, but much experimental work employs inbred laboratory animals that possess exactly the same genes as all other members of the colony. When donor and recipient are of the same species but different genetic characteristics, the tissue is an **allograft**. A graft transplanted across species lines (from mouse to rat or from baboon to human, for example) is called a **xenograft** or **heterograft**. Examples of these relationships are shown in Table 13–1.

Non-immunologic Problems

Autografts and syngrafts do not elicit immune rejection because no foreign genes are involved, but this does not guarantee that the graft will survive and function normally. Damage during removal, storage, and implantation may impair survival; there may be vascular problems at the recipient site that cause graft failure; or the condition that damaged the original tissue may persist and damage the grafted tissue as well. Genetic predisposition to disease will affect grafts from an identical twin or syngeneic experimental animal just as it damaged the host's original tissue.

In humans, allografts are the major area for immunologic concern, inasmuch as xenografts are performed only rarely and with full knowledge that the effects will be temporary.

ANTIGENS THAT AFFECT
ALLOGRAFTS

HLA antigens, the class I and class II products of the major histocompatibility complex (MHC), exert major effects on allograft survival,

---

TABLE 13–1. Descriptive Terms Applied to Grafts

Relation of Donor and Recipient	Noun	Adjective	Clinical Example
Tissue originates from the recipient	Autograft	Autologous, autogeneic	Frozen bone marrow infused after cytotoxic therapy Veins relocated during coronary artery bypass Skin taken from unburned site to cover raw burned area
Donor and recipient are different individuals with identical genes	Syngraft	Syngeneic	Kidney or marrow transplant in identical twins Experimental transplants with inbred animals
Donor and recipient are of same species but are genetically different	Allograft (Homograft is an older term)	Allogeneic, homologous	Human organ transplants from siblings, parents, or unrelated individuals
Donor and recipient are of different species	Xenograft (Heterograft is an older term)	Xenogeneic, heterologous	Baboon heart transplant in human Heart valve from pig inserted into human heart

---

but immune rejection occurs even when donor and recipient are HLA identical. The nature, the locations, and the genetic determination of these additional immunogens remain subject to intense investigation. Until it becomes possible to identify these features and to circumvent their effects, transplantation immunology must concentrate on recognizing and matching HLA antigens and applying the most effective and least dangerous means of immunosuppression.

Class I Antigens

Class I HLA molecules consist of one polymorphic chain determined by alleles of the MHC and a chain (called beta-2-microglobulin) that is the same on all human cells. Because virtually all nucleated cells express class I antigens, the antigens of the grafted tissue can be identified by testing white blood cells instead of cells from the organ itself. Class I antigens provoke both cellular and humoral immunity, but immune sensitization can more easily be documented in the humoral than in the cell-mediated arm of the system. The patient with preexisting or rapidly developing anamnestic antibodies against class I antigens of donor tissue may experience very rapid graft rejection. Early work in selecting donor-recipient pairs and predicting graft survival relied heavily on matching the class I antigens HLA-A and -B.

Class II Antigens

Class II antigens (HLA-DR, HLA-DQ, and HLA-DP) are not present on all cells, not even on all lymphocytes. Methods for identification and classification were developed only in the middle and late 1970s. Recognition of their importance in graft survival came relatively late, but it now appears that the HLA-DR series is the most significant HLA characteristic, followed by HLA-B and then by HLA-A. Circulating T lymphocytes do not express class II antigens. The blood contains relatively few B lymphocytes and monocytes, the cells that have strong and consistent expression of class II antigens, so examination for class II characteristics requires enriched cell preparations. It is important to know whether the recipient's cells react with the potential donor's class II antigens; cell-culture techniques, described below, are used for this.

Non-MHC Antigens

The term **major** histocompatibility complex implies that other histocompatibility determinants also exist; non-MHC characteristics are receiving increasing attention. Animals are more suitable for experimental investigations than human beings. Strains of mice have been bred for identity of MHC antigens but diversity in other respects. Transplantation within this system has clearly demonstrated the presence of **minor histocompatibility** (mH) antigens. Antigens termed H-Y, present in male subjects but not in female subjects, affect survival of tissue grafted from male donor to female recipient mice. Other antigens, present in both sexes and determined by sites on several different chromosomes, also affect graft survival in these highly specialized circumstances. It is not yet clear how significant such antigens are in outbred strains of mice, let alone in human beings, but the inevitable immune attack on MHC-identical tissue indicates a definite role for these "minor" antigens.

Vascular lining cells are strikingly involved in the tissue events of rejection, and there is growing conviction that molecules associated with these endothelial cells determine antigenic distinctions among individuals. Except for HLA-directed events, immune activity against endothelial elements is the most consistent site of tissue damage in allotransplantation.

Possible Role of Receptors

One possible area for non-HLA polymorphisms that affect histocompatibility is structural variation in receptor molecules of various sorts. Many proteins exhibit genetically determined variations; variant hemoglobins, immunoglobulin allotypes, and aberrant forms of enzymes are just a few examples. It is tempting to postulate subtle variations in receptor molecules, such that cell types with different receptors would express different polymorphisms. Polymorphisms of this type would be difficult to demonstrate by testing accessible specimens like blood or superficial epithelium, because only the tissue that possessed the specialized receptor would be capable of expressing the antigenic variability.

TYPES OF TISSUE

Therapeutically effective tissue grafting began long before immunologic mechanisms were understood; for certain types of graft, immunologic problems do not occur. The **cornea,** the clear part of the eye, has been successfully grafted since the 1940s. The cornea is transparent because it has no blood vessels. Because there are no blood vessels, engrafted corneal tissue lacks communication with immunologically active aspects of host tissue. No tissue typing or immunologic testing is necessary before the procedure, and no problems occur as long as the grafted tissue remains avascular. If blood vessels grow into the graft, however, the tissue loses its transparency and also its immunologic isolation. A vascularized cornea graft usually must be removed, and problems of inflammation and immune response seriously complicate replacement.

Temporary Grafts

Bone grafting also has a long history independent of immunology. In most procedures, engrafted bone serves a largely mechanical function and is not expected to provide actively metabolizing elements. In addition, procedures for storing and sterilizing bone render the cells nonviable and the protein elements less immunogenic than in unmodified tissue. Transplanted bone, whether autologous or allogeneic, provides structural support and stimulates ingrowth and proliferation of the host's own tissues; characteristically the grafted material is degraded and eliminated when the healing process is complete. In bone grafting, the major concerns are sterility of the transplanted material and the vascularity and regenerative capacity of the recipient site. Innovative new orthopedic techniques now use viable autologous bone for permanent modification of structure and function, but allografts are not used in these ways.

Similar considerations apply to **skin** grafting. Autografts provide permanent repair of surface defects, but allografts and sometimes even xenografts can be useful temporary measures to cover extensively damaged surfaces. The goal is to protect against infection and protein loss and to encourage regeneration of damaged tissue; as healing progresses, the graft becomes unnecessary and the foreign tissue is sloughed off.

Prolonged Survival of Renal Grafts

Kidneys provide the greatest opportunity for monitoring and manipulating immune events. Allografts from living donors are feasible because an individual with two healthy kidneys can donate one without adverse consequences. Most kidney grafts come from cadavers, however, and require careful attention to removal and preservation. The clinical condition of the recipient, the functional status of the donor organ, and many pharmacologic and clinical variables strongly influence success of renal transplantation. The best results are seen with grafts from HLA-identical sibling donors; 10-year survival of these grafts is nearly 70 percent. With all the many variables that affect outcome, including non-renal and non-immunlogic problems in the patient, 10-year survival of cadaver grafts averages 20 percent or better. When the donor is a living relative (described as a "living-related" graft), long-term success is directly proportional to degree of HLA matching. For grafts of cadaver origin, controversy exists as to the significance of HLA matching and the relative importance of class I versus class II MHC products.

Matching Antigens

Bone marrow of autologous or homologous origin may be subjected to transplantation. Autografting is useful in patients treated with intensely cytotoxic anticancer regimens, which would otherwise lethally damage hematopoietic tissue. Allogeneic marrow is used to replace marrow that harbors malignant or other disease that cannot be corrected medically. ABO blood groups need not be compatible for bone marrow allografts, but HLA matching, especially HLA-DR, is crucially important. Bone marrow transplantation is discussed in more detail in a later section.

The technical success of **heart** transplantation has created imbalance between supply and demand. The major indications for cardiac transplantation are inflammatory or metabolic disease of heart muscle (cardiomyopathy) and coronary artery disease; 5-year survival in the several thousand procedures now on record is better than 50 percent. Practical considerations often make it difficult to do much preoperative matching, although it is desirable to match for the ABO blood groups and for HLA-A, HLA-B and HLA-DR.

Experience with Liver Grafts

Success with **liver** transplants has been variable. Suitable donors are hard to find because metabolic and circulatory problems often damage the liver during terminal illness, and traumatic injury precludes use of many livers after serious accidents. When a suitable donor organ is found, little attempt is made to match antigens; it may be that the large mass of allogeneic tissue promotes a degree of immune tolerance. Graft and patient survival do improve with certain combinations of antigen matching and immunosuppression. In adults, the major indications for liver replacement are primary biliary cirrhosis, malignant tumors, inborn errors of metabolism, and cirrhosis from chronic active hepatitis. Except for metabolic deficiencies and congenital deformities, however, there is substantial likelihood that the disease that affected the original liver will recur in the transplanted organ. Children are usually treated for defective development of the biliary tracts or inborn errors of metabolism, and when the procedure is done before generalized deterioration has occurred, results can be very gratifying.

Problematic Procedures

Less widely practiced are procedures for transplanting **pancreas, other endocrine organs, lungs** (with or without the donor heart), and portions of the **intestines**. These organs present complex problems in surgical and medical management but no specific immunologic challenges unique to the tissue involved. Because immune dysfunction significantly affects insulin-dependent diabetes mellitus, attempts at transplanting pancreas to correct this condition carry a guarded long-term prognosis. In organ grafting for conditions other than diabetes, the usual alternative to transplantation is rapid progression of a known fatal process. In diabetes, however, the consequences of a difficult surgical procedure and a lifetime of immnosuppressive therapy must be weighed against the generally favorable clinical course and long life expectancy that accompany conventional therapy.

REJECTION PHENOMENA

More kidneys have been transplanted than all other organs added together. Immunologic mechanisms are universal, but the histologic details, the time sequence, and the clinical consequences of attempted grafting differ for different organs transplanted. For all vascularized grafts and in all donor-recipient pairs except monozygotic twins, the presence of transplanted tissue generates immunologic events that may lead to rejection. The events that accompany renal transplantation have been studied through several decades of biopsies from functioning grafts, examination of surgically removed failed grafts, and autopsies. The specific events described in this section summarize observations primarily from kidney transplants. Table 13–2 outlines the forms that rejection may take.

HYPERACUTE REJECTION

If the recipient already possesses antibodies against antigens of the donor tissue, irreversible damage can occur in the first minutes or hours after transplantation, an event described as **hyperacute rejection**. Circulating antibodies combine with tissue antigens in complexes that activate complement in vessels of the transplanted tissue. This provokes intense acute inflammatory phenomena that include accumulation of neutrophils and their proteolytic enzymes; aggregation of platelets, with release of vasoactive and coagulation-promoting substances; and activation of the coagulation cascade, leading to small-vessel thrombosis and disseminated intravascular coagulopathy. Blood supply to the transplanted organ is irreversibly compromised and the kidney undergoes ischemic necrosis.

HLA and ABO Antibodies

Hyperacute rejection is usually due to high-titered antibodies against class I antigens. The titer of such antibodies may wax and wane. Patients awaiting renal grafts are tested periodically for HLA antibodies, and there has long been the fear that transplantation could provoke anamnestic recurrence of antibody that had previously been identified but was absent at the time of grafting. Until recently, a history of previous antibody contraindicated transplanting a kidney with the corresponding antigens; accumulating data with current immunosuppressive strategies indicate, however, relatively little danger from antibodies undetectable at the time foreign tissue is introduced.

Vascular endothelium expresses ABO antigens, and kidneys incompatible with the recipient's ABO agglutinins are susceptible to hyperacute rejection. This is a problem especially for group O patients, whose serum contains both anti-A and anti-B. Some successes have been reported in reducing the level of antibody by plasma exchange and then administering immunosuppressives to prevent their untimely reappearance. Kidneys are the tissue most susceptible to damage from ABO incompatibility; liver and bone marrow transplants have been successful across ABO lines.

Unknown Specificities

Patients with no detectable HLA or blood group antibodies may experience hyperacute rejection, more often with second grafts than

TABLE 13–2. Ways that Recipients Reject Donor Tissue

Type of Rejection	Time Sequence	Mechanism	Tissue Events	Prognosis
Hyperacute	Minutes to hours	Antibodies to HLA or ABO antigens	Fibrin, complement in vessel walls Thrombosis of small vessels Acute inflammatory cells	Irreversible
Accelerated	1 to 5 days	Antibodies to HLA or ? vascular antigens Previously sensitized T cells	Lymphocytes as well as neutrophils Fibrin, complement in vessels Thrombosis of small vessels	Irreversible
Acute	5 days to years	Newly developing cell-mediated immunity	CD 4 and CD 8 cells Many macrophages Damage to parenchymal and interstitial elements	Usually reversed by increasing immunosuppression
Chronic	Years	Probably not immune	Progressive narrowing of blood vessels, with tissue damage from inadequate blood supply	Gradual irreversible deterioration

with first. An unsuccessful graft seems to provoke antibodies that cannot currently be identified; specificity against vascular endothelium is a prime suspect.

ACCELERATED REJECTION

Hyperacute rejection has extremely rapid onset. The grafted kidney may become swollen and ischemic before the eyes of the surgeons, who must acknowledge defeat by removing the graft through the incision made to implant it. When failure occurs several days after the primary procedure, the process is sometimes called **accelerated rejection**. Lymphocytes as well as neutrophils are seen in the tissue, but the resulting thrombosis and tissue necrosis are essentially the same as in the hyperacute process. Accelerated rejection may reflect previously established cell-mediated immunity, inasmuch as T lymphocytes already sensitized to the donor antigens require several hours to several days to produce their effects (compare with the tuberculin reaction, pages 116–117). Some accelerated episodes involve both antibodies and cellular events through the mechanism of antibody-dependent cell-mediated cytotoxicity (see pages 119–120). The targets of accelerated episodes are characteristically class I products, although many workers believe that activity against still-to-be-identified vascular endothelial components is also significant in this phenomenon.

Sensitive tests for preformed antibodies against HLA antigens have reduced the frequency of hyperacute and accelerated rejection episodes, but continued occurrence in 0.5 to 1 percent of transplants indicates that the entire story has not yet been told.

ACUTE REJECTION

The most common and prolonged problem with organ rejection seems to involve class II antigens and is largely cell mediated. Susceptibility to this phenomenon, called **acute rejection,** begins within a week and remains as long as the graft persists. The antigenic stimulus is thought to be both parenchymal and non-parenchymal cells present in the transplanted organ. Dendritic cells and monocytes are non-organ-specific cells that express class II antigens and are present in grafted tissue along with organ-specific elements; epithelial cells of the donor tissue may be stimulated to express class II antigens in the immunologically activated recipient setting. Inasmuch as rejection occurs even when donor and recipient are HLA identical and have been shown to cause no mutual stimulation when lymphocytes are cocultured, at least some of the antigens involved must be additional to the known MHC determinants and are not detected by present typing procedures.

Importance of Matching Antigens

Since the earliest days of pretransplant testing and posttransplant immunomodulation, it has been difficult to determine the degree to which HLA matching affects graft outcome. Variables include whether donor and recipient are from the same kinship or population group; what antigens are identified and by what techniques; what other criteria are used for recipient eligibility; and how antibodies are sought and evaluated. In all circumstances, immunosuppression is crucial in promoting graft survival. Less suppression is required with less antigenic disparity, but some degree of immunosuppression is always needed. Declining function in an established graft often heralds impending rejection. Although infection and non-immunologic vascular problems must be ruled out, intensifying the level of immunosuppression may reverse the functional deficit.

Tissue Events

Tissue undergoing acute rejection will be heavily infiltrated by macrophages and both CD4- and CD8-positive T cells, relatively few of which are antigen specific; most have been recruited by lymphokines secreted after antigen has stimulated cells with receptors for specific antigens. Macrophages of both donor and host origin produce interleukin 1 (IL-1), which causes T-cell multiplication and generalized inflammatory activation. Stimulated host T cells produce other mediators, including interleukin 2 (IL-2) and gamma interferon, which affect the number and the functional level of both lymphocytes and macrophages. Gamma interferon induces enhanced membrane expression of class I and class II antigens, which render the donor cells more susceptible to recognition and attack by host lymphocytes.

CHRONIC REJECTION

Previously functioning grafts sometimes deteriorate months or years after transplantation, owing to progressive vascular failure and gradual tissue hypoxia. Proliferation of cells lining the blood vessels narrows the lumen and reduces the volume of blood entering the tissue. Deficient oxygenation causes impaired functioning, loss of cell and tissue elements, and progressive fibrous scarring. Immune activity does not seem to be the problem; once the process begins, intensifying immunosuppression does not reverse it. Reducing the immunosuppression may even improve graft function if there is concomitant toxic damage from the agents given (see later section on immunosuppressive drugs).

It may be that growth factors from chronically stimulated platelets and IL-1 from activated macrophages combine to promote proliferation of endothelial cells. Proliferative changes are known to occur when vascular cells sustain such non-immune insults as physical trauma or exposure to abnormal lipids in atherosclerosis. Chronic activation might also, or alternatively, be due to interaction of endothelial or other cell antigens with antibody present at levels too low to be detected. No specific vascular disease or cause for damage has been consistently associated with this deterioration of previously successful grafts.

TESTING BEFORE TRANSPLANTATION

Although some element of immune rejection inevitably affects allografts, survival and function of grafted tissue are improved by selection of suitable donor-recipient pairs. Suppression of the immune response is discussed in the next section.

ANTIGENS OF DONOR AND RECIPIENT

Routine pregraft testing includes typing the recipient and the prospective donor for ABO blood group and for the HLA-A, HLA-B, and HLA-DR antigens. ABO antigens are present on many cell types, and it is important that the transplanted tissue be compatible with these high-titered complement-binding antibodies. This puts group O recipients, who possess both anti-A and anti-B, at a disadvantage; only the 45 percent of the population that is group O can be suitable donors for most tissues. Bone marrow is an exception to the ABO rule, as discussed later in this chapter, and some liver grafts have been successful across ABO lines.

Choosing Among Donors

HLA matching influences graft survival, but the magnitude and significance of this effect are controversial. In selecting among potential living-related donors, the best matching gives the best results. Members of a single kindred possess only a limited number of haplotypes. If HLA-A, HLA-B, and HLA-DR antigens are the same, the entire chromosomal segment can be assumed to be the same, including genes that determine the class III products and unidentified aspects of the MHC. Unrelated donor-recipient pairs who share two, three, or four HLA antigens are much less likely to have shared alleles in the remaining portions of the MHC. The allotypes of the class III complement-related proteins can be determined if close MHC matching is essential, as, for example, for bone marrow transplants. The advent of highly effective immunosuppressive regimens has improved survival of mismatched kidney and other grafts, but the best match possible in each clinical circumstance is still desirable.

For kidney grafts, the Lewis blood group system influences outcome. Overall statistics are less favorable for Lewis-negative than for Lewis-positive patients who receive Lewis-positive kidneys, but clinical circumstances usually preclude using Lewis types as a significant selection factor. If a Lewis-negative recipient needs regrafting after failure of the first graft, a Lewis-negative donor is definitely preferable.

THE SENSITIZED PATIENT

Recipients with established immunity to histocompatibility antigens may experience hyperacute or accelerated rejection of grafted tissue expressing those antigens. Serum from patients awaiting transplantation is tested periodically for antibodies that could compromise graft survival. The **lymphocytotoxicity** procedure tests serum against a panel of lymphocytes selected to express most of the significant HLA antigens. After serum is incubated with the target cells, complement is added; in the presence of complement, antibodies that have attached to the cell surface will lethally damage the membrane (Fig. 13–1). Antibodies reactive against most or all of the cells on the panel carry a worse prognosis than serum with limited

LYMPHOCYTOTOXICITY
TESTING BY DYE EXCLUSION

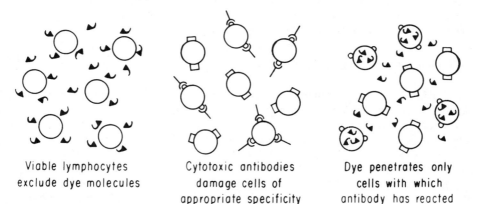

Viable lymphocytes exclude dye molecules

Cytotoxic antibodies damage cells of appropriate specificity

Dye penetrates only cells with which antibody has reacted

FIGURE 13–1. When serum contains cytotoxic antibody specific for antigens on lymphocytes, the immune interaction causes cell damage that can be detected by observing that dye ineffective against normal cells is able to enter the injured cells.

reactivity or no antibodies. Some patients have antibodies that react with all allogeneic cells on the panel and with their own cells as well. These panreactive autoantibodies tend to be IgM, to have a low thermal optimum, and to react with class II antigens; their presence does not correlate with hyperacute rejection. Dangerous antibodies are those that are IgG and react at 37°C with class I antigens. Patients with these antibodies must await a donor organ that lacks the corresponding antigens.

It is difficult to detect whether a patient has established cell-mediated immunity against some or many HLA antigens. *In vitro* tests that measure cellular reactivity cannot easily distinguish immunity that is already established from the genetic potential to mount an immune response after graft-related exposure.

CROSSMATCH PROCEDURES

Once a potential donor has been selected, suitability is confirmed by testing the recipient's serum in a lymphocytotoxicity assay against cells from the designated individual. This is done regardless of results in pretransplant antibody screening panels. The patient whose serum reacts with panel cells but not the specific donor's cells is a suitable recipient; the patient whose serum is negative for the panel but cytotoxic for the specific donor should not receive the planned graft. In the past it was customary to save serum samples that had been positive on screening procedures and to test the most highly reactive specimen against cells of the prospective donor. With current immunosuppressive therapy, however, good graft survival can occur in patients with a negative crossmatch against the current donor, even if serum had previously had strong reactivity.

Cellular Reactions

In selecting living-related donors, it is customary to use cell-culture tests against cells from the proposed donor, as well as serum testing. This is impractical for cadaver grafts because the culture procedure requires hours or days of delay that would damage an organ retrieved after death. The **mixed lymphocyte culture** (MLC) or **mixed lymphocyte reaction** (MLR) procedure tests the degree to which the donor's cells stimulate an immune response in the recipient's T lymphocytes. When cocultured with cells expressing foreign class II antigens, T lymphocytes undergo proliferation and activation. This response can be measured either through the increased synthesis of deoxyribonucleic acid (DNA) that proliferation requires or through cytotoxic actions directed against the target cells. Measuring heightened nucleic acid synthesis is faster and simpler, but under certain circumstances the **cell-mediated lympholysis** test is useful in measuring how much cell-mediated damage the patient can mount.

The One-Way MLC

When lymphocytes of different HLA phenotypes are cultured together, each proliferates after contact with foreign antigens on the other. The reaction significant for pretransplant testing is recipient against donor; donor against recipient is not an issue because solid tissue grafts contain few, if any, donor cells that might react against recipient's antigens. In the **one-way MLC,** the donor cells are irradiated to abolish their proliferative capacity, but the antigens remain immunogenic and capable of provoking the recipient's cells to proliferate (Fig. 13–2).

The one-way MLC is used to select the donor whose cells provoke the least response in the recipient. Mixed lymphocyte culture reactivity is to be expected whenever there is disparity of HLA-DR antigens, but some cells may be more immunogenic than others. Even when recipient and all potential donors are HLA identical, the MLC results may differ for different stimulating cells. Negative results on the one-way MLC do not guarantee prolonged graft survival, but the likelihood

MIXED LYMPHOCYTE CULTURE

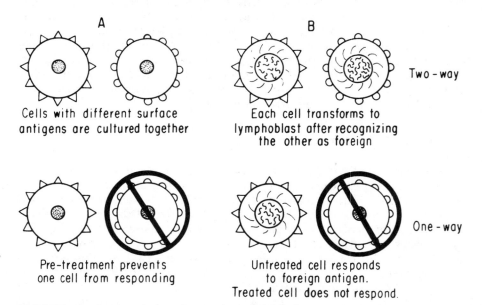

A

Cells with different surface antigens are cultured together

B

Each cell transforms to lymphoblast after recognizing the other as foreign

Two - way

Pre-treatment prevents one cell from responding

Untreated cell responds to foreign antigen. Treated cell does not respond.

One - way

FIGURE 13–2. Coculture of antigenically distinct cells, depicted in A, allows each cell to perceive the foreign characteristics of the other. Cells that are immunocompetent will undergo lymphoblast transformation, as shown in B. If, as shown in the lower drawings, one cell is prevented from responding, any blast transformation that occurs represents the response of the untreated cell to foreign antigens of the treated cell.

TABLE 13—3. Tests Performed Before Transplantation

To determine antigens of donor and recipient
ABO group
(Lewis blood group, for kidney grafts)
Class I antigens: HLA-A, -B
Class II antigens: HLA-DR
Family studies to distinguish haplotypes, in selecting living-related
    donors

To identify previous sensitization in recipient
Periodic tests for lymphocytotoxic antibodies against a panel of cells
    Usually suspensions of peripheral-blood lymphocytes
    Sometimes separate suspensions of T cells and B cells
    If autoantibody is suspected, test at 37°C and/or inactivate IgM with
        a reducing agent
Test recipient's serum for lymphocytotoxicity against lymphocytes of
    specific intended donor (lymphocytotoxicity crossmatch)
Not considered necessary to retain and to test the most highly reac-
    tive of previous serum samples

To determine whether donor's antigens stimulate recipient
One-way mixed lymphocyte culture, with donor's cells inactivated

of serious rejection problems increases with the degree of activity observed. Table 13–3 summarizes the usual battery of tests performed
before transplantation.

IMMUNOSUPPRESSION

As long as tissue that expresses foreign antigens remains in the
host, there remains a risk of immune-mediated rejection. The risk is
greatest in the first few years, but the need to suppress immune reactivity is life-long. Ideal immunosuppression would eliminate reactions
against the grafted tissue but leave all other immune actions intact.
This ideal donor-specific immunosuppression has not been achieved.
Strategies that prolong graft survivial by reducing activity against the
transplant also reduce the host's normal protective immunity. Immunosuppressive regimens rely heavily on pharmacologic agents, primarily drugs that impair cellular proliferation or alter inflammatory
or membrane-associated reactions (Table 13–4). Other approaches to
immunosuppression exploit immune events and products in an attempt to achieve a more physiologic way of modulating reactivity.

TABLE 13–4. Immunosuppressive Drugs Used in Transplantation

Drug	Action	Side Effects
Antiproliferative Agents		
Azathioprine	Interrupts DNA synthesis by inhibiting purine metabolism	Bone marrow depression Hepatotoxicity, hair loss
Cyclophosphamide	An alkylating agent Affects enzyme actions, nucleotide crosslinking	Depresses humoral immunity Bone marrow depression
Methotrexate	Folic acid antagonist Interferes with nucleotide synthesis	GI tract symptoms, liver damage, bone marrow depression
Anti-inflammatory Action		
Adrenal corticosteroids	Inhibits T-cell proliferation Reduces IL-2 production Reduces chemotaxis and activity of neutrophils and macrophages	Disturbs carbohydrate metabolism, bone metabolism, cardiovascular regulation Depresses wound healing, growth (in children), response to stress
Prevents Lymphocyte Activation		
Cyclosporine	Blocks proliferation of activated T cells; inhibits IL-2 production; depresses B-cell and macrophage actions by inhibiting production of lymphokines; modulates donor-tissue expression of class I and II antigens	Damage to kidneys Hyperplasia of gum tissue, hair growth Variable effects on liver, CNS, GI tract

IMMUNOSUPPRESSIVE DRUGS

Immune reactivity requires that antigen-specific cells multiply, both during activation and as part of effector events. Agents that limit cell proliferation will limit immune activity; drugs that affect mitosis and cell division will have more destructive effects on rapidly proliferating populations than on stable populations of functioning cells.

Antiproliferative agents are effective antitumor agents and, in somewhat smaller doses, are useful immunosuppressants. Unfortunately they also damage populations of normal cells that have a high turnover rate, especially cells of the bone marrow and the lining of the gastrointestinal tract. The goal in administering cytotoxic agents is to use the smallest dose that eliminates unwanted antigraft activity. Characteristically the dose will be high immediately after the procedure, with later reductions to a stable minimal level. Episodes of threatened rejection can be treated by increasing the dose or changing to more powerful but more dangerous agents. Episodes of infection often require reduction in immunosuppressive intensity.

Steroid Effects

Adrenal corticosteroids are powerful immunosuppressives that do not exert globally cytotoxic effects. Prednisone or prednisolone is routinely administered along with one or several cytotoxic drugs; the effects are additive, so that lower doses of each can be given. Corticosteroids exert a broad range of metabolic, anti-inflammatory, and anti-immune effects; high doses cause serious problems with infection, wound healing, hemodynamic balance, carbohydrate metabolism, and mineral regulation. Most patients receive low or moderate doses routinely, with high-dose therapy administered in response to acute rejection episodes. Corticosteroids affect cell-mediated immunity more than antibody production. Infections that result from this immunosuppression more often involve viruses, fungi, and intracellular organisms than pyogenic bacteria.

Actions of Cyclosporine

Since the mid-1980s, immunosuppression has been revolutionized by **cyclosporine**. This fungal metabolite exerts remarkable suppressive effects on helper T cells, thereby reducing both cellular and humoral responses to newly encountered antigens. Although B cells and suppressor and cytotoxic T cells are not directly affected, cyclosporine profoundly affects the activity of macrophages and other lymphocytes by reducing secretion of lymphokines. Cyclosporine interferes with activation of antigen-specific CD4 cells and prevents the secretion of IL-2 as well as secretion of many T-cell products and expression of receptors for these lymphokines. Cyclosporine not only diminishes active rejection but may allow or encourage a state of specific immune tolerance by allowing the proliferation of antigen-specific suppressor cells. Cyclosporine is not toxic to hematopoietic precursors or to the alimentary tract, thus avoiding a significant adverse effect of most cytotoxic immunosuppressives. Unfortunately, it causes significant dose-related damage to the kidney; effects on the liver and nervous system are less severe but still potentially troublesome.

Cyclosporine, despite its impressive therapeutic effects, has not made the immune problems of tissue transplantation disappear. It provides superior but non-specific immunosuppression; immunologic reactions to the transplanted tissue do continue, and normal immune actions against other foreign antigens are reduced. It has, however, significantly improved graft survival in virtually all series reported. With cyclosporine, imperfectly matched grafts give far better results than would previously be achieved. The survival of fully HLA-matched grafts has also improved. Most centers continue to observe better results with fully matched grafts than with mismatched grafts, but the overall consequence of cyclosporine use has been to make HLA matching less significant in selecting cadaver grafts.

IMMUNE MANIPULATION

An approach to avoiding globally cytotoxic agents is administration of antibodies directed against effector lymphocytes. **Antilymphocyte serum** (ALS) has proved unsuitable for long-term immunosuppression but works well for episodic treatment of acute rejection. A refinement is to use monoclonal antibodies against CD3, the T-cell receptor complex; this avoids damage to B lymphocytes. Selective, shielded **irradiation** causes a rapid fall in circulating lymphocytes; this seems to diminish the intensity of response to antigens newly encountered at that time. It may become possible to induce antigen-specific tolerance through combinations of cyclosporine, irradiation, and selective exposure to the relevant antigens. Table 13–5 presents several categories of immunomodulating therapy.

Certain tissues can be engrafted as individual cells, rather than as solid tissue. Introducing isolated cells avoids exposure to blood vessels of donor origin, and vascular endothelium appears to express non-HLA determinants that significantly affect graft survival. Endocrine cells, like those of the pancreas or the adrenal or parathyroid glands, can perform their physiologic roles after injection as free cells. Survival of these cellular implants improves over the results with fresh cells if the cells are **cultured** *in vitro* for several generations. There is less class II antigenic activity in the cultured than in fresh injected material, probably because culturing eliminates non-endocrine cells, like lymphocytes and macrophages, which have potent expression of class II determinants.

TRANSFUSION EFFECT

A remarkable application of immunomodulation is the **transfusion effect**. Because preformed antibodies prejudice graft survival, and because transfusion often stimulates antibodies, early workers tried to avoid transfusions to patients awaiting transplants. By the

TABLE 13—5. Immunobiologic Manipulations used in Transplantation

Immunosuppressive Approach	Target Action	Clinical Efficacy
Depletion of Effector Cells		
Antilymphocyte globulin	Rapid, profound loss of T and B lymphocytes	Short-term use to reduce initial immune response or to reverse acute rejection
Monoclonal anti-CD3	Prompt fall in T lymphocytes; newly produced cells lose ability to recognize specific antigens	Short-term use to reverse acute rejection; antibodies often develop, which reduce later efficacy and mediate sensitivity reactions
Total lymphoid irradiation	Rapid, profound loss of T and B lymphocytes	Useful in pretransplant conditioning to induce tolerance to grafted antigens
Transfusion Therapy		
Donor-specific transfusion	Depresses antigen-specific immune response	Given before planned renal transplant from living donor
Random-donor transfusion	Seems to depress overall immune responsiveness; may serve to screen out hyper-responders	Given during support period before cadaver kidney grafting
Modification of Graft		
Culturing pancreatic or other endocrine cells	Eliminates "passenger" cells with strong class II antigens	In recipient also receiving antilymphocyte globulin, reduces response to foreign tissue

mid-1970s, however, it became apparent that cadaver kidneys survived longer in those recipients whose clinical state had made transfusion unavoidable than in those who had never received red cells. Transfusion policy has come a full circle; red cell transfusions are now a routine part of pretransplantation conditioning.

The transfusion effect is most striking in two situations: random blood transfusions given to a patient receiving a cadaver graft unmatched for HLA, and pregraft transfusion from the specific individual who will donate a living-related graft. It is difficult to develop an optimum transfusion schedule, because the mechanisms for this graft-promoting effect remain unclear. Red-cell components are effective; leukocytes or platelet concentrates are not necessary or desirable. Benefit increases with increasing numbers of transfusions, up to about five or six in the weeks or months before transplantation.

Possible Explanations

Several explanations have been offered. One possibility is that transfusion imposes a selection mechanism upon patients designated to undergo transplantation. Individuals with antibodies often do not receive grafts; if a patient develops HLA antibodies after transfusion, this can be considered an indication of heightened responsiveness that might otherwise have become apparent only when the graft was rejected. If antibody formers do not receive grafts, the number of procedures with unfavorable outcome will decline. Those patients who do not develop antibodies would be precisely those in whom the graft is destined for better survival.

Unrelated to this selection effect is immunomodulation that occurs after contact with allogeneic material. Alloantigens in transfused blood seem to exert a generalized immunosuppressive effect that is widely acknowledged but difficult to define. Suggested mechanisms include stimulation of suppressor-cell clones or induction of antibodies that block either antigen recognition or communication among cell populations.

——— BONE MARROW TRANSPLANTATION ———

Transplanting bone marrow has consequences different from those of most other grafts. A successful graft does not merely replace a defective organ; it introduces an active population of immunologically unique cells into a recipient with different constitution. Marrow grafts were initially used to treat aplastic anemia, global immunodeficiency syndromes, or leukemias refractory to other therapy. With increasingly successful transplant techniques, the number of potential indications has widened to include a variety of enzyme-deficiency conditions and hematologic dysplasias.

DONOR SELECTION

HLA matching is more important for marrow transplant than for any other tissue. Until recently, only HLA-identical siblings were considered suitable donors, a restriction that made many patients ineligible for this form of treatment. Better immunosuppressive techniques now permit cautious use of one-haplotype matched relatives, opening the donor pool to parents and many additional siblings, and also use of HLA-matched unrelated individuals. Antibodies against donor ABO antigens can be removed by plasmapheresis; the profound immunosuppression used before marrow grafting prevents recrudescence of the recipient's anti-A or anti-B.

Bone marrow is renewable; the donor loses only a finite number of aspirated cells, not the solid mass of an irreplaceable organ. Approximately 20 percent of functioning marrow is removed from an adult, and this can be regenerated within a couple of months. Because donation creates no permanent deficiency, marrow donors can come from a wide range of size, age, and health status.

AUTOLOGOUS DONATION

Autologous transplantation is practical because bone marrow can be collected under optimal clinical conditions and be stored frozen for weeks or months with only moderate cell loss. Autologous marrow replacement is especially useful in treating non-hematologic malignancies. For such tumors as gonadal, breast, and certain lung cancers, permanent cure can be achieved by intensive radiotherapy and chemotherapy that destroys all traces of tumor; cytotoxic therapy of this magnitude also permanently destroys hematopoietic marrow. Provided the marrow does not harbor tumor, a generous hematopoietic specimen can be harvested before therapy begins. When the cytotoxic regimen is completed, the preserved hematopoietic elements are reinjected to replace blood-forming tissue destroyed by the ablative therapy.

Autologous marrow grafts can even be used in treating leukemia. If initial treatment produces complete blood and marrow remission, an aliquot of this restored normal marrow can be frozen for use if relapse occurs later. The relapse can be treated by intensive therapy intended to eliminate from the body every last, lingering malignant cell, and the non-malignant autologous marrow can then be infused to reconstitute the system. Besides the problems of infection and bleeding that inevitably accompany marrow ablation, this procedure carries the risk that undetected malignant cells may be present in the marrow retrieved during apparent remission.

CONDITIONING FOR ALLOGENEIC MARROW TRANSPLANTS

Before a patient receives allogeneic marrow, it is necessary to eliminate all existing marrow elements and to destroy immune capability. In autologous grafting, postgraft immunosuppression is unnecessary, but the need to eliminate all hematopoietic elements remains. More intense and complete immunosuppression is needed for allogeneic marrow than for grafts of other tissue, to avoid coexistence of residual host immunity along with activity derived from the transplanted allogeneic material. It is customary to use both radiotherapy and chemotherapy for several days before grafting is attempted.

The pregraft conditioning regimen leaves the patient with no immune, inflammatory, or hematologic resources. Red cells normally remain in the circulation for several months, so patients retain modest oxygen-carrying capacity after acute marrow destruction, but platelets and neutrophils drop to zero and remain absent until the grafted marrow establishes itself. This leaves the patient extremely susceptible to infection and bleeding. Prophylactic platelet transfusions are useful in preventing spontaneous bleeding, and potent antibiotics must be given to protect against infection. Neutrophils reappear within 2 to 4 weeks if the graft is successful, but platelets take much longer to achieve effective levels.

Immunomodulation with red-cell transfusion is not used before marrow grafting. Most patients have conditions for which they have already received many randomly selected transfusions, and donor-specific transfusion is risky because it might sensitize the recipients to antigens of the only suitable donor. Immune conditioning is not really needed, because the recipient's immune tissue is destroyed before the allogeneic material is introduced.

GRAFT-VERSUS-HOST DISEASE

The short-term risks of marrow transplantation are infection and bleeding. The most serious long-term complication of marrow transplantation is **graft-versus-host disease** (GVHD), in which immunocompetent cells from the donor recognize host antigens as foreign and attack the host tissues. Graft-versus-host disease can occur whenever viable T cells are transplanted into a recipient who is profoundly immunodeficient. Graft recipients who are only partially immunosuppressed retain capacity to recognize and to eliminate potentially aggressive donor T cells. For most transplants the goal is to preserve as much immune capacity as possible, but in bone marrow grafting, the recipient is deliberately and explicitly rendered unresponsive.

Because GVHD occurs after grafts from an HLA-identical sibling, it appears that HLA antigens are not the major target. Engrafted viable T cells initiate the process, but antibodies, macrophages, and natural killer cells may also have effector roles. Graft-versus-host disease can be either acute or chronic; although chronic changes may follow acute manifestations, the processes are different, and either can occur independently.

Clinical Events

Acute GVHD begins in the first few weeks after transplantation and lasts for several months, affecting most severely the gastrointestinal (GI) tract and the skin, along with the liver. Intractable diarrhea, necrotizing skin lesions, and depressed hepatic function occur in the most severe cases, and susceptibility to infection increases. Immunosuppressive therapy is variably effective in reversing the process. Eliminating viable T cells from the grafted material has been attempted as a way to prevent acute GVHD, but this has not demonstrably prolonged patients' survival.

Of graft recipients who survive for 3 months or longer, up to 50 percent suffer from **chronic GVHD,** which causes a kind of gradual damage to skin, joints, and mucous membranes that resembles the changes seen in autoimmune collagen-vascular diseases. Indolent liver damage is common, but the most conspicuous problem is progressive loss of immune defense. The number of suppressor T cells increases, and both humoral and cell-mediated functions decline, leaving the patient excessively vulnerable to both pathogenic and opportunistic organisms. The same agents used to treat autoimmune conditions are used, with varying degrees of success, for chronic GVHD.

Survival studies of leukemic patients treated with marrow transplants indicate that patients who experience chronic GVHD have fewer disease recurrences than those without this immune complication. Leukemic complications, graft rejection, and inappropriate lymphoproliferative responses to viral infection occur more often when allografts have been treated to eliminate T cells than when unmodified grafts are used. An aphorism summarizing these observations is that allogeneic marrow exerts a "graft-versus-leukemia" effect.

SUGGESTIONS FOR FURTHER READING

Bach FH, Sachs DH: Transplantation immunology. N Engl J Med 1987; 317:489–92

Cerilli J: Current trends in histocompatibility: clinical relevance versus laboratory phenomena. Am J Surg 1986; 151:716–21

Garovoy MR, Melzer JS, Gibbs VC, Bozdech M: Clinical transplantation. In: Stites DP, Stobo JD, Wells JV, eds. Basic and Clinical Immunology, 6th ed. Norwalk, CT: Appleton and Lange, 1987:420–34

Hao L, Wang Y, Gill RG, Lafferty KJ: CD4 T cells and allograft rejection. Transplant Proc 1988; 20:56–60

Keown PA, Stiller CR: Cyclosporine: a double-edged sword. Hosp Pract 1987; 22 (issue 5):207–20

Kerman RH: Effects of cyclosporine on the alloimmune response in vivo. Transplant Proc 1988; 20 (Suppl 2):143–52

Loveland B, Simpson E: The non-MHC transplantation antigens: neither weak nor minor. Immunol Today 1986; 7:223–28

Sanfilippo F, Amos DB: An interpretation of the major histocompatibility complex. In: Rose NR, Friedman H, Fahey JL, eds. Manual of Clinical Laboratory Immunology, 3rd ed. Washington, DC: American Society for Microbiology, 1986;874–80

Storb R: Graft-versus-host disease after marrow transplantation. In: Meryman HT, ed. Transplantation: Approaches to Graft Rejection. New York: Alan R Liss, 1986:139–56

Strom TB: The cellular and molecular basis of allograft rejection: What do we know? Transplant Proc 1988: 20:143–46

Williams GM: Transplant rejection: an overview from the clinical perspective. In: Meryman HT, ed. Transplantation: Approaches to Graft Rejection. New York: Alan R Liss, 1986:1–8

PART THREE

Laboratory Applications

CHAPTER 14

General Principles

END POINTS
 The Primary Immune
  Phenomenon
 Equivalence and Zone
  Phenomena
 Secondary Immune Reactions
 Tertiary Phenomena

MANIPULATING END POINTS
 Labeling Proteins
 Antibodies to Antibodies
 Separation Techniques
 Inhibiting an Indicator Reaction

With antibodies of suitable specificities, immune-mediated reactions can be exploited to measure innumerable materials. Ingenious applications of antigen-antibody interactions have long been used in analysis of chemical, physical, and clinical phenomena; the uniquely focused antibodies now available with monoclonal techniques have enormously expanded the information available through immunologic testing.

END POINTS

The end point of a test must signal occurrence and/or magnitude of the event under investigation. The simplest form of observation is enumeration: counting, weighing, or measuring. Magnification, fixation, denaturation, or staining of the target material often facilitates observation and quantification, but these manipulations distort evaluation of dynamic events. It is important that an end point reflect the interaction under study in a specific and unambiguous fashion, free of positive or negative artifacts. In immunologic tests, the fundamental concerns must be specificity of antigen-antibody recognition and stability of the reactants and the resulting complexes. These chapters cannot describe procedures for developing, concentrating, purifying, and evaluating reagent antibodies; the laboratory worker must, however, scrutinize the credentials of reagent antibodies before accepting results based upon them. Biologic materials like antibodies, enzymes, or proteins of any kind must be continuously monitored for expected potency, purity, and behavior.

Kinds of Observations

Immune reactions are conventionally classified as revealing primary, secondary, or tertiary phenomena. **Primary** immune phenomena involve only antibody molecule and the reactive epitope of antigen; they occur independently of any subsequent biochemical or biologic events. **Secondary** reactions reflect the physical and biologic state of the material that expresses the antigen, and the conditions in which the reaction occurs. These include phenomena like precipitation, agglutination, and complement activation, and such sequelae as cell lysis, cytotoxicity, and toxin neutralization. **Tertiary** manifestations occur in an intact host; these include such biologic phenomena as inflammation, vascular deposition of immune complexes, or enhancement of cellular function. In tertiary events, the *in vivo* interaction of antibody and antigen is modified not only by the biologic form of the reactants but also by variables of health and function in the host.

Tests that exploit immune interactions often use end points common to other laboratory tests, such as measuring transmitted, reflected, or scattered light; measuring physical properties like color, size, viscosity, or pressure; observing and quantifying movement; and quantifying electrical charge or radioactivity. Some procedures, however, employ techniques that directly reflect properties of the immune reactants.

THE PRIMARY IMMUNE
PHENOMENON

Union between antigen-binding (Fab) sites of antibody and individual epitopes of antigen is the primary phenomenon upon which all immune events depend. When antigen is part of a complex molecular or cellular entity, secondary phenomena may obscure the effects of the primary antigen-antibody encounter. Primary phenomena are best studied with a pure preparation of antibody and a preparation of soluble antigen that expresses only one active epitope. In a soluble system of this sort, union of antigen and antibody produces no readily detectable event, so the reactants must be manipulated to provide an indicator.

A classical procedure for demonstrating formation of soluble antigen-antibody complexes employs an agent, like ammonium sulfate or polyethylene glycol, that precipitates the combined complex but leaves the uncombined reactants in solution. More recent techniques label individual reactants in ways that allow distinction between bound and unbound material. These techniques are discussed in the chapter on receptor-ligand testing.

Association of Antigen and Antibody

Union of Fab site and epitope results from non-covalent bonds; these are much weaker than the covalent bonds that join amino acids into polypeptides, or sulfur-containing moieties into disulfide bonds. Distance between the reacting materials markedly affects non-covalent bonds; infinitesimally small differences in proximity significantly alter the strength of association. This is why the reciprocal configurations of antigen and antibody are so important. If the shapes fit together in a perfect lock-and-key relationship, all parts of both molecules have optimal proximity, so affinity is maximal. Shape changes induced by altered structure or by physical modification significantly diminish these bonds.

The attraction between the two molecules depends not only on configurational fit but also on intrinsic properties of the antibody. The binding forces between Fab site of an antibody molecule and its corresponding epitope are denoted by the term **affinity**. Except for monoclonal products, antibody preparations contain immunoglobulin molecules synthesized by a variety of individual cells; individual molecules exhibit different binding properties and respond somewhat differently to external events. The cumulative total of all attractive forces between antigen and the antibody molecules present in a specimen is described as the **avidity** of the serum.

Forces of Attraction

Many physical forces influence affinity of Fab site for antigen. Conspicuous among these are **van der Waals** forces, in which the presence of electrical fields in one molecule modifies electron distribution in another molecule, creating a reciprocal electrical field with attraction of opposite charges. **Electrostatic** forces depend on the attraction of opposites that occurs when molecules exist in ionized form at the pH of the medium, for example, NH_3^+ and COO^-. **Hydrogen bonding** depends upon attraction between electropositive and electronegative atoms present in the reactive site. **Hydrophobic bonds** arise from the properties of amino acids, which expel molecules of solvent water as they approach one another, generating an increment of energy that keeps the amino acids close to one another. The primary determinant of affinity is the molecular structure of the Fab site; the attractive forces described above vary in strength with changes in pH, in ionic strength of the medium, in temperature, and in the nature of the solvent.

Consequences of Interaction

To detect occurrence of the primary interaction, it is necessary to know the precise starting concentrations of antigen and antibody and to correlate the disappearance of free material with the consequent increase in combined product. Relative concentration of antigen and antibody do not affect the primary immune event; the concentrations of antigen, antibody, and combined complexes may, however, affect the means of detecting the reaction.

Some measuring techniques lose accuracy or sensitivity at different concentrations. **Precipitation** is the end point most significantly affected by the starting concentration of antigen and antibody. Strictly speaking, precipitation is a secondary immune phenomenon, but many antigens can be studied only in macromolecular form, and macromolecules often form precipitates after combination with antibody. The conditions that influence precipitation have been systematized into the quantitative principle of **equivalence**.

EQUIVALENCE AND ZONE PHENOMENA

When soluble antibody reacts with soluble antigen, the resulting immune complexes vary in size. The simplest complex is union of two separate hapten molecules with the two Fab sites of an immunoglobulin monomer. The antibody molecule remains discrete because it has no attachment, through shared antigen units, to any other Ig molecule. If a single antigen molecule expresses the same epitope at several sites, one epitope may combine with the Fab site of one Ig monomer, whereas another unites with the Fab of a separate molecule. Attachment to the same macromolecular expresssion of antigen brings two or more antibody molecules into complexes that contain both reactants. Very small complexes tend to remain in solution, undetectable by visual inspection. If numerous antigens and Fab sites combine, this generates a lattice of alternating antigens and antibodies that becomes too large to remain in solution. **Precipitation** means the formation of insoluble immune complexes after interaction between soluble antigen and soluble antibody. The size of the complex determines whether or not the precipitate becomes visible.

Excess of Antigen or Antibody

If antigen in preparations of varying concentration is added to multiple aliquots of antibody at a single concentration, precipitation characteristically occurs in the middle concentration range; little visible precipitate accumulates at low concentrations of antigen or with highly concentrated antigen. The specificity of configurations re-

ANTIGEN-ANTIBODY PROPORTIONS
AFFECT PRECIPITATION

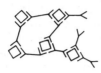

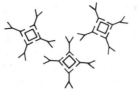

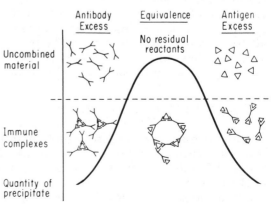

Maximum precipitation
at equivalence of
antigen and antibody

In antibody excess,
precipitates do not form

In antigen excess,
precipitation is scanty,
may be difficult to detect

FIGURE 14–1. Precipitation is greatest when antigen and antibody are present in approximately equal concentration, as shown on the left. At less than optimal proportions, shown in the other drawings, antigen-antibody reactions occur but produce much less visible precipitate.

mains the same, and epitopes continue to combine with Fab sites, but the size of the resulting immune complexes reflects concentration of the reacting materials (Fig. 14–1). With dilute antigen, there is **antibody excess,** and lattice formation is minimal because individual monomers compete for the few antigen epitopes available. When the number of multivalent antigen sites and divalent antibody molecules is approximately equal, lattice formation is optimal and visible precipitation occurs. As antigen concentration increases to a state of **antigen excess,** lattice formation again declines because relatively few antigen macromolecules succeed in simultaneously engaging several different antibody molecules. The relative concentration at which there is maximal lattice formation and minimal residual uncombined material is called the **zone of equivalence** (Fig. 14–2).

FIGURE 14–2. The curve shows the quantity of visible precipitate formed at differing concentrations of antigen and antibody. Residual uncomplexed material, depicted above the dotted line, comprises either antibody molecules or antigen epitopes when unequal proportions of reactants are in the starting material. Shown below the dotted line is the relative size of the immune complexes formed under differing conditions.

PRECIPITIN CURVE

Detecting Reactions

In experimental settings, absence of visible end point occurs more frequently with antibody excess than with antigen excess. When antibody in different concentrations is tested against a constant preparation of antigen, results are often negative when concentrated or unmodified antibody is used; if the antibody is diluted before addition to the standard antigen, precipitation promptly develops. Inhibition of visible end point by excess antibody is often called the **prozone** phenomenon. The reverse situation—failure to obtain a positive result until antigen is diluted—occurs much less frequently. Some workers use an analogous term, **postzone** phenomenon, to describe inhibition by antigen excess.

It is important to remember that absence of visible end point does not mean absence of immune reactivity. It is often possible to demonstrate that free antibody and free antigen have united to form immune complexes by showing reduced levels of unbound molecules. This requires removal of the complexed materials, so that remaining free reactant can be measured. In a prozone, uncomplexed antibody molecules are the residual reactant; in antigen excess, the suspending medium will contain unbound antigen but no antibody molecules.

SECONDARY IMMUNE REACTIONS

Formation of an antigen-antibody complex characteristically alters the physical, chemical, or immunoreactive state of the starting materials. Precipitation of insoluble immune complexes is the simplest such end point. Analogous to precipitation is **agglutination,** in which a lattice forms between soluble antibody and an antigen present in particulate form (Fig. 14–3). When Fab sites of several antibody molecules combine with antigens present on several particles, the resulting lattice brings the particles together into readily detectable clumps called **agglutinates**. Although this end point is affected by variables of antibody activity, particle composition, reaction conditions, and properties of the suspending medium, the size of the agglutinates reflects, in a crude fashion, the intensity of the antigen-antibody reaction. Proportions between antibody and antigen are much less critical for agglutination than for precipitation.

Applications of Agglutination

Agglutination is a more sensitive indicator system than precipitation, generating visible reactions at much lower antibody concentrations. It is often useful to convert a test system from precipitation to agglutination in order to exploit this increased sensitivity. A known preparation of either antibody or antigen can be coupled to inert particles, which are then tested against the unknown in soluble form. A

PRECIPITATION

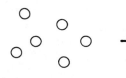 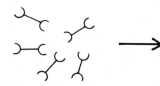 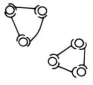

| Soluble antigen | Soluble antibody | Small, insoluble complexes form precipitate |

AGGLUTINATION

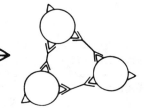

Particles with surface antigen   Soluble antibody   Particles are linked into readily visible agglutinates

FIGURE 14–3. As shown in the lower panel, agglutination involves particulate antigens, which are much larger than soluble molecules. When a lattice develops, the resulting complexes are larger and more easily detected than the macromolecules that constitute the precipitation end point, depicted in the upper panel.

combination of soluble unknown and solid-phase reagent forms agglutinates that give a readily detected end point. Soluble antigen and soluble antibody can also be manipulated to inhibit previously demonstrated agglutination, a variant procedure called **agglutination inhibition**. Laboratory tests based on precipitation are discussed in detail in chapter 15, and those based on agglutination in chapter 16.

Complement as an Indicator

Complement activation is a secondary phenomenon quite different from agglutination or precipitation. A complement-activating antibody must unite with its antigen before the first component of complement (C1) enters the recognition phase of the classical pathway. Complement activation, which can be documented in several different ways (see chapter 17), then serves as the indicator that the antigen-antibody reaction has occurred.

Measuring Reactants

Demonstrating disappearance, inactivation, or consumption of starting materials is another way to determine that antigen and antibody have combined. The antibody molecules do not disappear, but if their Fab sites have combined with antigen, no reactive markers remain to be measured. Antigenic material does disappear, in a functional sense; enclosure within Fab sites prevents interaction with other molecules of the same antibody. Molecules, cells, or particles may have numerous different epitopes, however, so that antigenic material fully combined with antibody of one specificity may remain accessible to antibodies that recognize other configurations.

TERTIARY PHENOMENA

Physiologic events initiated by reaction of antigen with antibody are considered tertiary immune reactions. Complement activation is a secondary event, but the phagocytic or inflammatory changes that follow in the living host are tertiary manifestations. Early immunologic tests used tertiary effects as end points because techniques to dissect and to demonstrate the initiating events were lacking. Examples of these observations include the skin changes used to demonstrate combination of cell-bound IgE with its antigen; and opsonic enhancement of phagocytosis in the presence of antibody to a specific organism. Biologic assays in current laboratory use include skin tests to demonstrate tuberculin-type cell-mediated immunity, several kinds of allergy tests, and administration of virulent organisms as a challenge to immunity induced in experimental animals.

─────── MANIPULATING END POINTS ───────

The remainder of this chapter describes, in general terms, some ways to enhance end points. If an immune reaction does not spontaneously generate a detectable secondary phenomenon, there is no immediate way to determine whether or not the reaction has occurred (Fig. 14–4).

LABELING PROTEINS

Proteins are complex molecules that can undergo independent interactions that involve different parts of the molecule; material can of-

IMMUNE INTERACTION
WITHOUT VISIBLE ENDPOINT

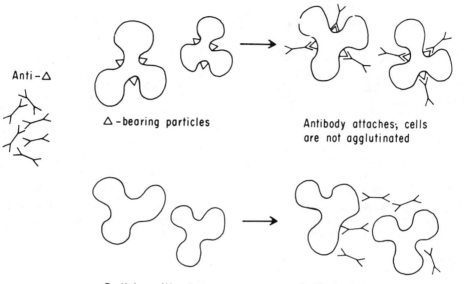

FIGURE 14–4. In the upper drawings, a specific antigen-antibody reaction has occurred, whereas in the lower drawings the antibody has not encountered its specific antigen. The steric configuration of the reactants is such, however, that both events have the same result: no visible change in the suspended material.

ten be added to or removed from a protein without affecting its remaining attributes. In laboratory immunology, antigens or antibodies can be labeled in ways that leave immune reactivity intact. Chemical stains are labels for denatured proteins; stains are useful in identifying location or intensity of an immune reaction after it has occurred but are unsuitable for ongoing reactions. Attaching a radioactive, enzymatic, or fluorescent label, however, marks the protein without interfering with reactivity (Fig. 14–5). The bond must be firm enough that label does not detach but gentle enough that the target protein is not altered. The labels most commonly used are radioisotopes, fluorescent compounds, and enzymes.

Major Forms of Labeling

Radioisotopes used as labels must emit levels of radioactivity susceptible to prompt and precise quantification but harmless to laboratory workers. Sometimes a radioisotope is substituted for an ele-

DETECTING AN END POINT

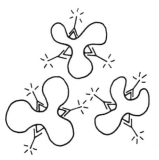

Antibody attachment
produces no
visible end point

Labeled antibody can
be detected by radio-
activity, fluorescence, etc.

FIGURE 14–5. Labeling the antibody molecules makes it possible to demonstrate whether or not antigen-antibody attachment has occurred in circumstances that produce no detectable secondary phenomenon.

ment in the natural molecule, such as ^{125}Iodine (^{125}I) in thyroid studies or ^{51}Cobalt (^{51}Co) in vitamin B_{12}; more often, an unrelated radionuclide is conjugated to the native compound. Most commonly used for proteins is ^{125}I, which binds to the amino acid tyrosine without affecting chemical or immunologic reactivity. Provided all molecules are uniformly labeled, counting radioactivity directly quantifies the amount of labeled protein present.

Fluorescence labeling is comparable, but uses a different physical principle for the end point. Compounds called **fluorochromes** experience excitation after absorbing light at certain wave lengths; excitation causes the substance to emit light at a different wave length, detectable with appropriate optical equipment. Fluorochromes can be bound to soluble proteins or to proteins on cells or other biologic surfaces.

A relatively new approach is labeling proteins with **enzyme** molecules, for measurement in multistage assays. The indicator enzyme must retain activity when conjugated to the immunologically reactive proteins. Once the enzyme-labeled material has completed its immune activities, substrate for the enzyme is added to the system; the still-active enzyme acts upon substrate to generate a measurable product. The concentration of product is directly proportional to the amount of enzyme, which is proportional to the amount of labeled immune reactant present (Fig. 14–6). Enzyme labeling avoids the problems of radioactive waste disposal, or of maintaining expensive equipment to count radioactivity or to measure fluorescence.

ENZYME AS INDICATOR

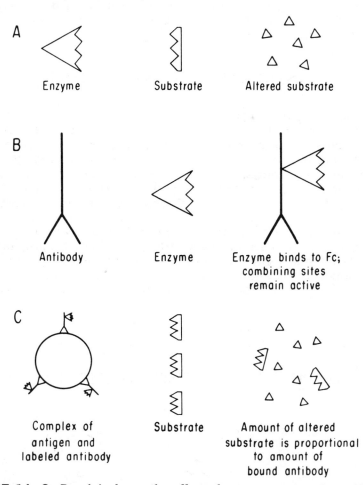

FIGURE 14—6. Panel A shows the effect of active enzyme on its substrate. Enzyme can be linked to an antibody molecule without altering the activity of either protein, as shown in panel B. When substrate is added to a system containing enzyme-labeled antibody, as shown in C, alteration of the substrate occurs at a level proportional to the number of enzyme-labeled antibody molecules present.

Overcoming Solubility

Measurement may be easier if proteins undergo alteration of physical state. Small individual molecules may be invisible in suspension but are readily observed if aggregated into a multimolecular mass. Another approach is to convert soluble molecules into solid phase by adsorbing them to an inert carrier surface. Tanned red cells; particles of various polymers; and the walls of tubes, plates, or wells are useful for this purpose.

ANTIBODIES TO ANTIBODIES

Antibodies against antibodies open an entirely new way to study immune events. Antibodies are proteins; proteins are excellent antigens; proteins from one species engender antibodies when injected into members of another species. Early workers injected whole human serum into rabbits, goats, and other animals, raising serum with a wide but unpredictable range of antihuman protein activity. Antihuman serum is often called **Coombs' serum,** in recognition of work done in the 1940s by Coombs and his coworkers in England. Subsequent refinements in processing antigen and in purifying and concentrating antibodies have allowed preparation of highly targeted antibodies against individual proteins and fractions of proteins. Especially important in analytical procedures are antiserums against individual classes and subclasses of immunoglobulins; against light

AGGLUTINATION OF ANTIBODY-COATED CELLS

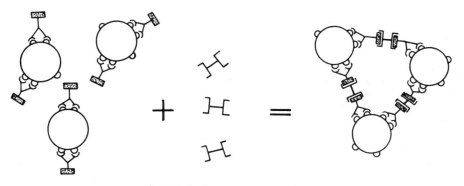

Antiglobulin serum reacts
with Fc of antibody

FIGURE 14–7. Combination of antibody with cell-surface antigens may leave the cells coated with antibody but freely suspended in the medium. Antibody againt Fc of the coating antibody links the bound immunoglobulin molecules and brings the underlying cells together into visible agglutinates.

chains, heavy chains, and portions thereof; and against the effector and regulator proteins of the complement system. Anti-idiotype antibodies are the ultimate refinement; they react with the antigen-specific portion of individual antibodies.

Antiantibody antibodies, called **antiglobulins,** find numerous uses. The earliest antiglobulin procedures were used in red-cell serology to induce visible agglutination after attachment of non-agglutinating antibody to surface antigens of red cells (Fig. 14–7). Antiglobulin antibodies can be used to identify immune precipitates dispersed in fluid, gel, or solid mediums. Fluorescence-labeled antiglobulins localize attachment of antibodies to various tissue sites in microscopic sections and to the surface of individual cells. Radio-labeled or enzyme-labeled antiglobulin antibodies are used in receptor-ligand assays for a wide variety of substances.

SEPARATION TECHNIQUES

Nature rarely provides materials in purified, concentrated form. Biologic specimens contain numerous components; specific assays attempt to measure individual constituents. It may be necessary to separate antigens from a diverse mixture, or to isolate antibodies from a multispecific serum, or to separate materials so that individual elements can be quantified. Many techniques for separating molecules are based on physical properties, including such procedures as ultracentrifugation, molecular sieving, and dialysis. **Electrophoresis** separates proteins according to their migration through an electrical field. The size, shape, and net charge of a protein determine the rate and direction at which it travels through a charged medium (see Fig. 6–3). Movement can be modified by altering the suspending medium or the duration, direction, and intensity of the current.

Antigen-antibody reactions can perform highly targeted separation procedures. Diverse mixtures can be separated by introducing an antigen or antibody that complexes with a single material. The resulting complex usually has different properties from the remaining materials and can be separated by physical manipulation, such as precipitation, filtration, or differential mobility. Antibody can be used to capture an antigen, or antigen can be introduced to isolate a specific immunoglobulin. Centrifugation and filtration are simple ways to separate immune complexes that have precipitated or agglutinated (Fig. 14–8). Adsorption is the separation procedure used in **affinity chromatography**. The reagent is immobilized on a solid-phase preparation, and the mixed solution is passed across the system; if concentrations and flow rate are appropriate, the immobilized agent captures its target material. The depleted effluent and/or the captured material can be subjected to further manipulation for isolation, concentration, or quantification (Fig. 14–9).

AGGLUTINATION USED TO
SEPARATE MIXED ANTIBODIES

 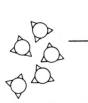 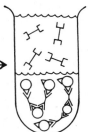

Mixture of   Particles with
antibodies   single specificity   Supernatant contains
                                          unattached antibody

FIGURE 14–8. Particles that express a single antigen can be used to separate specificities in a mixture of antibodies. The relevant antibody will link the particles into agglutinates, which can be removed from the medium by centrifugation; uncombined antibody remains in the supernatant fluid. The bound antibody can be harvested from the agglutinated material by subsequent manipulation.

ADSORPTION USED TO
SEPARATE MIXED ANTIGENS

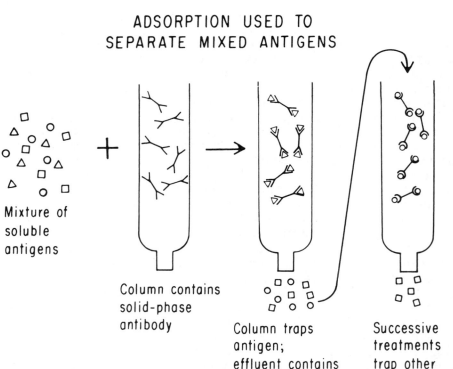

Mixture of
soluble
antigens

Column contains
solid-phase
antibody

Column traps
antigen;
effluent contains
unaffected antigens

Successive
treatments
trap other
specificities

FIGURE 14–9. When a mixed solution of antigens encounters an immobilized antibody specific for a single constituent, molecules of that antigen remain trapped, while the unaffected materials remain in solution. Columns containing antibodies against additional solutes can isolate other material from the effluent fluid.

VIRUS NEUTRALIZATION DEMONSTRATES
PRESENCE OF ANTIBODY

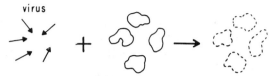

Virus infects, damages cells

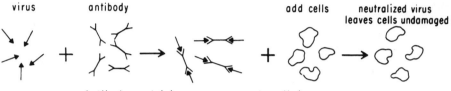

Antibody-containing serum prevents cell damage

FIGURE 14–10. The upper panel shows the damage that native virus inflicts on target cells. In the lower panel, incubation with antibody-containing serum neutralizes the virus and prevents it from damaging indicator cells added to the incubated mixture.

INHIBITING AN INDICATOR REACTION

Formation of soluble antigen-antibody complexes can be demonstrated through removal of material needed for an indicator reaction that has previously been standardized. Assays of this sort, called **neutralization** or **inhibition,** are useful end points in microbiology and in studying soluble antigens and antibodies. For example, a virus may consistently infect and kill cells under appropriate culture conditions. To demonstrate whether serum contains antiviral antibody, one aliquot of virus is incubated with the test serum and another with a control serum known to be inert. Test and control materials are then inoculated into preparations of sensitive cells. If the virus incubated with inert serum continues to kill the cells but incubation with test serum renders the virus harmless, the presence of antivirus antibody can be inferred (Fig. 14–10).

Inhibitory assays are useful when the test material is in soluble form or when an antibody reacts preferentially with non-particulate forms of the antigen. Many antibodies react more rapidly with soluble antigen than with the same material on a cell surface—a property that can be exploited to demonstrate presence of the soluble material in a test solution. The indicator system employs agglutination, at predetermined intensity, of antigen-coated particles. If incubation with the test material abolishes the agglutinating activity of the antibody, presence of soluble antigen has been demonstrated.

SUGGESTIONS FOR FURTHER READING

Larsen J, Odell WD: General principles of radioimmunoassay. In: Rose NR, Friedman H, Fahey JL, eds: Manual of Clinical Laboratory Immunology, 3rd ed. Washington DC: American Society for Microbiology, 1986:110–15.

Stites DP, Rodgers RPC: Clinical laboratory methods for detection of antigens and antibodies. In: Stites DP, Stobo JD, Wells JV, eds.: Basic and Clinical Immunology, 6th ed. Norwalk, CT: Appleton and Lange, 1987:241–84

CHAPTER 15

Laboratory Procedures Based on Precipitation

The union of soluble antibody with its specific antigen forms an immune complex that may or may not be apparent as a visible end point. One end point susceptible to observation and measurement is **precipitation** of insoluble immune complexes. Many factors affect precipitation of the immune complex; the relative concentration of antigen and antibody is the most significant, but the solvent medium is also important.

PHYSICAL ASPECTS OF PRECIPITATION

As the Fab sites of one or more antibody molecules join several molecules of antigen, the resulting lattice incorporates both participants. The initial state of antigen and antibody, the medium in which they are suspended, and the size of the complex that evolves determine whether or not the precipitate becomes visible.

EQUIVALENCE

When antibody molecules greatly outnumber antigen molecules, many antibody molecules remain uncombined, and each antigen unit binds so many antibody molecules that little crosslinking occurs. Complexes containing far more antibody than antigen are usually too small to precipitate. As antigen and antibody approach equivalent concentrations, the number and size of immune complexes increase to levels associated with visible precipitation. If antigen concentration continues to increase, the reverse phenomenon occurs; individual antibody molecules become so saturated with antigen that small or incomplete lattices form. The curve relating concentration and precipitation is parabolic, with maximum precipitation occurring at the point of equivalence (see Fig. 14–2). Analytic techniques exploit this quantitative relationship by controlling concentration of the known reagent material and measuring precipitation as a reflection of the unknown reactant.

Soluble antigen and soluble antibody that diffuse toward one another through an inert medium create their own zone of equivalence. As solutions of the materials diffuse from highly concentrated starting locations, precipitate forms where optimum concentration is achieved. Early immunologists layered solutions directly upon each other, generating a ring of precipitate called a **precipitin line** at or near the interface (Fig. 15–1). An unsupported ring at a fluid interface is easily disrupted and is difficult to observe and to quantify. Current precipitation methods incorporate the materials in a supporting medium such as agarose gel or cellulose acetate, or measure the precipitated material as it is dispersed in the medium.

MODIFYING CONDITIONS

The nature of the supporting medium and the physical properties of the reactants affect diffusion. From a well cut into a gel, a solution diffuses outward in a 360-degree arc (Fig. 15–2). Smaller molecules diffuse more rapidly than larger ones in the same gel; the viscosity,

PRECIPITIN RING WITH
ONE-DIMENSIONAL DIFFUSION

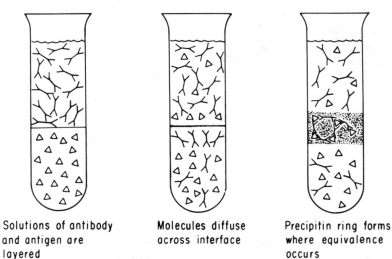

| Solutions of antibody and antigen are layered | Molecules diffuse across interface | Precipitin ring forms where equivalence occurs |

FIGURE 15—1. From left to right, antigen and antibody molecules in the layered solutions are shown diffusing toward one another. Where proportions are optimal, a ring of visible precipitate forms, usually at or near the interface between the solutions.

molecular size, hydration, and chemical composition of the gel affect the rate of diffusion. When solutions of antigen and antibody are simultaneously placed in suitably located wells, the outwardly moving molecules encounter each other, and immune complexes precipitate at the equivalence zone (Fig. 15—3). The size and intensity of the precipitin line reflect the quantity of precipitated immune complex. If the materials diffuse from wells of equal size, the precipitin line will be

MOLECULES DIFFUSE
THROUGH A GEL

FIGURE 15—2. The diagram on the left shows molecules in a highly concentrated solution beginning to diffuse from a central well into the surrounding gel. With the passage of time, all parts of the gel contain equal numbers of solute molecules, shown on the right.

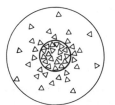

Molecules begin to diffuse from well into gel

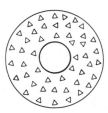

Eventually, molecules are evenly dispersed throughout gel

Antigen   Antibody

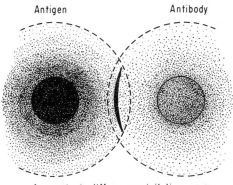

As reactants diffuse, precipitation occurs
where equivalence is reached

FIGURE 15–3. When solutions of antigen and antibody are placed in adjacent wells, molecules diffuse into the surrounding gel in all directions. Where the molecules encounter one another in optimal proportions, precipitation occurs, and a precipitin line is seen between the two wells.

arc shaped, concave to the well from which diffusion was slower. Higher molecular weight or lower concentration may slow diffusion rate (Fig. 15–4). Diffusion can be accelerated or slowed by modifying the supporting medium or by altering such physical conditions as electrical charge or temperature.

MOLECULAR SIZE AND CONCENTRATION AFFECT DIFFUSION RATE

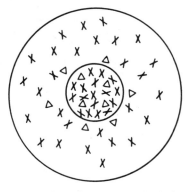

In a limited time, concentrated material moves farther than less concentrated material

In a limited time, smaller molecules move more rapidly than larger ones

FIGURE 15–4. If the central well contains a mixture of materials, shown on the left, the more concentrated material will travel through the gel more rapidly. In a mixture of small and large molecules, shown on the right, the smaller molecules reach the periphery more rapidly than the larger ones.

Significant Variables

Different materials diffuse at different rates. Proteins vary in size, charge, substituted side groups, and three-dimensional configurations, all of which affect their physical and immunochemical properties. All antibodies are immunoglobulins; despite differences in size and valence, they share many physical characteristics. Antigenic materials, on the other hand, embody a wide range of size, chemical composition, and reactive characteristics. Further variation may occur if reagents undergo changes in state; in some techniques, reagent properties are deliberately manipulated, but sometimes physical alterations occur unexpectedly and give results that do not reflect true analytic conditions. The nature and location of a precipitin end point must be evaluated in light of these considerations.

Diffusion Systems

Diffusion is a dynamic process; equilibrium is reached when solute molecules are uniformly dispersed throughout the medium. After antigen and antibody meet at the zone of equivalence, molecules continue to diffuse and to change the concentrations of both reactants. This can cause the quantity of precipitate to diminish or to disappear, so tests based on precipitation in gels must be read within a realistic time frame.

Analytical techniques that exploit diffusion can be classified as **single** or **double**. In **single diffusion,** the supporting medium contains one reactant at a uniform concentration, so only the added unknown manifests changing concentrations. Usually antibody is uniformly distributed, so diffusion of antigen molecules determines the location and intensity of the precipitate. In **double diffusion,** the gel is inert and both antigen and antibody molecules travel through the medium.

DOUBLE DIFFUSION

The earliest immunodiffusion procedure to enjoy wide use was developed by Ouchterlony and continues to bear his name. Although more rapid and more quantitative techniques have replaced it for many analytic procedures, it remains an important investigative tool.

OUCHTERLONY DOUBLE DIFFUSION

In the simplest double diffusion system, antigen and antibody solutions are placed in wells cut into an immunologically inert gel; as

DOUBLE DIFFUSION DEMONSTRATES
CONCENTRATION

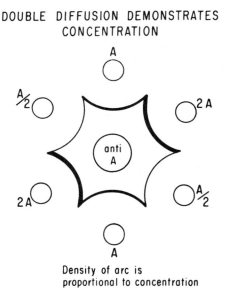

Density of arc is
proportional to concentration

FIGURE 15–5. With a constant antibody level, quantity of precipitate is proportional to the concentration of antigen. The peripheral wells shown above contain a single antigen at different concentrations. The precipitin arcs for the lowest concentration, A/2, are half as dense as those for A, which in turn are half as dense as those for the doubled concentration shown as 2A.

the molecules diffuse radially, a precipitin line forms where the moving fronts meet. Appearance of a precipitin line indicates that antigen and antibody of complementary specificity are present; density of the precipitin line reflects the amount of immune complex formed.

Most Ouchterlony plates have a central well surrounded by wells equidistant from the central well and from each other; material diffusing from the central well encounters the molecules diffusing from each of the peripheral wells. If the central well contains antibody and all circumferential wells contain the same antigen, lines of identical shape form between the central well and all surrounding wells. If the peripheral wells contain the same antigen at differing concentrations, the density of the precipitin arcs reflects the starting quantities of antigen (Fig. 15–5). If the peripheral wells contain different antigens, lines form only where antibody and antigen have the same specificity. If the central well contains several antibodies, each recognizing a different antigen, the appearance and location of the precipitin lines will reflect the specificity of antigens present in the surrounding wells (Fig. 15–6).

Ouchterlony double diffusion is a qualitative technique best suited to demonstrating specificity of antigen or antibody. Materials that give a "reaction of identity" have the same immunologic specificity, whereas a preparation that generates additional arcs with varied shape and location demonstrates the presence of antigen-antibody complexes with different properties. Absence of precipitation indicates that the unknown lacks any material reactive with the reagent in use.

SHAPE AND LOCATION OF ARCS
INDICATE SPECIFICITY

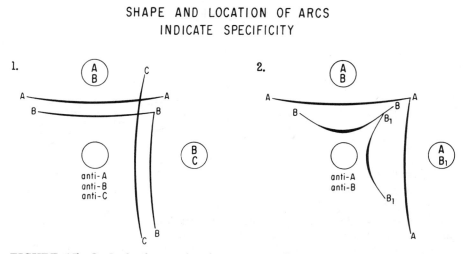

FIGURE 15—6. In both panels, the center well contains a mixture of antibodies, and each peripheral well contains two antigens. In panel 1, the crossed arcs for A/anti-A and C/anti-C indicate that the two antigens are unrelated. The perfectly matched B/anti-B arcs constitute a "reaction of identity" for the B antigen in each of the two wells. In panel 2, the A/anti-A arcs give a reaction of identity. The spur extending beyond the junction of the two B/anti-B arcs indicates "partial identity" of the B antigens present in the two wells.

COUNTERIMMUNOELECTROPHORESIS

Spontaneous diffusion through a gel characteristically takes hours. Applying an electric current speeds diffusion and induces movement that is linear rather than radial. In a suspending medium of constant properties, the speed and direction of migration vary with the composition of the protein. The net charge of many antigen preparations and antibody solutions causes them to migrate in directions opposite to one another. **Counterimmunoelectrophoresis** (CIEP), also called **countercurrent immunoelectrophoresis** and **electroprecipitation,** exploits this phenomenon.

In CIEP, the reagent material and the unknown are placed in side-by-side wells. Most procedures use a known antibody to determine whether or not antigen is present in the material under investigation. The supporting gel and the buffered pH are selected so that the antibody, which has a small net negative charge, moves toward the cathode while the antigen migrates toward the anode (Fig. 15—7). If antigen is present in the test material, a precipitin line forms between the two wells at a location determined by the concentration of antigen. Absence of a line indicates absence of the antigen being sought. Counterimmunoelectrophoresis is often used to demonstrate

COUNTERIMMUNOELECTROPHORESIS

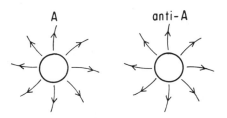

Unmodified reactants diffuse
slowly and radially

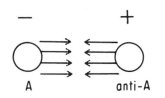

Electric current speeds movement, imparts direction

FIGURE 15–7. In counterimmunoelectrophoresis, electrical current passing through the gel affects the speed and direction of protein migration. Antigen and antibody molecules move more rapidly and more directly toward one another, as shown on the right, than they would in the simple diffusion shown on the left.

microbial antigens in the body fluids of a patient in whom infection is suspected; cultures take 1 or more days to give an answer, whereas documenting microbial antigens takes only an hour or so and is not affected by antibiotics or by viability of the organisms. Success of the procedure depends upon knowing which organisms are likely to be present and having available identifying antibodies of high specificity and affinity.

IMMUNOELECTROPHORESIS

Immunoelectrophoresis (IEP) is a two-stage procedure in which proteins are first separated by electrically stimulated migration and are then allowed to diffuse toward a preparation of precipitating antibody. First, gel is loaded with a mixture of proteins, and electrical current is applied; each protein migrates at its own rate and direction, generating individual protein bands distributed along the gel strip (Fig. 15–8, step 1). Antibody is then placed in a trough parallel to the line of separated proteins. Diffusion occurs from the trough and from the concentrated collections of individual protein molecules (see Fig. 15–8, steps 2 and 3). The trough may contain antibody of a single specificity or a mixture expected to react with several of the electrophoretically separated proteins.

Immunoelectrophoresis is often used for qualitative or semiquantitative demonstration of proteins in serum, urine, or cerebrospinal fluid. If the antibody trough contains a mixture of antibodies, numerous precipitin bands form that identify individual proteins, such as

IMMUNOELECTROPHORESIS

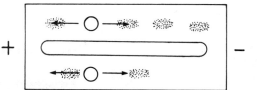

Electrophoresis separates antigens

FIGURE 15–8. The upper panel depicts migrated proteins of two different serum specimens, separated by electrophoresis. The middle panel shows the trough from which the selected antibodies diffuse outward. The lower panel shows the precipitin arcs formed. The migrated protein bands are invisible in the native gel, so only the precipitin arcs reveal the existence and location of reactive material. The upper serum contains several proteins that react with the reagent antibodies; the lower specimen contains only one. The fact that the arcs are in different locations indicates that the two specimens contain reactive proteins of different compositions.

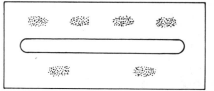

Trough contains mixture of antibodies

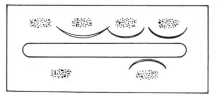

Arcs form where antibody meets corresponding antigen

albumin, transferrin, alpha-1-antitrypsin, or various classes of immunoglobulin. Failure to develop an expected band suggests a protein deficiency; bands of abnormal location, shape, or intensity indicate abnormalities of protein composition or concentration.

In other applications, the antibody trough may contain a single antibody; antibody to an immunoglobulin light-chain isotype is a common example. This induces bands at any site where there are immunoglobulin molecules with that light chain; an abnormal precipitin arc develops if the fluid contains unpaired light chains, as occurs in multiple myeloma (see page 209).

IMMUNOFIXATION ELECTROPHORESIS

Proteins that have been separated by migration can be exposed to antibody directly, rather than by diffusion. In **immunofixation electrophoresis** (IFE), antibody is layered onto the gel where proteins

IMMUNOFIXATION ELECTROPHORESIS

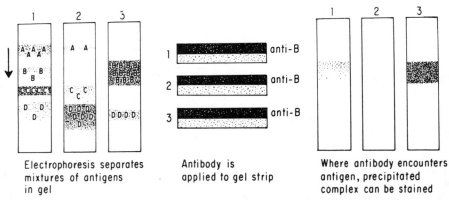

Electrophoresis separates mixtures of antigens in gel

Antibody is applied to gel strip

Where antibody encounters antigen, precipitated complex can be stained

FIGURE 15-9. The migration patterns of three different protein mixtures (designated 1, 2, and 3) are shown on the left. The protein bands would not be visible under test conditions. In the center, a single antibody (anti-B) is applied to each strip. The strips are then stained to show protein precipitated at those sites where antibody complexes with antigen. The results at the right show that serum 1 had a small amount of B antigen, serum 2 had none, and serum 3 had a large amount. To test for A, C, or D antigen, additional strips would have to be tested with the corresponding antibody.

have migrated. Combination occurs more rapidly and results are more sharply defined than when antibodies diffuse from a trough, but only one antibody can be used per strip and proportions of antigen and antibody are less flexible. Immunofixation electrophoresis with an antibody of known specificity is often used to detect whether antigenic material with characteristic migration properties is present in a specimen. After antibody is placed on the gel strips, immune complex will precipitate at whatever site the migrating antigen has reached. Non-precipitated proteins are washed away, leaving only precipitated immune complexes that can then be stained or labeled (Fig. 15-9). Immunofixation electrophoresis is useful in demonstrating antigens present at low concentrations, because the antibody is highly specific and electrophoretic migration leaves the antigenic material isolated and fully accessible. Immunofixation electrophoresis is often used to demonstrate abnormal proteins in spinal fluid or proteins present in serum at low concentrations, like complement degradation fragments or other abnormal immune products.

WESTERN BLOTTING

The **Western blot** (WB) procedure is conceptually similar to IFE, but the material under investigation is antibody rather than antigen.

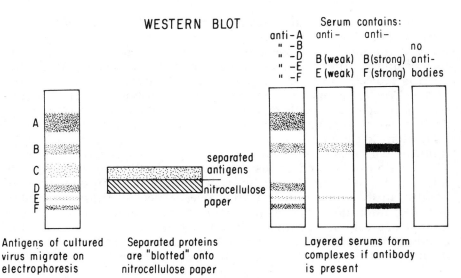

FIGURE 15–10. The first step in Western blot testing is electrophoretic separation of a protein mixture into bands of individual antigen, shown on the left. "Blotting" the proteins onto nitrocellulose, shown in the center, leaves each antigen in a distinctive location. The strips on the right show staining patterns achieved when four different serums are reacted with the separated antigens. The serum on the left contains moderately strong antibodies to 5 of the 6 antigens present. The second serum generates weak precipitin bands against two antigens. The next serum contains much stronger antibody against the B band, and also strong activity against F. The last serum contains no antibodies against any of the antigens in this preparation.

The first step in Western blotting is electrophoretic separation of the complex antigenic material used as the known reagent; this is usually a mixture of proteins or glycoproteins prepared from virus or other microorganisms. The separated components are transferred from the initial gel to a nitrocellulose medium by "blotting" from one surface to another. The term "Western blot" is a scientific joke. Blot transfer of electrophoretically separated material from one surface to another was developed by Dr. Edward Southern, who transferred fragments of deoxyribonucleic acid (DNA); DNA transfer thus became known as "Southern" blotting. A later application of the technique was to transfer ribonucleic acid (RNA); this was dubbed "Northern" blotting. Transfer of migrated proteins was named for one of the two remaining compass points, to become "Western" blotting.

Procedure and Interpretation

In Western blot procedures, the proteins are separated in one medium and then blotted to a nitrocellulose support where antigen-antibody complexes can be demonstrated. The test is done to show whether a serum contains one or more antibodies to any of the antigenic bands. For each antibody present, immune complex precipitates at the site where the individual antigen has blotted onto the nitrocellulose. After unprecipitated proteins are washed away, the strip is labeled to reveal the presence and intensity of precipitated bands. The test is most often used to detect antibodies against organisms of complex antigenic composition. Material from a purified preparation of microorganism is blotted to the support medium after migration. If the serum contains antibodies to any of the antigens, immune complexes precipitate in bands at characteristic locations. The location of stained bands reflects the specificity of the antibody (Fig. 15–10). The most familiar application of Western blotting is to identify antibodies to human retroviruses, especially those involved in acquired immunodeficiency syndrome (AIDS). These viruses provoke a range of antibodies against well-characterized antigens; the number and location of precipitated bands indicates the specificity of the infecting organism that host antibodies have identified.

SINGLE DIFFUSION

Single diffusion procedures may use spontaneous or electrically modified movement through the medium. Because concentration of one reactant remains constant, the position and nature of the precipitation reaction reflect the quantity of the other reactant.

SINGLE RADIAL DIFFUSION

In **radial immunodiffusion,** antibody is uniformly distributed in the supporting gel, and antigen diffuses outward from a single well. The proportions between antigen and antibody change continually as the diffusion front moves radially; antigen-antibody complexes form at the zone of equivalence. After a predetermined interval, the radius of the precipitin ring is measured as an indication of antigen concentration. If the initial amount of antigen was small, the ring will be small. The more material initially present in the well, the greater the distance the material must travel to reach the zone of equivalence (Fig. 15–11). A standard curve is constructed from the size of rings produced by control preparations of known concentrations; the concentration of the unknown can be determined by comparison. Complete diffusion may take as long as 72 hours, but calculation is possible from observations taken at a fixed interval after loading the well.

Radial immunodiffusion allows simple, accurate measurement of relatively low protein levels; it is used to quantify serum levels of immunoglobulins or haptoglobin. Unfortunately, it is subject to a number of artifacts. If proteins polymerize or form aberrant complexes,

RADIAL IMMUNODIFFUSION

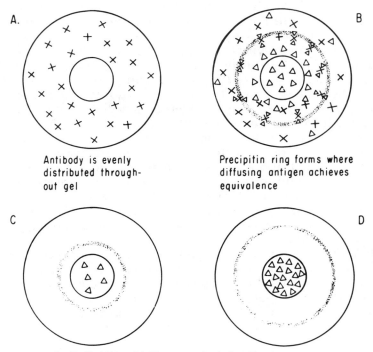

A.

Antibody is evenly
distributed through-
out gel

B

Precipitin ring forms where
diffusing antigen achieves
equivalence

C

D

In limited time, highly concentrated antigen moves
farther, forms precipitin ring with larger radius

FIGURE 15—11. Radial immunodiffusion starts with a single antibody evenly dispersed throughout the gel, shown in A. Antigen placed in the well diffuses radially, forming a visible ring wherever equivalence is reached, shown in B. The radius of the ring formed after a limited interval is proportional to concentration of the antigen, because diffusion is more rapid from a solution that is highly concentrated (shown in D) than from one that is less concentrated (shown in C).

the resulting macromolecular aggregates diffuse more slowly than the native protein; this makes the precipitin ring smaller and causes underestimation of total concentration. Conversely, low-molecular-weight variants of normally polymerized proteins migrate faster and give falsely high results. Abnormally reactive serum constituents— such as rheumatoid factor, which has intrinsic reactivity with IgG— may create misleading precipitation patterns.

ONE-DIMENSIONAL
ELECTROIMMUNODIFFUSION

In **one-dimensional electroimmunodiffusion** (also called **rocket electrophoresis** or **Laurell's rocket procedure**) electric current stimulates movement of antigen through antibody-containing gel. Mixtures of proteins can be examined without special preparation because the reagent antibody incorporated in the medium reacts only with its target antigen. As the antigen moves by electrical stimulation, the zone of equivalence changes continually, relative to the fixed concentration of antigen incorporated in the medium. Precipitation occurs at the leading edge of the band, leaving reduced quantities of antigen in the trailing material. The zone of equivalence moves more and more toward the center as antigen is depleted, giving a pointed (rocket-shaped) contour to the resulting precipitin line (Fig. 15–12). Antigen concentration is proportional to the distance the rocket travels; absolute values are calculated from a standard curve constructed with known concentrations of control material. Rocket electrophoresis is especially useful for measuring materials too concentrated for receptor-ligand assays (see chapter 18) but below the accuracy threshold for light-scattering (see below) or other analytic techniques; examples include alpha-fetoprotein in amniotic fluid and immunoglobulins in cerebrospinal fluid.

Variations of the rocket technique provide comparison of protein behavior and allow identification of abnormal protein derivatives or contaminating proteins. In the **fused-rocket** technique, separate antigen preparations are placed side by side; if the elements in both materials are the same, the rocket curves fuse in a manner analogous to the "reaction of identity" on an Ouchterlony plate (see earlier section

ROCKET ELECTROPHORESIS

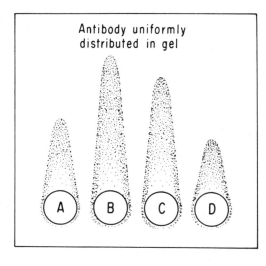

Antibody uniformly
distributed in gel

A   B   C   D

Migrating antigen forms
precipitin arcs

FIGURE 15–12. In rocket electrophoresis, the precipitin arc is shaped by electrical current, which causes the antigen to move in a single direction through the antibody-impregnated gel. Height of the rocket reflects the relative concentration of antigen; absolute quantities must be extrapolated from comparison with controls of known concentration. Relative concentrations, in the example shown above, are B>C>A>D.

on Ouchterlony double diffusion). In **crossed immunoelectrophoresis,** the materials in the mixture are separated by initial electrophoresis in an immunologically inert medium; the separated proteins are then subjected to electrical stimulation at a right angle to the original current, to carry them into antibody-containing gel where rockets can form.

——— TECHNIQUES THAT MEASURE LIGHT ———

When immune complexes precipitate out of solution, the behavior of light traveling through the medium will change; the concentration, size, and shape of the immune complexes determine the effect upon transmission. The physics of these interactions are exceedingly complex, and quantitative relationships are confounded by different rates of formation and dissipation at differing concentrations of antigen and antibody. In biological systems, relationships are further confused by materials like dispersed lipids or abnormal pigments that independently absorb or scatter light.

Nephelometry and **turbidimetry** are photometric techniques widely used in laboratory analysis. Turbidimetry measures changes in light transmission; nephelometry measures scatter at one or more defined angles. Both techniques can be used to measure immune-complex formation in a fluid medium. Most procedures start by introducing a monospecific antibody into the antigen-containing test material; the resulting immune complexes alter the behavior of light in a measurable fashion. If the physics of the instrument and the properties of the individual antigen-antibody system are carefully controlled, the technique allows accurate quantification, at microgram or milligram levels, of proteins such as complement components and their degradation products, normal and abnormal immunoglobulins, and variant immune products, such as C-reactive protein.

—————— SUGGESTIONS FOR —————— FURTHER READING

Johnson AM: Immunoprecipitation in gels. In: Rose NR, Friedman H, Fahey JL, eds: Manual of Clinical Laboratory Immunology, 3rd ed. Washington DC: American Society for Microbiology, 1986:14–24

Mehl VS, Penn GM: Electrophoretic and immunochemical characterization of immunoglobulins. In: Rose NR, Friedman H, Fahey JL, eds: Manual of Clinical Laboratory Immunology, 3rd ed. Washington DC: American Society for Microbiology, 1986:126–37

CHAPTER 16

Methods Based on Agglutination

In agglutination, the antigen-antibody lattice incorporates particles, whereas the visible end result of precipitation is formation of macromolecular complexes; the difference is in state of suspension. Agglutination can usually be observed with the naked eye, although discrimination is enhanced with a magnifying lens or low-power microscope. The relative concentration of antigen and antibody is less critical for agglutination than for precipitation, and agglutination techniques detect reactants at lower concentrations. Initially used to detect antibodies against bacterial or blood-cell antigens, agglutination procedures are applied to demonstration and sometimes quantification of a wide range of antigens and antibodies.

324

—————— PRINCIPLES OF THE REACTION ——————

Agglutination occurs in two stages. In the first stage, immunoglobulin molecules attach to the antigen-bearing surface; crosslinking into the visible lattice is a separate phenomenon. Specificity and reactivity of the antibody determine whether or not the first stage occurs; the second stage depends primarily upon physical conditions.

ANTIBODY ATTACHMENT

Attachment of antibody to antigen on a particle surface is called **sensitization** of the particle. Sensitization occurs only when specific antigen and antibody are present simultaneously. If the serum lacks antibody or if the antigens present are not recognized by the antibodies present, attachment will not occur (Fig. 16–1). Even with the necessary elements present, however, characteristics of the antibody and the reaction conditions influence the rate and magnitude of sensitization (Fig. 16–2). With antigen-antibody systems of the same specific-

SPECIFICITY OF AGGLUTINATION

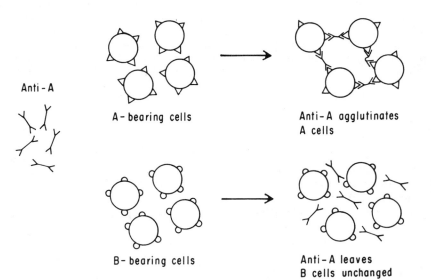

Anti-A

A-bearing cells

Anti-A agglutinates
A cells

B-bearing cells

Anti-A leaves
B cells unchanged

FIGURE 16–1. Agglutination occurs only when antibody encounters particulate antigen of the correct specificity. With a known antibody, agglutination reveals antigen specificity, as shown above. If the antigen is known, the procedure can identify antibodies in an unknown serum.

FACTORS AFFECTING SENSITIZATION

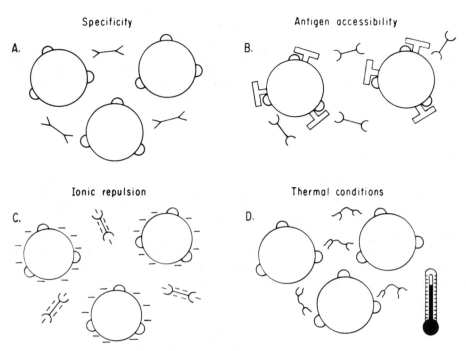

FIGURE 16–2. Antibody may not unite with particulate antigen under several circumstances. Specificity, shown in A, is the primary determinant. Reaction conditions also affect the combination of antibody with surface antigens. Steric interference by other molecules, shown in B, may impair immunoglobulin attachment. In a highly charged medium, shown in C, mutual repulsion may prevent antibody from uniting with surface proteins. If temperature is above (shown in D) or below thermal optimum for the antibody, reaction may not occur.

ity, antibody molecules of higher affinity bind more rapidly than those with a lower binding constant. Temperatures other than the thermal optimum of the antibody may reduce or prevent association of antigen with antibody.

The nature of the antigen-bearing surface also affects sensitization. Antigenic sites may be inaccessible if overlaid or obscured by other surface molecules or if the epitopes are very sparse or very dense on the particle surface. Erythrocytes, bacteria, and other carrier particles express a net negative surface charge which may be sufficient to prevent effective steric interaction with antibody molecules. Surface charge can be modified by changing the ionic composition of the medium or by modifying the charge present on the particles (Fig. 16–3). Some agglutination procedures routinely include treating the particles with enzymes or other agents to modify surface properties.

ALTERING CHARGE ALTERS REACTIONS

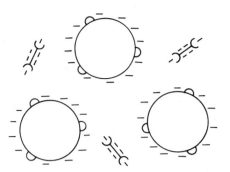

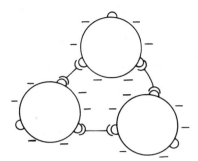

Surface charge keeps particles
and antibodies separated

Agglutination occurs with
reduced surface charge

FIGURE 16–3. If ionic forces prevent engagement of antigen and antibody, lowering the ionic strength of the medium or altering the surface properties of the particles may permit sensitization and agglutination to occur.

FORMATION OF THE LATTICE

Sensitization of particles does not guarantee agglutination. Before a lattice can form, antigen-combining (Fab) sites of antibody molecules must combine with antigen expressed on different particles. If antigen sites are sparsely distributed on the particle surface, antibody molecules attached to one particle may fail to encounter, by chance association, epitopes on another particle. Conversely, if epitopes are densely present, the Fab sites of each antibody molecule may unite with several epitopes on a single particle, thus failing to engender a lattice. Centrifugation is a physical process used to increase proximity of antibody and antigen-bearing surfaces. Even after centrifugation, however, residual surface charge causes particles to preserve a certain space around themselves. Like charges repel, and individual units suspended in a medium remain measurably separate. Antibody with the same charge as the particle may succeed in combining with surface epitopes but, after attachment, may be unable to bridge the distance maintained between the particles. The IgG monomer, which is only 250 Ångstrom units long, often fails to agglutinate particles after sensitizing surfaces that express the appropriate antigen. The IgM pentamer, with a diameter of about 1000 Ångstrom units and five active combining sites, is far more effective in inducing agglutination than IgG molecules of the same specificity (Fig. 16–4).

Failure of Agglutination

Early serologists who observed this failure of agglutination theorized that such antibodies possessed only one combining site, and

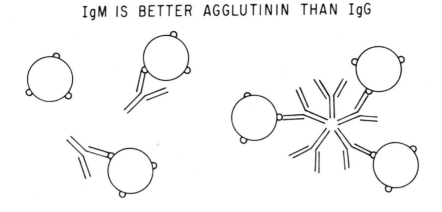

IgG IS BETTER AGGLUTININ THAN IgM

IgG is unable to link
widely separated particles

Larger IgM easily spans
distance between particles

FIGURE 16—4. Antigen-specific IgG antibodies often attach to surface antigen but fail to bridge the distance between suspended particles, shown on the left. IgM antibodies, with more combining sites and a greater diameter, readily agglutinate target material, as shown on the right.

they described antibodies that caused sensitization but not agglutination as "incomplete." This interpretation was incorrect; non-agglutinating antibodies are complete in all respects, but, unable to bridge the distance between antigen-bearing particles, they do not induce an effective lattice. Agglutination can sometimes be promoted, after there has been sensitization without agglutination, by altering the ionic strength or viscosity of the suspending medium, the temperature of the reaction, or the non-antigenic surface properties of the particles.

If excessive numbers of antibody molecules attach to each particle, agglutination may not occur; antibody excess can cause a prozone (see page 298) in agglutination procedures as well as in precipitation. If individual antibody molecules attach to every available antigen site, no single molecule can combine with several particles to draw them into a lattice; the heavily sensitized particles remain suspended separately in the fluid medium. Diluting the serum to reduce the antibody concentration corrects the problem and allows agglutination to occur.

USE OF ANTIGLOBULIN REAGENTS

Sensitization can be converted to visible agglutination by superimposing an additional antigen-antibody reaction. Immunoglobulin molecules coating sensitized particles engage their Fab sites, but the constant portion of the molecules remains exposed and accessible.

Antibodies against the Fc portion of heavy chains or against constant domains of the light chain can unite with these surface-bound molecules. These antiglobulin antibodies combine with target sites on separate immunoglobulin molecules and link them together. Because the target immunoglobulins are attached to particles, crosslinking the surface-bound target proteins brings the underlying particles together in visible agglutinates (see Fig. 14–7). The antiglobulin reagent must be standardized to react only with globulin molecules and to have no effect on the particles or their antigens.

Unbound Globulins

Antiglobulin antibodies react with immunoglobulin wherever they encounter their target molecules. Immunoglobulin molecules that are not bound in immune complexes combine more readily with antiglobulin antibodies than do immunoglobulins attached to a cell surface. If unbound immunoglobulin molecules are present in the medium that contains antibody-coated particles, an antiglobulin reagent may unite so promptly with unbound immunoglobulin that little or no reactivity remains to crosslink the sensitized particles (Fig. 16–5). In procedures that use antiglobulin reagents, it is crucially important to remove all unbound proteins before adding antiglobulin serum.

NEUTRALIZATION OF ANTIGLOBULIN SERUM

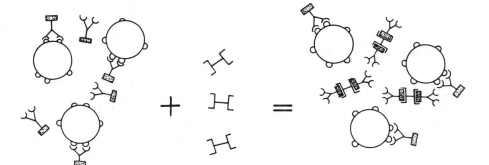

Unbound globulins react
preferentially with antiglobulin

FIGURE 16–5. Antiglobulin antibodies combine more rapidly with unbound than with bound immunoglobulin molecules. If all combining sites of the reagent antiglobulin are occupied by free immunoglobulin molecules, as shown above, indicator particles will not be agglutinated, whether or not there is antibody bound to their surface.

QUANTIFICATION

Agglutination is inherently qualitative; the end point is a reaction that occurs or fails to occur but cannot be quantified accurately. When temperature, suspending medium, and centrifugation are held constant, the rapidity with which agglutination occurs and the size of the clumps are roughly proportional to the intensity of the antigen-antibody reaction. These variables are often recorded on a scale of trace, $+/-$, $1+$, $2+$, $3+$, and $4+$, or by assigning numerical values. To compare strength of several different preparations, the antigen or antibody used as indicator material must be held stringently constant. With an antibody of known properties, reaction strength reflects antigenic characteristics of the cells or particles tested. Conversely, progressively stronger agglutination of standardized antigen-bearing particles occurs as antibody concentration increases, unless and until a prozone occurs.

Performing and Interpreting Titration

Titration is a semiquantitative technique in which differential dilution allows approximate estimation of concentration. In comparing activity levels of specimens collected at different times or from different sources, titration can demonstrate relative differences for which precise units of measurement are unnecessary. Each dilution is reacted against an indicator of reproducible properties; as the test material becomes less and less concentrated, agglutination diminishes and disappears. The result is reported as the titer, defined as the reciprocal of the highest dilution that causes agglutination. If reaction occurs at 1:64 and not at 1:128, the titer is 64 (Fig. 16–6). It is not correct to report titer as dilution; in this example, the titer is 64, not 1:64.

The major problem with titration—besides its necessarily inferential approach to quantity—is difficulty of performing accurate dilutions and achieving precisely comparable results. Dilution intervals must be selected so that the expected results fall in an informative part of the range. If, for example, doubling dilutions go from 1:128 to 1:256, and the critical distinction in concentration lies between 1:100 and 1:150, the test loses much of its sensitivity. A more frequent problem is accuracy of dilution and reproducibility of results. As dilution proceeds, increment or loss of very small volumes can produce enormous inaccuracy in concentration. Because of this imprecision, results in titrating two different specimens are considered significantly different only if end points differ by more than two dilution levels. With doubling dilutions of 1:8, 1:16, 1:32, and 1:64 and precision no better than plus or minus 1 dilution, an antibody truly detectable at 1:16 might, in three replicate tubes, give results at 1:8, 1:16, and 1:32. To be significant, there would have to be a difference of more than two tubes; for example, between 1:8 and 1:64. Prozones can present an artificial problem in titration. With highly concen-

TITRATION AND SCORING

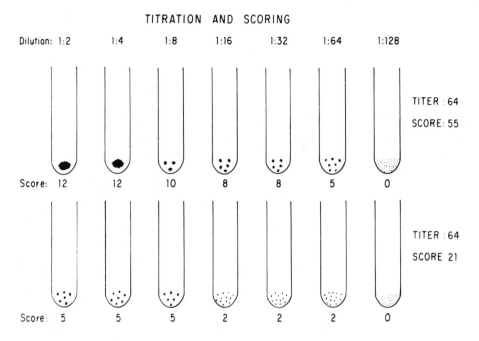

Dilution: 1:2   1:4   1:8   1:16   1:32   1:64   1:128

TITER : 64

SCORE: 55

Score: 12   12   10   8   8   5   0

TITER : 64

SCORE 21

Score: 5   5   5   2   2   2   0

Antibodies with same titer may have different activity.

FIGURE 16–6. Both panels show dilutions of antibody going from 1:2 to 1:128. The upper specimen causes intense agglutination (score of 12) at the first 2 dilutions, and reactivity decreases sharply with increasing dilution. The lower specimen causes only modest agglutination (score of 5) at 1:2, but this reactivity changes relatively little at much higher dilutions. In both specimens, the highest dilution to show agglutination is 1:64, so both have a titer of 64.

trated antibody, serum that is undiluted or at the 1:2 dilution may cause little or no agglutination, whereas strong agglutination can occur at 1:4, 1:8, and so on.

Differences in Behavior

Combining titration with numerical scoring can give additional information. Antibodies that recognize the same antigens may express clinically significant differences in serologic behavior. The biologic properties of an antibody that gives 4+ agglutination when undiluted and declines progressively with increasing dilution are often different from those of a serum that gives persisting low levels of agglutination at every dilution over a wide range. Both might have the same titer, but the differences in intensity of agglutination suggest differences not only in serologic but also biologic behavior. Figure 16–6 illustrates this distinction.

─────────── **AGGLUTINATION PROCEDURES** ───────────

Agglutination was first used to demonstrate activity of antibody in unmodified serum, directed against unmodified red blood cells or bacterial cell bodies. This direct agglutination of natural materials continues useful in immunohematology and microbiology, but procedures that use processed antigen or antibody or both have greatly expanded the applications of agglutination testing. In **passive agglutination** procedures, antigenic material is processed onto carrier particles; this allows antibody to encounter in particulate form an antigen that would otherwise be soluble (Fig. 16–7). In **reverse passive agglutination,** the material linked to the carrier is antibody; the test is done to demonstrate presence of soluble antigen, which induces agglutination of the particle-linked antibody (Fig. 16–8).

Agglutination as an end point can be determined by visual inspection or with suitably calibrated instruments. With carrier particles of precisely reproducible characteristics and instrument-assisted test conditions, agglutination tests can give quantitative results. The particle-enhanced reaction can be quantified by measuring how agglutination affects the transmission or scatter of light; by counting the number of freely suspended particles before and after the immune reaction; or by observing that the size of suspended material changes as individual particles agglutinate into cohesive clumps.

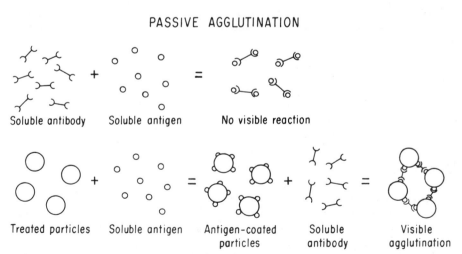

PASSIVE AGGLUTINATION

Soluble antibody   Soluble antigen   No visible reaction

Treated particles   Soluble antigen   Antigen-coated particles   Soluble antibody   Visible agglutination

FIGURE 16–7. In the upper panel, reaction between soluble antigen and soluble antibody produces immune complexes too small to be detected. The lower panel shows how attaching soluble antigen to indicator particles converts immune complexes into particulate lattices readily detected as agglutination.

REVERSE PASSIVE AGGLUTINATION

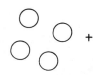 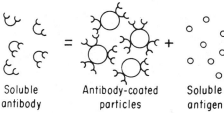 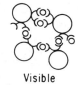

Treated particles   Soluble   Antibody-coated   Soluble   Visible
              antibody   particles   antigen   agglutination

FIGURE 16–8. In reverse passive agglutination, soluble antibody is rendered particulate by adsorption to inert indicator particles. Contact with specific antigen brings the particles together into lattices visible as agglutination.

DIRECT AGGLUTINATION

Direct agglutination is most useful in the immunohematology and microbiology laboratories. Agglutination gives prompt, accurate, and reproducible information about surface antigens on blood cells and about blood group antibodies in serum. For ABO antigens and antibodies, immediate agglutination is characteristic. To demonstrate antigen-antibody reactions in the Rh system and the so-called "minor" systems like Kell, Duffy, and others, antiglobulin serum is often necessary. Agglutination tests are also used to demonstrate abnormal antibodies, like those in cold-agglutinin disease or infectious mononucleosis.

THE "COOMBS' TEST"

Modern antiglobulin testing began with Coombs and coworkers, who injected whole human serum into rabbits and used the resulting antihuman reagent to demonstrate anti-red-cell antibodies that sensitized target cells but did not agglutinate them. Immunohematologists continue to find antiglobulin reactions invaluable, and several blood banking procedures bear the informal name **Coombs' test**. The reagents now used differ enormously from the anti-whole serum first used by Coombs and his colleagues, and the more correct term is **antiglobulin test**.

Antibody Attached to Cells

In blood bank serology, antiglobulin serum has two quite different applications. The **direct antiglobulin test** demonstrates whether antibody or complement globulins have attached to blood cells in the circulating blood of the living host (Fig. 16–9). Normal individuals do

DIRECT ANTIGLOBULIN TEST

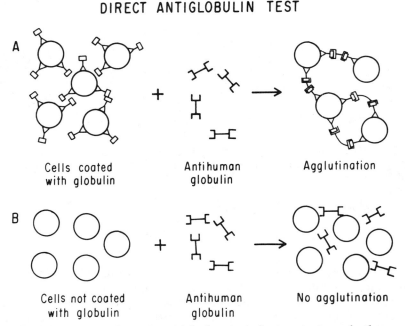

FIGURE 16–9. The direct antiglobulin test demonstrates whether or not cells are coated with globulin. In panel A, antiglobulin reagent that combines with globulin molecules complexed to the cell surface causes agglutination of the underlying cells. In panel B, uncoated cells do not engage the antiglobulin antibody and remain unagglutinated.

not have globulin-coated cells. The event usually indicates an autoimmune process, and the direct antiglobulin test is used to diagnose hematologic or immunologic abnormalities. The test is called "direct" because cells are tested directly as they come from the body, processed only by washing to remove proteins that might neutralize the antiglobulin reagent.

Antibody Present in Serum

A different application of antiglobulin testing is not a single test but, rather, a general procedure used to examine antibodies in serum. The **indirect antiglobulin technique** is a two-stage procedure. First, the serum is incubated with antigen-bearing cells so that antibody, if present in the serum, can combine with surface antigen and sensitize the cells. The incubated cells are then separated from the original serum, washed, and mixed with antiglobulin serum. If the original serum contained antibody that attached to antigens on the cell surface, the antiglobulin reagent will combine with the sensitizing immunoglobulin and agglutinate the coated cells. If the serum

INDIRECT ANTIGLOBULIN TECHNIQUE

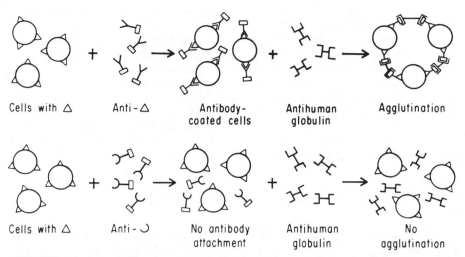

Cells with △   Anti-△   Antibody-coated cells   Antihuman globulin   Agglutination

Cells with △   Anti-◡   No antibody attachment   Antihuman globulin   No agglutination

FIGURE 16–10. Indirect antiglobulin procedures require two steps: combination of antibody with specific antigen, followed by combination of antiglobulin reagent with cell-bound antibody. In panel A, antibody specific for the surface antigen sensitizes the cells, which are then agglutinated by antiglobulin serum. In panel B, the antigen-antibody reaction does not occur, leaving the cells unsensitized and unaffected by the antiglobulin serum.

did not contain antibody against antigens on the test cells, addition of antiglobulin serum has no effect on the indicator cells (Fig. 16–10). The test investigates the properties of serum, but the end point is indirect, namely agglutination of indicator cells. The indirect antiglobulin technique is used to demonstrate and to identify blood group antibodies and to crossmatch red cells for safe transfusion.

MICROBIOLOGY TESTS

Microbiology employs direct agglutination in two different diagnostic approaches. Reagent antibodies of known specificity can be used to identify **antigens on bacteria**. Agglutination is also the end point in **serodiagnosis** of infection, which depends upon identifying antibodies in serum samples. An immunocompetent individual exposed to an organism characteristically develops antibodies against the infecting agent. The most accurate way to diagnose infection is to culture the organism, but sometimes this is difficult or impossible. It may be that suitable material cannot be obtained, the patient is studied only after the organisms have left the body, the organism is difficult to grow, or handling the organism constitutes a threat to laboratory personnel. Under these conditions, demonstrating antibodies against the suspected agent provides important diagnostic information. Agglutination tests are most often used to diagnose typhoid, brucellosis, tularemia, and leptospirosis.

Cross-reactive agglutination is exploited in serodiagnosis of certain rickettsial diseases—Rocky Mountain spotted fever, typhus, and several others. Infections with these rickettsiae provoke antibodies that, coincidentally, agglutinate suspensions of *Proteus* bacteria, a completely different organism. It is difficult to prepare rickettsial antigens but easy to make suspensions of various strains of *Proteus*. This examination for cross-reactivity, called the **Weil-Felix** test, is used to diagnose rickettsial infections in which it is otherwise very difficult to identify the causative organism.

PASSIVE AGGLUTINATION

Passive agglutination is the same as direct agglutination except that the antigen has been manipulated to achieve a particulate expression. Suitably purified solutions of many hormones, drugs, bacterial metabolites, and serum proteins can be adsorbed to indicator particles with little difficulty. Red blood cells are useful carrier particles because many proteins adhere spontaneously to the cell membrane. Treating the cells with tannic acid, with various enzymes, or with certain organic agents enhances the binding event.

Alternatively, carrier particles of uniform size and physical characteristics can be prepared from latex, charcoal, clay, and other subtances. These inert particles circumvent one problem that carrier red cells may create: the possibility that unsuspected antibodies may react against red-cell elements. Human serums sometimes contain heterospecific antibodies that can agglutinate non-human red cells used in some test systems.

Clinical Applications

Rheumatoid factor is an autoantibody directed against the Fc portion of IgG (see page 255). Serum that contains rheumatoid factor agglutinates indicator particles to which IgG has been attached. The original test for rheumatoid factor, the **Rose-Waaler** test, employed sheep erythrocytes to which rabbit antisheep antibodies had attached. Present tests for rheumatoid factor use latex particles coated with human IgG, a test system that is more sensitive and less liable to artifacts than the sheep-cell system.

Other tests that employ red cells passively coated with antigen include those for antibodies to **thyroglobulin,** the hormone-containing storage protein of the thyroid; and antibodies to bacterial toxins, notably those involved in **diphtheria** and **tetanus**. Penicillin, cephalosporins, or other pharmaceuticals can be adsorbed to allogeneic red cells to demonstrate **drug antibodies** that cause immune-mediated red-cell destruction.

Latex particles are used in test kits for diagnosis of many **autoimmune conditions**. Besides the latex test for rheumatoid factor mentioned above, there are preparations to detect autoantibodies against DNA, nucleoproteins, and a variety of cytoplasmic proteins. In many autoimmune conditions, antibodies develop against circulating hormones, and many assays are available that use hormone-coated particles. Other applications include testing for the group of liver-derived proteins characterized as **acute-phase reactants** and for antibodies against streptococcal enzymes and against a variety of fungal and protozoal antigens.

REVERSE PASSIVE AGGLUTINATION

An effective means to demonstrate presence of soluble antigen is to coat carrier particles with antibody and to allow the antigen to induce lattice formation. This kind of agglutination procedure is useful as a screening test for various materials that do not need to be measured precisely. It has found wide acceptance as a rapid way to demonstrate infection, in place of the time-consuming but definitive technique of culturing the invading organism. When multiplying organisms are present, soluble antigenic material often enters body fluids, where it can be detected through agglutination of particles coated with appropriate antibodies. This provides highly suggestive diagnostic information available within a few minutes and useful for beginning treatment while more definitive diagnosis is being undertaken.

Reverse passive agglutination is also suitable for semiquantitative assay of substances in body fluids. Cleavage products of fibrinogen, for example, are not present at measurable levels under normal conditions. Presence in serum of these abnormal products can be demonstrated through agglutination of particles coated with antibodies against fibrinogen-related peptides. The same approach can be used to detect threshold levels of drug in body fluids. The coated carrier particles must be standardized so that agglutination occurs only at or above the desired concentration; possibilities of cross-reactivity and non-specific agglutination must be rigorously excluded.

INHIBITION OF AGGLUTINATION

Soluble antigen and soluble antibody often form complexes without leaving visible evidence; one way to demonstrate this combination is to show that material originally known to be present has been consumed or eliminated. **Agglutination inhibition** procedures require

AGGLUTINATION INHIBITION

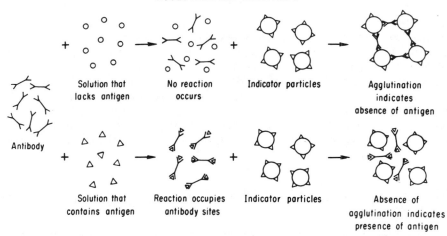

FIGURE 16–11. Antibody, shown at far left, that is specific for antigens on the indicator particles will cause agglutination under standard conditions. Incubating the antibody with antigen in soluble form, shown in the lower panel, engages available Fab sites and prevents the antibody from causing agglutination. The upper panel shows undiminished agglutination occurring after incubation with material that lacks the specific antigen.

several steps. The first step is establishment of an indicator system: Reagent antibody and reagent antigen are standardized to produce agglutination of demonstrated intensity. Usually the reagent antibody is soluble and the indicator antigen is in particulate form, but the reverse conditions can be used. After establishment of baseline agglutination, the next step is to incubate the test material and the soluble reagent, to allow formation of immune complexes. The last phase is addition of the indicator particles. If incubating the test material with the known reagent abolishes agglutination, the inference is that soluble molecules are present in the specimen that have combined with and inactivated the active agent. If incubation does not affect the baseline level of agglutination, absence of soluble activity can be inferred (Fig. 16–11). Appropriate controls are essential, to rule out the possibility of non-specific interference.

SOLUBLE ANTIGENS

A familiar application of agglutination inhibition is in **pregnancy tests,** which measure raised levels of human chorionic gonadotropin (hCG) in urine or blood. The test consists of particles coated with hCG and a solution of anti-hCG antibodies. First, urine or blood is incubated with the antibody; then the incubated mixture is added to the indicator particles. Persistence of agglutination at the previously established level indicates that the test material contained insufficient hCG to inactivate the reagent antibody. Abolition or pronounced reduction of agglutination indicates a level of soluble hCG sufficient to neutralize agglutinating activity of the reagent antibody and constitutes a positive result.

Agglutination inhibition can be used to estimate drug levels in body fluids. After establishment of baseline agglutinating action of reagent antibody on drug-coated particles, inhibitory effect of diluted serum samples can be determined. Titration of this sort gives semiquantitative results, but comparison against levels observed with known drug concentrations often provides clinically useful information.

Agglutination-inhibition procedures have been used to detect antigens and antibodies associated with hepatitis B infection, but these have largely been supplanted by receptor-ligand methods (see chapter 18).

Applications in Immunohematology

Many blood-cell antigens exist in soluble form as well as on cell membranes. The ABO antigens, for example, are an integral part of cell membranes but are also present in plasma and other body fluids. Other antigens—such as Le^a, Le^b, Sd^a, and the MHC class III proteins—exist primarily in body fluids and attach only passively to cell surfaces. It is sometimes desirable to demonstrate the presence or the concentration of these materials in body fluids, and agglutination inhibition is useful for this purpose. Because there are so many variables in concentration, in antibody behavior, and in cell-membrane properties, each test system must be carefully standardized before conclusions are drawn.

SOLUBLE ANTIBODIES

Certain antiviral antibodies can be demonstrated by their capacity to inhibit agglutination; the test depends upon the biologic behavior of the virus involved. Viruses may agglutinate suspensions of red cells that have specific receptors for their proteins. Different viruses manifest hemagglutination against cells from different animal species, so the tests have to be carefully selected and standardized. The principle of the test is simple: Antibodies stimulated by contact with the organism combine with the proteins of the virus and interfere with its attachment to red-cell receptors. The two-stage test involves, first, incubating test serum with the virus preparation and, second, adding red cells that the unmodified virus is known to agglutinate. Reduction or abolition of agglutination indicates presence of antibodies against the virus (Fig. 16–12). This technique is used for antibodies to a wide range of viruses: rubella, measles, mumps, influenza,

HEMAGGLUTINATION INHIBITION

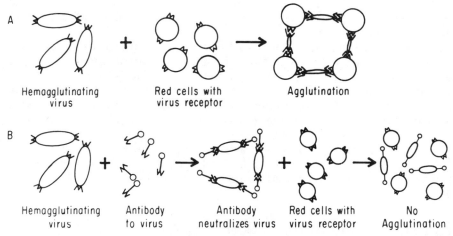

A

| Hemagglutinating virus | Red cells with virus receptor | Agglutination |

B

| Hemagglutinating virus | Antibody to virus | Antibody neutralizes virus | Red cells with virus receptor | No Agglutination |

FIGURE 16–12. Panel A depicts agglutination of indicator red cells by a preparation of active virus. The presence of antibody specific for the virus can be demonstrated, as shown in panel B, by incubating serum with virus and then observing failure of the incubated virus to agglutinate the indicator cells.

adenoviruses, and several others. Controls are necessary to detect artifacts that affect the results, especially loss of agglutinating potency in the reagent virus, and presence, in the test serum, of antibodies capable of agglutinating the indicator cells.

Streptococcal infection often induces antibodies against the bacterial metabolite called streptolysin O; the antibody, **antistreptolysin O** (ASO), is useful as an indicator of recent streptococcal infection. The classic test for ASO demonstrates that antibody-containing serum can neutralize effects of the metabolite, but an immune procedure is far simpler. The reagent system includes a soluble preparation of streptolysin O and particles coated with the antistreptolysin antibody. The test serum and the soluble bacterial product are incubated; if the serum contains antibodies against streptolysin O, the protein enters immune complexes and is unable to combine with the antibody-coated particles. Because normal serum characteristically contains low to moderate levels of ASO, the test must be standardized so that inhibition occurs only at a concentration that is clinically significant.

QUALITY ASSURANCE

Agglutination tests are rapid, require relatively little specialized training to perform, and appear misleadingly simple. Both false-positive and false-negative results may occur if there are insufficient controls to detect common pitfalls.

THE SYSTEM ITSELF

Basic to agglutination testing is the behavior of the suspended particles. They must remain in a stable suspension, without spontaneous aggregation or excessive mutual repulsion. Particularly with red blood cells, membrane characteristics that change with physiologic or artificial events may alter serologic behavior of the indicator particles. This is important both in immunohematology procedures that employ unmodified red cells and in passive systems that use red cells as carriers. Changes in the ionic composition or the viscosity of the medium will affect agglutination, as will changes in temperature, incubation period, or the quantity or concentration of the substances tested. It may be difficult to distinguish spontaneous association of particles caused by altered physical conditions from a low level of true agglutination. Using known positive and negative controls illuminates many artifacts, but the observer must always be alert to problems in interpretation.

When several specimens are to be compared, stringently uniform test conditions must be maintained. Variation in preparing reagents or timing the reactions can introduce errors of interpretation that are easy to overlook. With titration, especially, comparisons are most valid when all specimens are tested simultaneously by a single interpreter observing a single indicator system. Automated pipetting and diluting significantly improve reproducibility over manual manipulation.

PROBLEMS IN INTERPRETATION

Difficulty in observation and interpretation is more conspicuous and more significant in blood bank serology than in most other agglutination procedures. Known or unsuspected disease states often alter the behavior of serum and/or cells, and it may be difficult to distinguish subtle but significant disturbances from artifacts of the suspending medium, the incubation process, or the effect of centrifugation.

It is important to remember that several independent immune responses can occur simultaneously; an apparent positive result in an immunologic test may, in fact, reflect an event completely different from the one under investigation. Several pitfalls apply especially to agglutination procedures. In serum from patients with inflammatory and/or immunologic diseases, abnormalities of protein composition and concentration occur frequently; these changes often affect the behavior of suspended particles. Serum with increased globulins, decreased albumin, or various abnormal proteins may cause suspended particles to come together in stacked or clustered aggregates called **rouleaux.** Rouleaux formation occurs independent of antibody in serum or antigen on cell surface; it is simply the effect that the protein-containing fluid has on the charged particles.

Separate from rouleaux formation is the problem of antibodies that agglutinate cells intended as inert indicator particles. Some patients have antibodies that agglutinate virtually all human cells— their own and those from nearly any other adult human. Other patients have antibodies that react with red cells from other species. Tests that use carrier red cells should include uncoated red cells as a control, to detect whether the test serum causes non-specific agglutination.

Cross-reactivity is a problem in serodiagnosis of infections. Exposure to one organism may promote antibodies capable of agglutinating material from other organisms that share surface configurations. Sometimes antigen reagents prepared from cell cultures express characteristics of the cells in which the organisms were grown. The test serum may have antibodies against this cellular material and thus give an apparent positive reaction against the microbial preparation.

Rheumatoid factor, an antibody directed against human IgG, can cause agglutination in any test that uses a human IgG reagent, either adsorbed to a carrier particle or as part of an agglutination inhibition system.

The preceding discussion, although far from exhaustive, should highlight the need for continuous care in performing agglutination tests and judgment in interpreting them. A vast array of test kits are available; the most important safeguard to accurate results is careful attention to the manufacturer's instructions.

SUGGESTIONS FOR FURTHER READING

Nichols WS, Nakamura RM. Agglutination and agglutination inhibition assays. In: Rose NR, Friedman H, Fahey JL, eds. Manual of Clinical Laboratory Immunology, 3rd ed. Washington DC: American Society for Microbiology, 1986:49–56

Widmann FK, ed. Technical Manual of the American Association of Blood Banks, 9th ed. Arlington VA: American Association of Blood Banks, 1985:91–101 (The antiglobulin test)

CHAPTER 17

Complement in Laboratory Testing

Laboratory tests involve complement in three different contexts. The oldest technique is to induce complement-mediated biologic events as a way to detect antibodies. Development of a complement-mediated end point is essential, but the purpose of these tests is **demonstration that antibody is present**. The usual end points are red-cell hemolysis in complement fixation tests and complement-mediated killing of lymphocytes in lymphocytotoxicity testing. A second way in which complement enhances laboratory testing is **identification of complement components** at the site of immune reactions. This usually involves C3 cleavage fragments on cell membranes or complement-containing immune complexes in biologic fluids. The third role is determination of the **quantity** or the **characteristics of complement** components themselves, either in the entire cascade or as individual components.

343

—— **COMPLEMENT IN THE DEMONSTRATION** ——
OF ANTIBODIES

Activation of the entire complement cascade generates the "membrane attack unit," which lethally damages cell membranes. If red blood cells are the target, liberated hemoglobin provides an end point that is easy to observe and to measure. Demonstrating lethal damage to lymphocytes requires a different, inherently semiquantitative, end point.

THE COMPLEMENT FIXATION
TECHNIQUE

When they combine with antigen, all IgM antibodies and many IgG antibodies activate the first component of complement. Union with antigen is an independent event, but if C1 is present and functional, it will attach to the Fc portion of the bound immunoglobulin molecule. If a membrane was the site of antigen-antibody reaction, C4 and later components attach to the surface; if the antigen-antibody combination generates a fluid-phase aggregate, complement components accumulate in or on the macromolecular complex. Neither the specificity of the antibody nor the nature of the antigen affect the cascading activation of complement proteins.

In complement fixation (CF) testing, the end point is hemolysis; the indicator system requires (1) red cells already coated with a complement-activating antibody, (2) a preparation containing reagent complement, and (3) reaction conditions that allow the antibody under investigation to combine with its antigen. Antibody action alters the baseline level of hemolysis generated when reagent complement is added to the coated reagent cells. Most CF procedures test for the presence of a specific antibody, and the reagent system includes a standardized preparation of known antigen. Figure 17–1 illustrates the principle of CF testing.

Two-Stage Procedure

After the indicator system has been standardized for baseline level of hemolysis, the test requires two steps. First, the unknown serum and the known antigen are allowed to interact in the presence of complement. If complement-activating antibody is present, it combines with the antigen and causes C1 to enter the immune complex; this is described as "fixing" complement components. Antibody present in the unknown material reacts with antigen and causes the level of free complement in the system to drop significantly. If the serum

COMPLEMENT FIXATION TEST

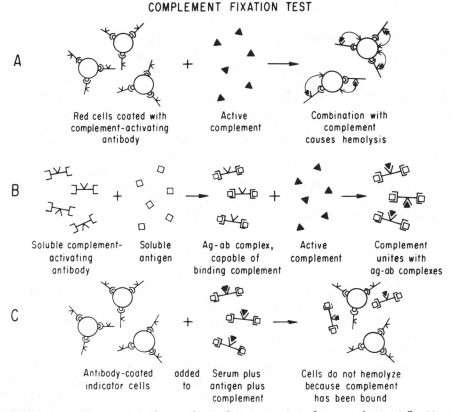

FIGURE 17–1. Panel A shows the indicator system for complement fixation tests: hemolysis when reagent complement is added to red cells sensitized with a complement-activating antibody. Panel B shows the first step of the test, in which serum containing soluble antibody is allowed to complex with soluble antigen. When reagent complement is added, C1 binds to the complexed antibody. Panel C shows that the complement, now "fixed" in the soluble complexes, is no longer available to unite with the sensitizing antibody on the indicator cells. Absence of hemolysis thus indicates that an antigen-antibody reaction occurred in the soluble phase depicted in Panel B.

contains no antibody, no immune reaction occurs, no complement is fixed, and the level of available complement remains unchanged.

The second step is addition to the incubated mixture of indicator red cells already coated with a complement-fixing antibody. The reagent antibody that coats the indicator cells must not agglutinate the cells but must strongly and invariably interact with complement. If the sensitized reagent cells are exposed to free complement, C1 interacts with the bound immunoglobulin and the hemolytic cascade proceeds; the sensitized cells will not hemolyze in the absence of complement.

Interpretation

If antibody is present in the test serum, it combines with reagent antigen in the first step; the resulting immune complexes bind complement, which is then unavailable for subsequent reactivity. If the unknown specimen contains no antibody, the complement present in the incubation mixture persists at its previously calibrated level. In a positive test, the complement-depleted incubation mixture lacks the factors needed to hemolyze the sensitized indicator cells; a positive end point is absence of hemolysis, as shown in Figure 17–1. In a negative test, the serum lacks antibody, no complexes form, and no complement is removed from the medium; sensitized cells are hemolyzed at the same intensity as in the baseline control. The degree to which complement is fixed and hemolysis diminished is directly proportional to the concentration of antibody in the test serum.

Potential Problems

Most CF procedures use guinea pig complement and antibody-coated sheep red cells as the indicator. The range of potential problems is enormous; accurate CF testing requires numerous painstaking steps to standardize all reagents and to avoid artifacts and misinterpretation. The complement preparation must be tested each time because several components are labile on storage. Reactivity of the indicator red cells may change over time and may, additionally, be affected by environmental conditions. The sensitizing antibody must behave consistently. The concentrations of all materials, including the ionic and macromolecular composition of the suspending medium, must be stringently reproducible.

Variables exist not only in the indicator system but also in the test materials. The reagent antigen must have uniform specificity and reactivity. The serum must be examined for effects on complement that occur without regard to antibody presence. Serums that impair complement reactivity are described as "anticomplementary." Immune complexes or aggregated immunoglobulins in serum are anticomplementary because they bind complement through the alternative pathway. Chelating agents bind the cations necessary for complement interactions, and heparin, if present in even small amounts, will inhibit the complement cascade. Complement fixation procedures must include a control of serum and complement without added antigen, and of complement and antigen without added serum.

Applications

Although complement fixation tests demand a high level of time and technical proficiency, they are highly sensitive and are useful in detecting antibodies difficult to demonstrate with other systems. The earliest serologic test for syphilis was a CF procedure, the **Wasserman** test. Syphilis testing has long employed other techniques, and routine tests for many other antibodies have switched from CF testing to simpler procedures. Complement fixation testing is still used as a reference, however, against which newer and less demanding techniques are compared, and it remains useful in identifying and quantifying antibodies against certain viral, fungal, and protozoal antigens.

LYMPHOCYTOTOXICITY

Lymphocytotoxicity tests are used to demonstrate antibodies against HLA antigens. These antibodies mediate various serologic effects, but lymphocytotoxicity gives consistent and accurate reactions for serums with a wide range of specificities. In the presence of complement, the union of cytotoxic antibody with HLA antigen irreversibly damages the cell membrane, which cannot then perform its barrier functions. This lethal damage is detected by showing that materials normally excluded from the cell interior can cross the damaged membrane and penetrate the cell.

Three-Stage Procedure

Cytotoxicity testing is a three-stage procedure. Serum and cells must first be incubated together. After optimal opportunity for antibody to attach to surface antigens, a standardized preparation of complement is added. If antibodies have bound to the cell membrane, the added complement unites with the bound immunoglobulin, the cascade is activated to completion, and the cell is irreversibly damaged. The last step is to introduce a dye that penetrates the membrane of nonviable cells but cannot enter intact cells. Viable cells remain unstained, but cells to which the complement-binding antibody attached will be suffused with the intracellular dye. This principle is illustrated in Figure 13–1 on page 279.

The proportion of viable to damaged cells indicates the magnitude of antigen-antibody reaction. Reactivity is affected by the concentration and avidity of the antibody and the intensity with which antigen is expressed on the membrane, as well as by the specificity of antibody for membrane antigen.

Biologic Variables

The test is easier to explain than to interpret. Variations in serum-cell reactivity are much greater for HLA antibodies and their antigens than for red-cell antigens and antibodies. Individuals who form HLA antibodies seldom produce a single, monospecific reactivity; a serum specimen often reacts to a variable degree with many different cells. Conversely, cells of a single phenotype may show variable reactivity with a number of different serums. Even reagent antiserums licensed for typing purposes give results that are not clearcut. Lymphocytotoxicity tests are usually performed in trays that contain numerous microtiter wells, allowing reactivity patterns of different cell suspensions and different serum samples to be observed and to be compared.

DEMONSTRATION THAT ANTIGEN-ANTIBODY REACTION HAS OCCURRED

Many events initiate the complement cascade but do not provoke membrane attack and do not cause immediate cell damage. Activation of classical or alternative pathways often causes cleavage products of C3 to accumulate, either on cell membranes or in the fluid-phase complex of antigen and antibody. In these settings, the presence of C3b or other C3 fragments indicates that an immune reaction of some sort has occurred. In immunohematology, cell-bound C3 indicates that there has been reaction between antibody and cellular antigens. When soluble antigen and antibody form complement-containing immune complexes, the complexes may behave in various ways. They may remain free in body fluids; they may adhere to circulating blood cells; or they may settle out on membranes of blood vessels, renal glomeruli, pulmonary air spaces, or other locations.

ANTIBODIES AGAINST BLOOD-CELL ANTIGENS

Antibodies that react with blood-cell antigens often activate the complement cascade through cleavage of C3, but inhibition then outstrips activation and the process stops. Only for activation of C1 is the physical presence of immunoglobulin molecule essential; even after antibody dissociates from the complex, subsequent complement interactions can continue on the cell membrane. The presence of C3 or its conversion products can be demonstrated with an antiglobulin specific for these cleavage products. Whether or not antibody has dissociated, the presence of residual C3 fragments signals that antibody had previously combined with antigen. The action of antibodies active against red cells, granulocytes, or platelets can be demonstrated in this way. The technique is easiest for red-cell antibodies but can be adapted for platelets and neutrophils through measurements adapted for low levels of complement fragments.

Antiglobulin Testing

When suitably specific, anticomplement serum does not react with any membrane antigen or any part of the immunoglobulin molecule; its sole target is the complement protein. Anticomplement serum agglutinates red cells that have complement attached to their membrane but has no effect on unmodified cells or on cells sensitized only with immunoglobulin. Tests for platelet antibodies cannot use agglutination as an end point because platelets tend to agglutinate spontaneously; a radioactive label or an immunofluorescent system is often used to demonstrate complement bound to platelets by previous antibody activity.

Anticomplement globulin is used to demonstrate either *in vivo* or *in vitro* events. A direct antiglobulin test (see pages 333–334) positive with anticomplement demonstrates that a complement-activating autoimmune reaction has occurred within the patient's circulation. Autoantibodies with a low thermal optimum characteristically activate complement but do not persist in their attachment to the cell surface; examining the cell membrane for bound antibody is unrewarding after these reactions. Even transient antibody attachment, however, causes irreversible attachment of complement. Finding complement on circulating cells thus indicates that antibody activity has been directed against antigens of the individual's own cells.

Tests for Antibody in Serum

Anticomplement antiglobulin also can be used in an indirect antiglobulin procedure to demonstrate *in vitro* antibody activity. Most blood group antibodies that react with cellular antigens either cause agglutination or remain as sensitizing adherent molecules; a few, however, interact so briefly or in such small numbers that they cannot be detected with anti-immunoglobulin reagent. If the brief antigen-antibody encounter has caused complement attachment, it is possible to demonstrate that serum contains antibody by demonstrating complement components on the cell membrane after serum has been incubated with cells (Fig. 17–2).

DETECTING IMMUNE COMPLEXES

Immune complexes are etiologically significant in such type 3 hypersensitivity diseases (see page 255) as the rheumatic or collagen-vascular diseases, many hematologic disorders, and some forms of glomerulonephritis. Tissue changes result from the inflammation-promoting effects of complement incorporated in deposited immune complexes. Tests for immune complexes characteristically use an indicator system that exploits the presence of complement, using anti-

USE OF ANTICOMPLEMENT ANTIGLOBULIN

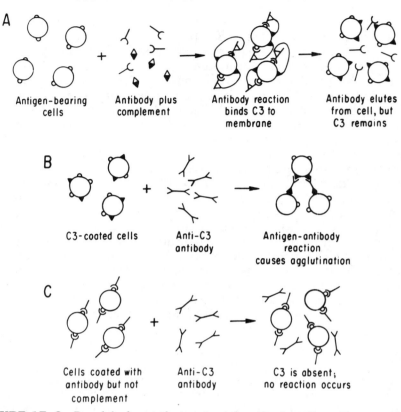

FIGURE 17–2. Panel A shows that union of antibody with antigen can bind C3 to the cell membrane, even if the immunoglobulin dissociates after interacting with C1qrs. Panels B and C show how antiglobulin serum with specificity for C3 can demonstrate that this has occurred. The surface-bound C3 demonstrated by agglutination with anti-C3 is evidence that a complement-binding reaction has occurred, whether or not the immunoglobulin remains attached to the cells.

serum specific for C3 fragments or for earlier components in the classical pathway.

Tissue versus Serum

It is easy to apply fluorescent-labeled anticomplement serum to sections of tissue; if complement has been deposited in the tissue, attachment of the labeled indicator identifies the location. The presence of complement in tissue undergoing acute inflammation is considered diagnostic for immune-mediated inflammatory disease. Demonstrating complement-containing complexes in body fluids is less definitively diagnostic. Immune complexes initiate type 3 hypersensitivity conditions, but serum or other fluids may contain complexes when there are no manifestations of disease, and active type 3 disease can exist when the fluids available for testing contain no demonstrable complexes. Many ingenious techniques can demonstrate soluble immune complexes, but they are not universally accepted as useful diagnostic procedures.

Tests for immune complexes exploit two properties of complement: interaction of free C1q with the Fc of bound immunoglobulin molecules, and the interaction of C3 fragments with complement receptors on the membrane of indicator cells. The first application uses the same principle as the complement fixation procedure described earlier in this chapter. Test serum is incubated with reagent serum known to contain hemolyzing quantities of complement. If the test serum contains antigen-antibody complexes, they incorporate available C1q, which is then unavailable for participation in the standardized cascade provoked by sensitized reagent cells. A positive result is reduction in previously established hemolytic activity, through consumption of C1q by immune complexes in the test material.

Exploiting C3 Receptors

Many cells—including red blood cells, B lymphocytes, macrophages, and many tumor cells—have membrane receptors for C3b or its degradation products (see pages 142–143). Tests use suspensions of these cells to adsorb immune complexes that may be present in the test material; any of several different indicator systems can then demonstrate this adsorption. One procedure uses peripheral-blood B lymphocytes, with inhibition of membrane-receptor events as the indicator. Another uses a line of tumor cells called **Raji cells** to adsorb complexes; radiolabeled antiglobulin serum is used to measure the immunoglobulin present in the captured complexes.

─────── **MEASUREMENT OF COMPLEMENT** ───────

Serum complement activity can be low because of rare congenital deficiencies of individual component proteins or because of acquired pathophysiologic events. Congenital deficiencies are usually encountered during investigation of aberrant immune function or defective antibacterial defenses. Acquired conditions are usually evaluated during investigation of immune-mediated diseases. Events that may depress functioning complement include consumption of components during immune-complex formation, increased levels of protein destruction with or without decreased protein manufacture, and development of inhibitors. Overall complement function is screened by measuring either the hemolytic properties of native serum or other complex physiologic events, such as opsonization or chemotaxis. Assay of individual proteins can be undertaken if screening indicates significant abnormality.

THE CH_{50} ASSAY

Hemolysis is the end point of the entire complement cascade. Demonstrating reduced hemolytic capacity cannot indicate the nature of the defect, but demonstrating that normal hemolytic activity exists suggests functional integrity of the entire system. Wide latitude exists, however; minor deficiencies in C4, C5, C8, or C9 do not affect overall hemolytic activity, and major deficiencies (up to 50 percent) in factors C1, C2, C3, C6, or C7 may not depress overall hemolysis. The curve that relates complement activity to observed hemolysis is S shaped. Tests for overall hemolytic activity use 50 percent hemolysis (CH_{50}) as the indicator because changing levels of complement exert maximal visible effect at the midpoint of the curve.

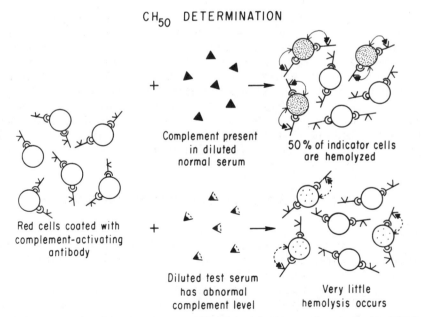

CH_{50} DETERMINATION

Red cells coated with complement-activating antibody

+

Complement present in diluted normal serum

50% of indicator cells are hemolyzed

+

Diluted test serum has abnormal complement level

Very little hemolysis occurs

FIGURE 17–3. Sensitized red cells used as indicator in the CH_{50} test will hemolyze if complement is added. The upper drawings show that complement present in diluted normal serum induces hemolysis at the 50 percent level. The lower drawings show that a similar dilution of abnormal serum contains reduced amounts of complement and induces very little hemolysis.

Technical Considerations

The CH_{50} assay uses red cells presensitized with an antibody that strongly initiates hemolysis when complement is present (Fig. 17–3). Different dilutions of test serum are added to the sensitized cells, and the amount of hemoglobin that the test serum releases is compared with hemolysis induced by pooled normal serum at the same dilutions. Collection and storage of test serum and control pools must be stringently standardized because *in vitro* events can rapidly damage the balanced system. Other artifacts that may affect reproducibility include the condition of the sensitized red cells; the activity of the indicator antibody; and the time, temperature, and ionic conditions of the reaction.

When CH_{50} is reduced, the assay can be modified to pinpoint the factor at fault, provided preparations of individual components are available. This cumbersome approach is seldom employed, however, and individual components are better evaluated by specific assays.

INDIVIDUAL COMPLEMENT COMPONENTS

When there is congenital or, more often, acquired deficiency of overall function, it may be useful to measure levels of specific proteins. Components normally present in large quantities are most easily measured. C3 is most often measured; it is not only the most abundant component but it is also associated with both activation pathways and plays a pivotal role in most complement-mediated activities. Other components that can easily be quantified are C2, C1q, and factor B of the alternative pathway. Nephelometry (see page 323) is often used for these milligram-level measurements. Radial immunodiffusion (see pages 320–321) is useful for these proteins as well as for others present at or above 25 μg/ml. A low-concentration product that can provide useful information about systemic events is C5a, the anaphylatoxin cleaved from C5 by either classical- or alternative-pathway generation of C3b. Bioassay is used to demonstrate elevated levels of this product, thought to be the cause of abnormal vascular conditions and neutrophil activity in many shocklike states.

Protein Polymorphisms

In addition to quantitative measurement, qualitative evaluation of complement components is achieving increasing importance. The genes that regulate manufacture of complement components exhibit allelic variation, and significant polymorphism has been noted for the proteins. Structural variants of some components may depress overall complement activity, but a more significant finding is that immune dysfunction of various sorts, especially predisposition to autoimmune diseases, often accompanies these abnormal products.

Both immunologic and functional techniques are used to identify these protein polymorphisms. Ouchterlony double diffusion (see chapter 15) is used to compare the patient's proteins with the precipitin arcs given by normal components. Immunoelectrophoresis allows similar direct comparison against patterns characteristic of normal proteins. In multistage assays, proteins are first separated by electrophoresis, and then overlaid with antibody-containing gels that allow both qualitative and quantitative characterization. An interesting variant is to overlay the separated proteins with a gel containing sensitized cells that undergo hemolysis at the migration sites of functional components.

When polymorphism is suspected or demonstrated, molecular techniques can be used for precise characterization; endonucleases (see page 68) are used to cleave the nucleoproteins, and a library of probes are used to characterize the variant forms present. The proteins that manifest the highest degree of polymorphism are associated with genes of the major histocompatibility locus, namely the class III products C2, C4, and factor B of the alternative pathway.

SUGGESTIONS FOR FURTHER READING

Cooper NR: Assays for complement activation. Clin Lab Med 1986; 6:139–65

Fligel SEG, Johnson KJ, Ward PA: The role of complement in immune complex induced tissue injury. In: Rother K, Till GO, eds: The Complement System. New York: Springer-Verlag, 1988:487–504

Laurell A-B: Complement determinations in clinical diagnosis. In: Rother K, Till GO, eds: The Complement System. New York: Springer-Verlag, 1988:272–326

Ruddy S: Complement. In: Rose NR, Friedman H, Fahey JL, eds: Manual of Clinical Laboratory Immunology, 3rd ed. Washington DC: American Society for Microbiology, 1986:175–84

Whaley SD, Palmer DF: Complement fixation test. In: Rose NR, Friedman H, Fahey JL, eds: Manual of Clinical Laboratory Immunology, 3rd ed. Washington DC: American Society for Microbiology, 1986:57–66

CHAPTER 18

Receptor-Ligand Assays

Receptor-ligand assays use interaction with a specific binding molecule to detect and to measure target material. Immune reactions, with their exquisite sensitivity and the close steric association of antigen and antibody, are ideal for this form of assay, but other binding proteins and receptor molecules are effective for selected measurements. Receptor-ligand immunoassays employ only the first stage of antigen-antibody interaction; an artificial end point substitutes for second-stage phenomena.

INTERACTION OF RECEPTOR AND LIGAND

The definitions of receptor (or binder) and ligand are somewhat circular: A **receptor** is material with one or more sites that bind a specific target molecule; a **ligand** is a molecule capable of complexing

355

with its specific binder. In this usage, the term receptor goes far beyond the concept of receptor molecules on cell membranes and encompasses many diverse chemical and biologic materials.

NECESSARY CONDITIONS

The receptor-ligand reaction must have high affinity and specificity. **Specificity** of receptor means reaction with a single ligand and absence of reaction with similar but non-identical molecules; **cross-reactivity** connotes the tendency to bind molecules other than the primary ligand. **Affinity** is the strength of the forces that maintain association between the ligand and the receptor. In cross-reactions, when receptor interacts with material other than its primary ligand, the affinity is much lower than that of the primary interaction. In general, the higher the affinity between receptor and ligand, the greater the specificity and sensitivity of the assay system.

Analytic Use of Antibodies

Antibodies have many desirable properties as receptors: They can be raised against selected targets; they exhibit high specificity and affinity; they can be prepared to a high degree of purity and stability; and they can be manipulated, labeled, and otherwise modified without loss of reactivity. Some analytic techniques use, instead of antibodies, binding proteins naturally present in serum, notably those for corticosteroids, thyroglobulin, estrogens, vitamin D, and intrinsic factor. Only a few binding proteins occur naturally, however, and their affinity is often too low for optimum sensitivity at low concentrations. Analysis by receptor-ligand interaction was independently developed in the late 1950s and early 1960s by Yalow and Berson, who used anti-insulin antibodies for an immunoassay; and Ekins, who used naturally occurring thyroid-binding globulin to measure thyroid hormone.

Combination of antigen with antibody in the first stage of an immune reaction characteristically generates no immediately detectable effect. For adaptation as an assay, reacting elements must be labeled to make the end point visible. Either binder or ligand can be labeled, but specificity and reactivity must be preserved intact. For quantitative results, the magnitude of binder-ligand reaction must correlate with concentrations of the analyte. Correlation is accomplished by constructing an activity curve from results with control preparations of known concentration. Test results should accurately reflect concentration over a wide range, and the reagent material used to construct the curve must have the same behavioral characteristics as the material naturally present in biologic specimens.

Reactivity without Biologic Function

One problem with immunoassay is that immunologic behavior is not always the same as biologic behavior. A molecule may express the epitope recognized by reagent antibody but lack the configuration necessary for biologic activity. Examples of this dissociation abound: Immunoassays for fibrinogen can measure dysfunctional fibrinogen molecules or degradation fragments that lack coagulation activity; partially cleaved complement components may combine with reagent antibodies but lack elements necessary to perpetuate the cascade; tissue fluids may contain antigenic material from previously infective microorganisms despite current absence of viable organisms.

DIRECT ASSAYS

Direct union of binder and ligand is the simplest test system. If labeled binder reacts with ligand in a known volume of material, the quantity of ligand can be calculated directly from the quantity of labeled material that is bound. The principle is simple, but it can be very difficult to control volume, concentration, and the conditions of the reaction; limits must be imposed so that units of measurement can be derived. Frequently, one reactant is immobilized on a solid phase, such as inert particles or the walls of a tube, well, or column. Most often the binder is immobilized and the material containing ligand is added as the unknown. It may be difficult to demonstrate union of ligand with the immobilized binder, so a second binding agent can be added in a "sandwich" technique. After ligand completes its interaction with immobilized receptor, the system is washed to remove everything except those ligand molecules that have bound to the receptor. The "sandwich" indicator must react only with the ligand, not with the receptor or any of the solid-phase elements; and its reaction with bound ligand must not disturb the original receptor-ligand bond. When these conditions are met, the amount of labeled indicator that attaches will be directly proportional to the quantity of previously bound ligand (Fig. 18–1).

If the ligand is fixed in quantity and location, receptor can be labeled and added directly. This is done to demonstrate antigens on cell surfaces or in sections of tissue (Fig. 18–2). The label can be a fluorochrome, an enzyme, a radionuclide, or some material visible on electron microscopy. Either the specific antibody can be labeled, for direct demonstration, or a labeled antiglobulin serum can be used in an indirect technique to identify where unlabeled reagent antibody has attached. This is discussed more fully on pages 372–373.

COMPETITIVE BINDING

Competitive binding assay is an indirect technique that uses, as a baseline, a measured interaction between reagent binder and reagent ligand. The end point is the change imposed upon this interaction by addition of the unknown. The degree to which the unknown alters the indicator reaction is proportional to the quantity of un-

SANDWICH TECHNIQUE
DEMONSTRATES BINDING

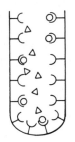 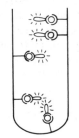

Fixed receptor binds
specific ligand

Labeled indicator
forms "sandwich" with
bound ligand

FIGURE   18–1. When mixed antigens are incubated with a single receptor, only the corresponding ligand binds to the solid-phase material, as shown on the left. Presence of the ligand can be demonstrated by "sandwiching" with a labeled indicator material that recognizes a separately accessible binding site, as shown on the right.

known. Competitive binding depends upon random interaction of individual receptor and ligand molecules according to the laws of mass action. In a system containing ligand molecules that are identical in every respect except that some are labeled and some are not, the number of labeled and unlabeled molecules that bind to the receptor depends entirely on the number of labeled and unlabeled molecules in the starting material (Fig. 18–3). It is essential that the label not bias the interaction either positively or negatively. If 75 percent of ligand molecules are unlabeled and 25 percent are labeled, the receptor will

LABELED RECEPTOR BINDS TO FIXED LIGAND

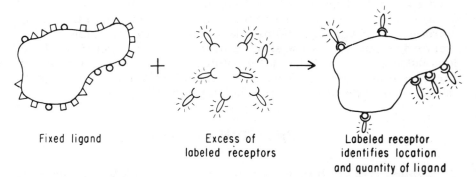

Fixed ligand

Excess of
labeled receptors

Labeled receptor
identifies location
and quantity of ligand

FIGURE 18–2. If the ligand is present in a fixed tissue preparation, direct application of a labeled receptor demonstrates the location and the quantity of the target ligand.

COMPETITIVE BINDING

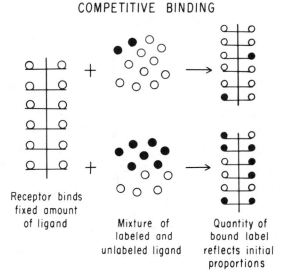

FIGURE 18–3. Competitive binding procedures require that the limited amount of receptor, shown at left, bind labeled and unlabeled materials equally. Provided there is no preferential binding, the number of labeled and unlabeled molecules that fix to the receptor will be exactly proportional to the number present in the starting material, as shown at center and at right.

Receptor binds fixed amount of ligand

Mixture of labeled and unlabeled ligand

Quantity of bound label reflects initial proportions

bind 75 percent unlabeled molecules and 25 percent labeled. If the starting proportion changes to 50 percent labeled and 50 percent unlabeled, the bound material will be 50 percent labeled and 50 percent unlabeled, regardless of absolute concentration.

Measuring the Analyte

A limited quantity of receptor can bind only a limited quantity of ligand. Competitive binding procedures are standardized by determining how much label is bound after the receptor interacts with ligand that is 100 percent labeled. Ligand molecules in the unknown specimen will necessarily be unlabeled. In the test, the unknown specimen is added to a system containing a limited quantity of binder and an excess of labeled reagent ligand. The receptor binds labeled and unlabeled ligand molecules in proportion to their concentration in the starting mixture (Fig. 18–4). Unlabeled ligand molecules in the specimen reduce the number of labeled molecules that attach to the receptor. If the unknown contains no ligand at all, the receptor will bind as much label as it did under control conditions. If the unknown contains small numbers of ligand molecules, the quantity of label binding to the receptor will be modestly reduced; if the unknown contains large amounts of the ligand, unlabeled molecules will occupy so many of the available binding sites that fixation of labeled material is markedly reduced. Competitive binding tests employ a wide range of labels, of materials that receive label, of receptors, fixation procedures, and ways of measuring the end point.

INTERPRETING
COMPETITIVE BINDING

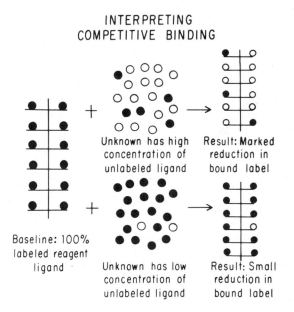

Baseline: 100%
labeled reagent
ligand

Unknown has high
concentration of
unlabeled ligand

Result: Marked
reduction in
bound label

Unknown has low
concentration of
unlabeled ligand

Result: Small
reduction in
bound label

FIGURE 18–4. The baseline is quantity of label bound when the receptor is saturated with labeled reagent ligand, as shown at left. Labeled reagent is mixed with the unknown, in which ligand is unlabeled. In the upper drawings, the unknown contains a large amount of unlabeled ligand, which severely dilutes the labeled material. The lower drawings show that a low concentration of unlabeled ligand dilutes the reagent material very little and causes little reduction in the amount of bound label available for measurement.

PROPERTIES OF THE LABEL

A wide choice of labels can be used for either receptor or ligand. Three major categories are in use, each with advantages and disadvantages. Essential features are that the label remain attached throughout the entire test, that it not alter reactivity of the native material, and that it retain its activity throughout the shelf life of the reagents.

Radioisotopes as Label

Radioactivity was the label used in the first immunoassays; end point is determined by counting emissions. The nature and number of emissions vary with the isotope employed, but measurement affords a high degree of precision and sensitivity. Variables significant in selecting radioactive labels include the half-life of the radioactive element; the specific activity, which is the number of emissions per unit mass of the material; and the nature of the emission, either gamma or beta. It is usually easier to measure gamma emissions. Perhaps the most frequently employed isotope is ^{125}Iodine (^{125}I), a gamma emitter with a half-life of 60 days and a relatively high specific activity. ^{125}Iodine can be linked to a variety of proteins in a stable association that damages the protein relatively little. Another gamma emitter with narrower applicability is ^{57}Cobalt (^{57}Co), which has a half-life of 270 days. The beta emitters ^{3}Hydrogen (^{3}H) and ^{14}Carbon (^{14}C) have much lower specific activity than ^{125}I, and half-lives of 12.3 years and

5730 years, respectively. All radiocounters are expensive and require detailed maintenance and controls.

Disadvantages of radioactivity as a label are that reagents lose potency as radioactivity decays; radioactivity may alter the test materials; and disposal of spent or unused materials creates problems in waste management. Fixed material must be separated from unbound material before tests are counted, because the counter cannot distinguish whether emissions come from complexed or residual label. Equipment to quantify radioactivity is expensive, and the procedures require that personnel be knowledgeable in the principles of physics and capable of stringent adherence to safety requirements.

Fluorochromes as Label

Fluorescent labels are stable, inexpensive, and pose no health threat. Detection instruments are not unduly expensive, but fluorescence immunoassays have relatively low sensitivity, and optically active material in serum or body fluids may affect determinations. Fluorescence assays have an advantage that separation of bound from unbound ligand is often unnecessary, because binding state often alters fluorescence properties. The dose-response curve for such systems is not linear, however, and they are useful over only a restricted range of concentration.

Enzymes as Label

In **enzyme** labeling, enzymically active protein is conjugated to the reactive material; after the immune reaction occurs, the quantity of enzyme-labeled material is determined by adding substrate and measuring the intensity of enzyme effect. The enzyme must have specific activity that persists after conjugation and must not act upon the material to which it is conjugated. The enzyme-substrate reaction must be one that is easy to observe and to quantify. Enzymes are stable, inexpensive labels that can be attached to many antigens and antibodies, and they provide an end point suitable for measurement by readily available photometric equipment. One potential problem is difficulty of conjugating one protein to another without altering either. Enzymes are large molecules; in some cases, their mass imposes a physical obstacle between antigen and antibody. Enzymes are highly sensitive to conditions of temperature, pH, substrate concentration, and the presence of other materials—variables that may affect accuracy and reproducibility of the quantitative assay.

SEPARATION SYSTEMS

The point of most immunoassays is to discriminate between bound and unbound reactants. Often these must be physically separated before the end point is measured, but in some cases, immune

HETEROGENEOUS ASSAY

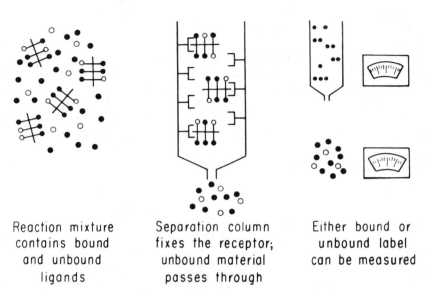

Reaction mixture contains bound and unbound ligands	Separation column fixes the receptor; unbound material passes through	Either bound or unbound label can be measured

FIGURE 18–5. After receptor fixes both labeled and unlabeled ligands, as shown on the left, it is often necessary to separate ligand that remains unbound from the molecules attached to the receptor. A separation column, shown in the center, is one way to effect physical separation. Labeled material will be present in both the bound and the unbound fractions, as shown at the right. The magnitude of the receptor-ligand interaction can be determined by measuring either fraction.

complex formation sufficiently alters the characteristics of the label that bound and unbound constituents can be discriminated without separation. Procedures that determine the end point without separating the reactants are called **homogeneous** assays; those requiring separation are described as **heterogeneous**. An example is shown in Figure 18–5.

Physical Manipulation

Bound and unreacted materials may have different physical properties that facilitate separation. Bound material characteristically forms larger complexes and can often be isolated by centrifugation. Some assays measure unbound label remaining in the supernatant, whereas others measure the quantity of label incorporated in the bound material sedimented by centrifugation. More elaborate separation techniques exploit differences in molecular size, as in gel filtration, or differences in charge and configuration, as in electrophoresis.

Either the complexed or the unreacted materials may preferentially adhere to solid-phase material like charcoal, resins, or silicates, which facilitate removal by centrifugation or filtration. Physical differences can sometimes be induced if they do not occur spontaneously, as, for example, by precipitating proteins with non-specific agents like ammonium sulfate or various alcohols.

Immune Manipulation

A common technique is to introduce a second antibody, which engages either a bound or unbound phase of the reaction mixture. Sometimes soluble antibody is introduced to induce precipitation or agglutination, but more often the separating antibody is in a solid phase, coupled to particles or to the walls of a column, tube, well, or disk. Staphylococcal protein A, which has receptors specific for the Fc portion of IgG, can be used as a separatory binder if IgG is one of the reactants (Fig. 18–6).

STAPHYLOCOCCAL PROTEIN A AS BINDER

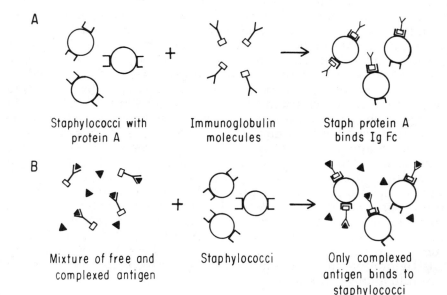

FIGURE 18–6. Protein A of the staphylococcal cell wall binds the Fc of IgG in a non-immune fashion, shown in panel A. This can be exploited as a separation technique. As shown in panel B, immunoglobulin adheres to the organisms, bringing with it antigen bound to the Fab sites. Removing the particulate organisms removes the antigen-antibody complexes and leaves behind antigen that has not combined with antibody.

───────── **SOME SELECTED PROCEDURES** ─────────

Immunologists and immunochemists have displayed remarkable ingenuity in adapting receptor-ligand interactions to analytic purposes. This section considers a few widely employed techniques, but the list is far from exhaustive.

RADIOIMMUNOASSAY

Radioimmunoassay, abbreviated RIA, is a general term comprising several different applications. Radioimmunoassay is used for competitive-binding techniques and for direct demonstration of antigen-antibody attachment.

Labeled Ligand

The most common RIA is a **competitive-binding procedure** in which the unknown is measured as ligand. The test system consists of a limited amount of antibody and a radiolabeled reagent ligand (Fig. 18–7). The baseline is the radioactivity bound when the limited number of antibody sites combine fully with labeled ligand. Because antibody binds labeled and unlabeled molecules in whatever proportions exist in the reaction mixture, adding unlabeled unknown to the reaction mixture reduces fixation of radioactivity. After the reaction reaches equilibrium, bound and unbound material are separated.

Measurement can determine either the level of radioactivity complexed to antibody or the activity that remains unbound. If bound material is measured, radioactivity count will vary inversely with the amount of ligand in the unknown; small amounts of unlabeled ligand allow large amounts of activity to remain as captured reagent label, whereas high levels in the unknown compete successfully for most of the binding sites. If the end point is radioactivity left unbound, the number of counts is directly proportional to the quantity of the unknown; increasing levels of unlabeled material occupy increasing numbers of binding sites, causing progressively more activity to remain unbound and to be counted. It must be possible to relate absolute concentrations of the material to counted activity results; ideally, this calibration curve should be linear or susceptible to transformation into a linear function.

Labeled Antibody

If label is attached to antibody rather than to ligand, the term **immunoradiomimetric assay** (IRMA) is sometimes used. The competitive-binding principle is the same, but the baseline is the amount of

COMPETITIVE RADIOIMMUNOASSAY

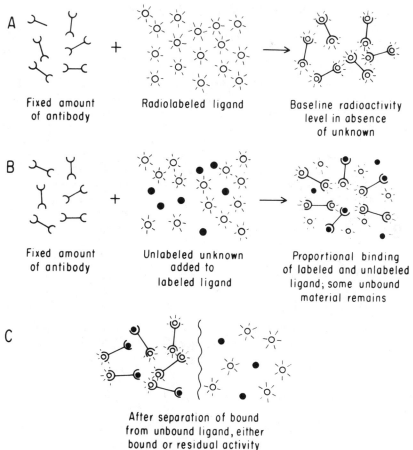

FIGURE 18-7. The first step in competitive radioimmunoassay is determining baseline radioactivity when receptor antibody is saturated with labeled ligand, shown in panel A. Panel B shows how incubation with a mixture of labeled and unlabeled ligand alters the level of bound radioactivity. As depicted in panel C, the result can be expressed as the change in level of bound label or as the quantity of label left unbound.

labeled antibody that fixes to a limited amount of solid-phase antigen. The test begins by incubating soluble labeled antibody with soluble unknown ligand. If there is antigen in the unknown, it will bind to Fab sites of the labeled antibody. The incubated mixture is then added to the immobilized reagent antigen; only those labeled antibody molecules that have not already bound antigen present in the un-

IMMUNORADIOMIMETRIC ASSAY
(IRMA)

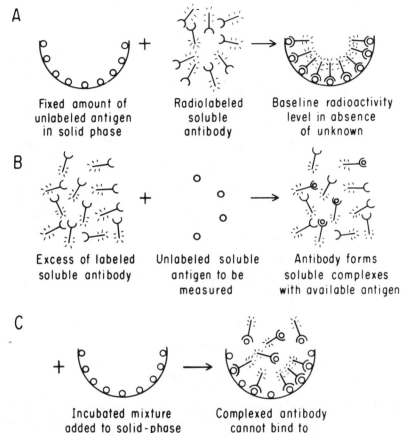

A

Fixed amount of
unlabeled antigen
in solid phase

Radiolabeled
soluble
antibody

Baseline radioactivity
level in absence
of unknown

B

Excess of labeled
soluble antibody

Unlabeled soluble
antigen to be
measured

Antibody forms
soluble complexes
with available antigen

C

Incubated mixture
added to solid-phase
unlabeled antigen

Complexed antibody
cannot bind to
solid-phase antigen

FIGURE 18—8. In immunoradiomimetric assay, the receptor is labeled and both the reagent ligand and the ligand present in the unknown are unlabeled. Panel A shows the baseline level of radioactivity when labeled antibody combines with a limited quantity of fixed, unlabeled ligand. In panel B, the antibody reacts with unlabeled material in the unknown solution. All the antigen present will unite with Fab sites of the labeled antibody. Panel C shows that antibody molecules complexed with ligand from the unknown are unable to react with the solid-phase material. The reduction of bound radioactivity reflects the amount of soluble ligand in the unknown.

known can combine with the fixed antigen. Labeled antibody is allowed to bind with the solid-phase antigen and unbound material is washed away. The radioactivity bound to the solid-phase antigen is inversely proportional to the amount of ligand that was present in the unknown (Fig. 18–8).

The **sandwich** form of RIA characteristically starts with unlabeled antibody immobilized to a solid phase. The unknown specimen is added, and any ligand present binds to the solid-phase antibody. After attachment of ligand molecules and removal of unbound material, a radiolabeled second antibody is added. The ligand must have at least two epitopes, one that binds to the solid-phase antibody and the other available to react with the labeled indicator antibody. Indicator antibody adheres wherever a ligand molecule has attached to the original antibody; the amount of radioactivity bound is directly proportional to the level of analyte. Two separation steps are necessary: one after incubation of ligand with solid-phase antibody and the other to remove indicator antibody that has not attached to the immobilized ligand.

Sandwich RIA can be used to measure unknown antibody by reversing the positions of the reagents. Unknown serum is incubated with unlabeled antigen prepared as the solid phase. Antibody molecules present in the serum unite with fixed antigen. Immunoglobulin that binds to the solid-phase antigen can be detected with radiolabeled antiglobulin serum. If the test is performed twice—once with labeled anti-IgM and once with anti-IgG—the levels of each antibody class can be compared.

ENZYME-LABELED PROCEDURES

The two principal applications of enzyme labeling are **enzyme-linked immunosorbent assay** (ELISA) and **enzyme-multiplied immunoassay test** (EMIT). In the ELISA, enzyme performs exactly the same labeling function as the radioactivity in RIA. Enzyme is coupled to one of the immune reactants; addition of substrate after the primary reaction indicates how much labeled material has entered the complex (Fig. 18–9). Enzyme-linked immunosorbent assay procedures are heterogeneous; unbound labeled material must be removed before measuring the end point. The procedure called EMIT is homogeneous. The enzyme used is one that changes reactivity depending upon the bound or unbound state of the underlying molecule. Alteration in enzyme function thus reflects the degree of immune binding, and the materials need not be physically separated.

ELISA Techniques

Like RIA, ELISA can be used for competitive-binding or direct reactions. In competitive-binding assays, the reactant in limited quan-

PRINCIPLE OF ENZYME-LABELED IMMUNOSORBENT ASSAY
(ELISA)

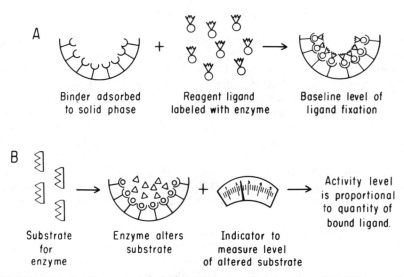

FIGURE 18–9. Enzyme-labeled immunosorbent assay (ELISA) employs a solid-phase receptor and uses enzyme to label the reagent ligand. The baseline condition, shown in panel A, is saturation of all binding sites with labeled ligand. The quantity of ligand is measured by introducing substrate on which the enzyme acts and measuring the end product, as shown in panel B.

tity is usually antibody. Enzyme-labeled reagent ligand and unlabeled ligand in the unknown are incubated with a limited quantity of antibody; after immune reaction occurs, unbound material is removed. Enzyme is thus immobilized on the solid phase at sites where reagent ligand has combined with antibody; substrate is then added to determine how much enzyme-labeled ligand is present (Fig. 18–10). The end point of the enzyme-substrate reaction must be readily quantifiable, usually a color change but sometimes a change in state of fluorescence.

Sometimes the solid-phase material is antigen, the unknown to be measured is antigen, and antibody carries the enzyme label. The baseline is the binding of labeled antibody to the limited quantity of immobilized antigen. The labeled antibody is incubated with a solution of the unknown material, providing an opportunity for antigen molecules to complex with Fab sites of the labeled antibody. After incubation, only unoccupied Fab sites are left to bind with the reagent antigen; the amount of enzyme bound to solid-phase antigen is inversely proportional to antigen concentration in the unknown.

COMPETITIVE BINDING ELISA

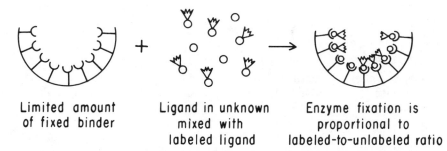

| Limited amount of fixed binder | Ligand in unknown mixed with labeled ligand | Enzyme fixation is proportional to labeled-to-unlabeled ratio |

FIGURE 18–10. In competitive binding ELISA, the end point is the degree to which admixture with unlabeled ligand reduces the previously established level of enzyme activity. Only two steps are necessary: incubating the fixed receptor with a mixture of reagent and unknown ligand, and adding the substrate to determine the level of enzyme present.

Enzyme-Labeled Antiglobulin Serum

A sandwich ELISA is widely used to demonstrate the presence of antibodies. Unlabeled antigen constitutes the solid phase. Antibody molecules in the unknown serum unite with the immobilized antigen; these complexed antibody molecules can then be measured by addition of enzyme-labeled antiglobulin serum. Enzyme activity in the indicator antiglobulin serum is directly proportional to the number of antibody molecules combined with solid-phase antigen (Fig. 18–11).

EMIT Techniques

The term enzyme-multiplied immunoassay (EMIT) is misleading; the antigen-antibody reaction is not multiplied. The enzyme-multiplied immunoassay test is a competitive-binding assay in which the enzyme label is applied to reagent antigen. Its widest use is in measuring drug levels. Enzyme is coupled to the reagent drug in a configuration that allows the enzyme to remain active when drug molecules are free in solution but causes it to lose activity if the underlying drug molecule complexes with its antibody. The material present in limited quantity is unlabeled antibody specific for the drug. Competition for antibody sites occurs between the labeled reagent drug and unlabeled drug molecules in the unknown. As with all competitive assays, binding of labeled reagent diminishes as the concentration of ligand in the unknown increases.

In EMIT, binding of labeled drug can be measured without a separation step because enzyme on the bound molecules loses its ability

SANDWICH ELISA

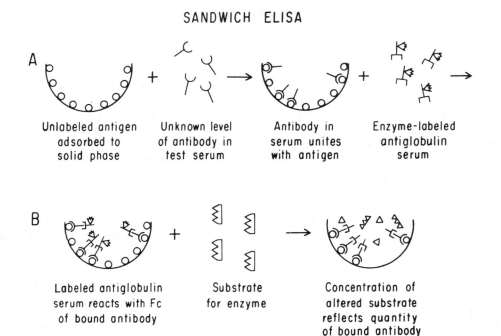

A

| Unlabeled antigen adsorbed to solid phase | Unknown level of antibody in test serum | Antibody in serum unites with antigen | Enzyme-labeled antiglobulin serum |

B

| Labeled antiglobulin serum reacts with Fc of bound antibody | Substrate for enzyme | Concentration of altered substrate reflects quantity of bound antibody |

FIGURE 18–11. A sandwich ELISA measures antibody in an unknown specimen, using unlabeled reagent antigen fixed to a solid phase. As shown in panel A, when antibody in the unknown binds to the limited quantity of antigen, the Fc portions remain accessible for combination with enzyme-labeled antiglobulin. Panel B shows that the quantity of antiglobulin reacting with complexed antibody molecule can be measured through its effect on added substrate.

to convert substrate (Fig. 18–12). Enzyme activity declines with increasing fixation of labeled reagent; increasing levels of drug in the unknown diminish fixation of labeled reagent, so the measurable level of enzyme activity is directly proportional to the drug level in the unknown. If the unknown has low concentration, most of the labeled reagent unites with antibody, loses its reactivity, and exhibits low substrate conversion. A high level of unknown prevents reagent drug from entering a complex, so the numerous unbound molecules retain ability to convert large amounts of substrate.

FLUORESCENCE-LABELED PROCEDURES

Fluorescence is emission of light at one wavelength after electrons of the susceptible substance have been excited by exposure to light at

BINDING STATE AFFECTS LABEL ACTIVITY

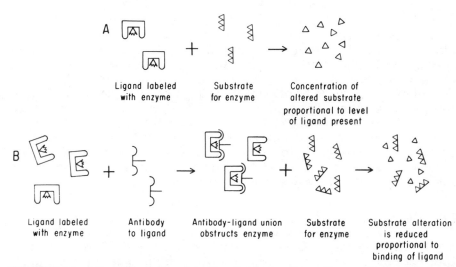

FIGURE 18–12. With molecules of suitable configuration, activity of the enzyme changes if the underlying molecule enters an immune complex. Panel A depicts an enzyme-labeled molecule that retains full activity. Panel B shows how antibody to the ligand molecule can hinder activity of the attached enzyme. In the example above, two thirds of the labeled ligand molecules have united with antibody, and a corresponding proportion of substrate remains unaffected.

a different wavelength. In fluorescent compounds, called **fluorophores** or **fluorochromes,** the electrons oscillate to produce energy detectable as emission of longer wavelengths than the light absorbed. The exciting wavelengths are usually in the ultraviolet spectrum, and emitted light is in the visible spectrum. Fluorophores useful in the laboratory include **fluorescein isothiocyanate** (FITC), which emits a green light, and **rhodamine,** which emits red light. Equipment for detection and measurement uses filters to remove all but the desired excitation wavelength and to provide optimum detection of the emitted light.

Kinds of Tests

Fluorochrome can be conjugated to antibody so that fluorescence will be directly proportional to the number of antibody molecules present. Antibody-mediated fluorescence can be evaluated in qualitative, semiquantitative, or quantitative fashion, depending upon the fluorometric devices used. Quantitative fluorescence procedures use sandwich or competitive principles that are the same as those for radioactive or enzyme-labeled assays. Fluorescence often varies with physical conditions and with the configuration of the underlying protein; these variables can be exploited to develop homogeneous assays, in which bound and unbound materials need not be separated before measuring the end point. Fluorometric assays are less widely employed for quantification than tests using other end points, but in specialized applications they provide highly flexible and sensitive measurements.

Fluorescent-labeled antibodies are particularly useful in qualitative procedures to identify and to locate antigens in tissue or on microorganisms. For example, immune complexes deposited in tissue can be demonstrated and characterized with fluorescent-labeled antibodies to immunoglobulin or to complement. Labeled antibody attaches wherever the proteins have deposited, and the fluorescence microscope makes it easy to observe location.

Direct versus Indirect

It is customary to classify fluorescence microscopy into **direct** and **indirect** techniques. In direct procedures, the fluorescent label is attached to the specific antibody directed against target antigen. These are one-step tests: fluorescent antibody is layered on the slide preparation where it combines with its target antigen. Because the antibody recognizes no other target, no other tissue elements will be labeled and fluorescence outlines exactly where antigen is present (Fig. 18–13). This requires a separate labeled antibody specific for each target antigen. Indirect fluorescence procedures require two steps. First, unlabeled antibody is applied to the slide where it can

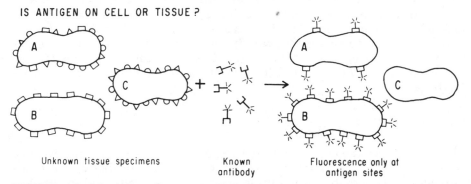

FIGURE 18–13. When fluorescent-labeled antibody is incubated with fixed cells or tissue, it attaches where its antigen is expressed in the specimen. In the drawing above, fluorescence completely outlines structure B but adheres at only a few locations to structure A. Structure C has many surface antigens, but none has the specificity recognized by the labeled antibody.

INDIRECT IMMUNOFLUORESCENCE

IS ANTIGEN PRESENT IN TISSUE?

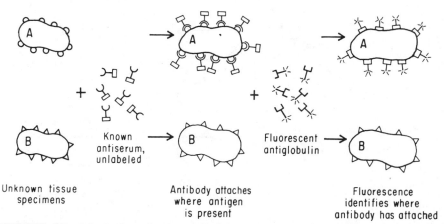

| Unknown tissue specimens | Known antiserum, unlabeled → Antibody attaches where antigen is present | Fluorescent antiglobulin → Fluorescence identifies where antibody has attached |

FIGURE 18—14. Indirect immunofluorescence employs two steps. Adding fluorescent-labeled antiglobulin serum is the second; the first is incubating unknown material with unlabeled antibody of known specificity. In the example above, the antibody combines, in a reaction that cannot be observed, with antigen present on structure A but not on structure B. The reaction is made visible when fluorescent antiglobulin serum unites with antibody bound to A but fails to react with structure B.

recognize and combine with specific antigen. The slide is then washed to remove unbound antibody and all other extraneous proteins. The second step is addition of fluorescence-labeled antiglobulin serum, which combines with the Fc portion of bound antibody molecules. Only one reagent need be labeled, the fluorescent antiglobulin, which will react with any antibody that has bound to antigens on the slide (Fig. 18—14).

Characterizing Antigens

Direct fluorescence is used in diagnosing conditions characterized by antibody attachment or deposition of immune complexes or abnormal proteins. Testing requires knowledge of which proteins are likely to be present, so as to select labeled antibodies of those specificities. Most commonly used are antibodies against immunoglobulin isotypes; against complement components; and against fibrinogen, amyloid, and other materials associated with inflammation. Direct fluorescence microscopy is also used to diagnose and to identify microorganisms. Because the fluorescent label is easy to locate, the technique is helpful in demonstrating small numbers of organisms

DIRECT IMMUNOFLUORESCENCE

WHAT IS THE ORGANISM ?

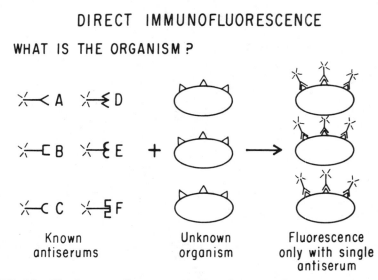

| Known antiserums | Unknown organism | Fluorescence only with single antiserum |

FIGURE 18–15. Immunofluorescent identification of unknown microorganisms employs a battery of known antiserums, each labeled with fluorochrome. Separate preparations of the unknown are incubated with each antiserum. In the example above, the organism is strain A. The other antibodies do not encounter antigens with which they can react.

present in tissue preparations or in mixed microbial populations. Direct fluorescence microscopy also identifies individual strains of organisms by their reactions with a battery of selected specific antiserums (Fig. 18–15).

Identifying Antibodies

Indirect fluorescence is used to examine serum for the presence of antibodies, especially those associated with autoimmune conditions. Specificities often studied include antibodies against tissue-specific antigens like pancreas, colon, or thyroid, or against internal cellular elements like deoxyribonucleic acid (DNA), ribonucleic acid (RNA), mitochondrial constituents, or smooth muscle antigens. Indirect fluorescence for antibody testing requires a preparation of tissue or fixed cells on which antigen is expressed. Serum is incubated with the slide to allow antibodies, if present, to combine with their antigen; unbound proteins must be washed away before antiglobulin serum is added. If the serum contained antibodies against antigens on the slide, the fluorescent antiglobulin reagent finds bound immunoglobulins with which to unite. If no antibodies were present, the antiglobulin serum finds no suitable target and no fluorescence will adhere (Fig. 18–16).

INDIRECT IMMUNOFLUORESCENCE

DOES SERUM CONTAIN ANTIBODY?

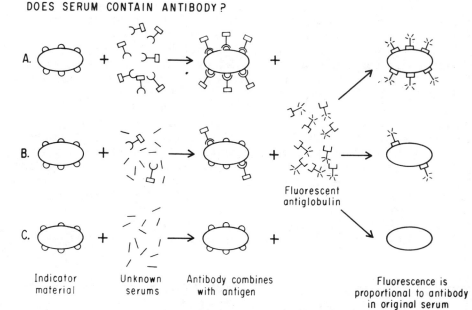

| Indicator material | Unknown serums | Antibody combines with antigen | | Fluorescence is proportional to antibody in original serum |

FIGURE 18–16. Indirect immunofluorescence can demonstrate and quantify antibody in an unknown serum. After serum is incubated with an indicator preparation of known antigen, fluorescent antiglobulin serum unites with whatever antibody has attached to the reagent material. In the example above, serum A contains a large amount of antibody, serum B contains a small amount of antibody, and serum C contains no immunoglobulin that reacts with the reagent material.

The **fluorescent treponemal antibody** (FTA) test, a serologic test for syphilis, uses indirect immunofluorescence. The reagent slide containing a fixed suspension of organisms is incubated with the patient's serum. Fluorescent antiglobulin serum adheres to any antibody molecules that have bound to the organisms. Problems with this, as with all indirect fluorescent tests, are non-specific adherence of unwanted proteins and the possible presence of antibodies that cross-react with the intended antigen or organism.

Fluorescence in Flow Cytometry

Direct and indirect immunofluorescence techniques have proven very useful in **flow cytometry**. In flow cytometers, large numbers of cells pass through an aperture, where they are exposed to light or electric current and are enumerated by the changes they induce on electrical transmission or the behavior of light waves. Flow cytometers can quantify the fluorescence emitted as individual cells flow through the aperture; with appropriate wavelengths and filters it is possible to measure two different emission spectrums at the same time, allowing simultaneous use of two different fluorescent reagents.

Direct fluorescence is extremely useful for characterizing cell-surface and cytoplasmic properties. Cell suspensions can be prepared from body fluids or from solid tissues carefully dissociated into individual cells. The most common application of fluorescent flow cytometry is enumeration of CD4 and CD8 lymphocytes, but virtually any antigen can be studied if a specific antibody exists and the target cells can be suspended in a carrier fluid. For indirect techniques intended to demonstrate abnormal serum antibodies, flow cytometry has less advantage over fluorescence microscopy. Because the specific antibody need not be labeled, however, the indirect approach can be useful if reagent antibodies are in limited supply. The antibody can be reacted with the indicator cells, in a manner analogous to direct examination, but the presence or absence of antibody attachment is confirmed by adding fluorescent antiglobulin serum.

SUGGESTIONS FOR FURTHER READING

Dauphinais RM: Solving and preventing problems in ligand assay. In: Rose NR, Friedman H, Fahey JL, eds: Manual of Clinical Laboratory Immunology, 3rd ed. Washington DC: American Society for Microbiology, 1986:88–98

Valenzuela R, Deodhar SD: Tissue immunofluorescence. In: Rose NR, Friedman H, Fahey JL, eds: Manual of Clinical Laboratory Immunology, 3rd ed. Washington DC: American Society for Microbiology, 1986:923–25

Voller A, Bidwell D: Enzyme-linked immunosorbent assay. In: Rose NR, Friedman H, Fahey JL, eds: Manual of Clinical Laboratory Immunology, 3rd ed. Washington DC: American Society for Microbiology, 1986:99–109

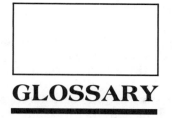

GLOSSARY

Absorption: Removal of antibody from fluid by causing it to bind antigen-bearing material and then separating the solid-phase complex from the fluid phase.

Accessory cells: Cells that enhance immune interactions but do not express antigenic specificity. Usually monocyte/macrophages or antigen-presenting cells.

Activation: 1. For lymphocytes, stimulation by antigen or mitogen, leading to immunoblast transformation and, often, to clonal expansion and synthesis of antibodies or lymphokines. 2. For complement components, cleavage or configurational change leading to altered functional state. 3. For macrophages, heightening of functional state after stimulation by cytokines.

Acute-phase reactants: Serum proteins that exhibit altered concentration in systemic inflammatory states. Fibrinogen and C-reactive protein are examples.

Adjuvant: Material that does not elicit an independent immune response but does, when given with a specific antigen, enhance immune reactivity.

Adsorption: Adherence of material to a solid surface, especially the association between antigen-bearing particles or surfaces and specific antibody.

Affinity: The strength of interaction between a single antigenic determinant and a single immunoglobulin combining site. Expressed as K, the association (or binding) constant.

Agglutination: Clumping of antigen-bearing particles by formation of a lattice in which combining sites of the corresponding antibody incorporate previously suspended particles.

Agglutination inhibition: Abolition of agglutination by soluble antigen molecules that complex with combining sites before the immunoglobulin can bind to solid-phase antigen.

Allele: Any of the two or more alternative forms of a gene that can occupy a single chromosomal locus.

377

Allelic exclusion: The phenomenon whereby active expression of an allele on one member of a chromosome pair prevents the corresponding allele on the other chromosome from generating a product.

Allergen: An antigen that provokes hypersensitivity reactions in a susceptible individual. Often, especially, those agents that provoke immediate-type hypersensitivity.

Allergy: A harmful immunologic reaction to extrinsic material; often applied to immediate-type hypersensitivity reactions.

Allogeneic: Material originating from individuals of the same species but different genetic constitution.

Allograft: Grafted or transplanted tissue from a donor of the same species but different genetic constitution from the recipient.

Allotype: The form of a protein synthesized under direction of any single allele determining that polypeptide; connotes antigenic difference among products made by different individuals of the same species.

Alternative pathway: Activation of the complement cascade by interaction of C3, factors B and D, and properdin; initiated by contact with appropriate surfaces and occurs independently of antigen-antibody reactions. Also called **properdin** pathway

Analyte: Material that is measured or analyzed.

Anaphylatoxins: In the complement cascade, cleavage fragments that promote release of cellular products that induce increased vascular permeability, enhanced inflammatory reactivity and increased smooth-muscle and epithelial-cell activity.

Anamnestic: Pertaining to immunologic memory, whereby second or subsequent contact with an antigen provokes an immune response different in nature or intensity from that elicited by the first contact.

Anaphylaxis: Systemic manifestation of immediate-type hypersensitivity, mediated by widespread release of cellular mediators following interaction between antigen and cell-bound antibody.

Anergy: Loss of previously present immune reactivity; usually disappearance of delayed-type hypersensitivity against antigens that previously induced a positive skin test.

Antibody: An immunoglobulin capable of specific combination with an identifiable antigen.

Antibody-dependent cell-mediated cytotoxicity: Damage inflicted upon antibody-coated cells by lymphocytes that do not recognize specific antigen but have Fc receptors that combine with the Fc portion of antibody already bound to the target cell.

Anticomplement activity: Capacity to inhibit activation of the complement cascade in a complement fixation test.

Antigen: A material capable of provoking an immune response when introduced into an immunocompetent host to whom it is foreign.

Antigen binding site: The portion of the immunoglobulin molecule, comprising the variable domains of heavy and light chains, that expresses a configuration complementary to that of antigen.

Antigenic determinant: The configuration of antigen material that elicits a specific immune response; the site that interacts with the idiotypic portion of the antigen receptor.

Antigen-presenting cell: Any cell capable of retaining, on its membrane, processed antigen in a form accessible to the receptors of T or B lymphocytes. Primarily cells of epithelial or of monocyte/macrophage origin.

Antigen receptor: Molecules, present on membranes of T and B lymphocytes, that express a configuration complementary to that of a specific antigen and through which the appropriately presented antigen initiates immune activation.

Antiglobulin serum: A preparation of antibody for which the specific target is globulin, either a wide range of globulins (e.g., polyspecific antihuman globulin serum) or a single molecule (e.g., anti-C3b or antitransferrin). An informally used synonym is **Coombs' serum.**

Arthus reaction: Localized complement-mediated acute inflammation induced when injected antigen unites with circulating antibody to form complexes that precipitate at the injection site.

Atopic: Pertaining to immediate-type hypersensitivity reactions induced by contact with widely distributed environmental antigens such as pollens, yeast, and animal proteins.

Atopy: A constitutional state of predisposition to immediate-type hypersensitivity reactions.

Autograft: Grafted or implanted tissue that originates from the individual in whom it is placed.

Autologous: Deriving from self.

Autoimmunity: Immune manifestations directed against self (autologous) antigens.

Avidity: The cumulative strength of interaction between all the antigen combining sites in a preparation of antibody and all the epitopic determinants of a complex antigen.

B lymphocytes: The lymphocyte population that possesses the membrane characteristics of class II MHC products and immunoglobulin molecules that serve as antigen receptor.

Bence-Jones protein: Monoclonal immunoglobulin light chains, either kappa or lambda, characteristic of several neoplasms of B-cell origin, especially multiple myeloma. Usually found in urine but sometimes also present in serum.

Beta-2-microglobulin: A small (11.6 kD) glycoprotein that constitutes one chain of the major histocompatibility complex (MHC) class I heterodimers and is synthesized under the control of a gene on chromosome 15.

Blocking antibody: Antibody present in body fluids that interferes with other manifestations of immunity; especially IgG antibodies that prevent association of antigen with cell-bound IgE, and antibodies that inhibit the cytolytic reaction of NK cells with tumor cells.

Bradykinin: A small polypeptide (nine amino acids) that evolves from a plasma precursor during activation of the kinin system and induces increased vascular permeability, contraction of smooth muscle, and perception of pain.

Bursa equivalent: The tissue or organ in mammals that performs the function served by the bursa of Fabricius in birds; probably the fetal bone marrow and, possibly, also the fetal liver.

Bursa of Fabricius: An outpouching of lymphoid tissue, in the cloaca of immature birds, that is the site at which avian B lymphocytes differentiate and mature.

CALLA: Common acute lymphoblastic leukemia antigen.

Cardiolipin: A phospholipid present in mitochondrial and bacterial enzymes, against which autoreactive antibodies develop in syphilis and in many of the dysfunctional conditions known as "collagen-vascular diseases"; it is the antigen used in non-treponemal serologic tests for syphilis.

Carrier: A macromolecule that combines with a smaller molecule, called a **hapten,** to render the hapten immunogenic.

Carrier particles: Otherwise inert particles to which either antigen or antibody can be adsorbed, to induce agglutination as an end point for union of otherwise soluble immune reactants.

Cell-mediated immunity: Immune reactivity for which the participation of viable T lymphocytes is essential, manifested either by secretion of lymphokines or exercise of direct cell-to-cell toxicity.

CH$_{50}$: Complement-mediated hemolysis of 50 percent of a preparation of indicator red cells. Used to evaluate hemolytic complement level in whole serum.

Chemotaxis: Migration of cells in response to a stimulus, often to the presence of cytokines, anaphylatoxins, or cell-derived mediator substances.

Class: 1. For immunoglobulins, the category determined by identity of the heavy chain. 2. For products of the major histocompatibility complex (MHC), the structural characteristics of the complex proteins synthesized under direction of individual alleles.

Class I: Products of the major histocompatibility complex (MHC) that constitute the HLA-A, HLA-B, and HLA-C series; all class I products are dimers containing the beta-2-microglobulin chain in addition to a large, polymorphic alpha chain.

Class II: Products of the major histocompatibility complex (MHC) that constitute the HLA-DP, HLA-DQ, and HLA-DR series; class II products are heterodimers in which both polypeptides are determined by alleles in the MHC.

Classical pathway: Activation of the complement cascade by enzymic and steric interactions initiated after reaction with antigen by an antibody that expresses a site to which Clq can bind.

Clone: A population of genetically identical cells derived from successive divisions of a single parent cell.

Cluster determinants: The term CD (see **clusters of differentiation**) is sometimes interpreted to denote **cluster determinant**.

Clusters of differentiation: Antigenic features (abbreviated **CD**) characteristic of leukocytes of various types and maturational phases, identified by groups (clusters) of monoclonal antibodies that express common or overlapping reactivity.

Codon: The set of three adjacent bases in a segment of deoxyribonucleic acid (DNA) that codes for individual amino acids and for initiation and termination signals.

Collagen: The dense white protein that constitutes the bulk of connective tissue and scar tissue.

Competitive binding: An assay principle in which two different forms of the same material, usually labeled and unlabeled, compete for binding sites on a limited quantity of receptor.

Complement: A system of serum proteins that interact in a prescribed sequence to initiate many effector functions of immune reactions and other events that involve the inflammatory and coagulation systems.

Complement fixation: An assay principle in which occurrence of an antigen-antibody reaction is revealed through binding of complement components to the immune complex.

Constant region: The carboxy-terminal portion of immunoglobulin heavy or light chains, comprising the unvarying polypeptide sequence characteristic of all chains of a given class or subclass.

Contact sensitivity: A form of cell-mediated hypersensitivity manifested by redness, itching, and other symptoms at the site where allergens have been in contact with skin.

Coombs' serum: An informal designation for antiglobulin preparations, especially those used in agglutination procedures.

Coombs' test: An informal designation for agglutination procedures that use antiglobulin serums to demonstrate prior attachment of antibody or complement to antigen-bearing cells.

Cortex: The outer portion of an organ or structure.

Counterimmunoelectrophoresis: A precipitation assay in which the diffusion of antigen and antibody through the supporting medium is given speed and direction by an applied electrical field.

CR proteins: The diverse group of plasma and membrane proteins that serve as receptors for individual components or cleavage fragments of the complement system.

Crosslink: In immunology, the simultaneous engagement of several adjacent receptors by multiple examples of a single ligand.

Crossing-over: Interchange of genetic material between the two members of a single chromosome pair.

Crossmatch: A procedure to detect previously established immune reactivity between serum or cells of a recipient and the antigens present in tissue or blood of a prospective donor.

Cross-reactivity: Reactivity of an antibody with material other than the antigen that elicited its secretion.

Cytokine: A non-antibody protein, secreted by a stimulated cell, that affects the function or activity of other cells.

Cytophilic: The property of antibodies, especially IgE but sometimes also IgG, to bind to receptors on the membrane of certain cells, especially basophilic granulocytes.

Cytotoxic T lymphocytes: CD8-positive T cells that exert lethal contact effects on target cells expressing the correct MHC I products and the appropriate antigenic specificity.

Degranulation: Release of preformed materials from cytoplasmic granules, as occurs, for example, after antigen recognition by IgE bound to a basophilic granulocyte.

Delayed-type hypersensitivity: A cell-mediated immune response that reflects the actions of lymphokines released when CD4-positive T cells encounter their specific antigen.

Dendritic cells: A diverse population of cells with branching cytoplasmic processes, lying close to aggregates of B lymphocytes and serving to present antigens.

Diffuse: To spread through a medium, from an initial site of high concentration.

Diploid: Characterized by two complete sets of chromosomes, as found in normal somatic cells.

Direct antiglobulin test: A procedure that demonstrates *in vivo* attachment of antibody or complement to circulating blood cells; performed by adding antiglobulin reagent directly to a preparation of washed cells.

Disulfide bond: A strong covalent bond formed by oxidation of two contiguous sulfhydryl (SH) groups. Can be cleaved by reduction; that is, restoring the electrons so that the S-S bond breaks down to two separate SH groups.

Domain: A segment of the immunoglobulin light or heavy chain composed of approximately 110 amino acids and held in a globular configuration by disulfide bonds.

Double diffusion: A precipitation technique in which preparations of both antigen and antibody diffuse through an inert supporting medium.

DR antigens: Major histocompatibility complex (MHC) class II antigens, identified by serologic reactions and originally noted to be related, but not identical, to HLA-D antigens, which can be identified only by cell-culture techniques. Now believed to be the most important histocompatibility antigens for most tissue allografts.

Effector: A cell, protein, or other agent that produces a specific effect.

Effector cells: The cells that mediate a specific activity, as distinct from accessory cells that enhance a variety of effects.

Electrophoresis: A procedure to separate mixed molecules by differences in migration patterns during application of an electrical field.

ELISA: Enzyme-linked immunosorbent assay.

End point: The detectable event that demonstrates occurrence of a given interaction.

Enzyme-linked immunosorbent assay: An assay procedure in which either antigen or antibody is adsorbed to a solid phase and the end point is determined by the activity level of an enzyme label bound to one of the reactants.

Enzyme-multiplied immunoassay: A homogenous immunoassay in which the bound or unbound state of the labeled reactant is measured by changes in the activity level of the enzyme used as label.

Epitope: A single, discrete configuration with antigenic activity.

Equivalence: The proportion between antigen and antibody concentration at which maximal precipitation occurs.

Fab: The fragment, generated by papain cleavage of an immunoglobulin monomer, that contains one antigen-binding site. Original term meant **f**ragment, **a**ntigen-**b**inding, but now often used as an adjective, as in the terms **Fab fragment** or **Fab segment**.

Fc: The fragment, generated by papain cleavage of an immunoglobulin monomer, that consists of the hinge region and the linked C-terminal ends of both heavy chains. Original term meant **f**ragment, **c**rystallizable, but often used as an adjective, as in the terms **Fc fragment** or **Fc region**.

Fc receptor: Any receptor molecule that binds with the Fc region of immunoglobulin molecules. Often modified by designating the heavy-chain isotype for which the receptor is specific.

Flow cytometry: Any procedure that counts cells or particles by subjecting the fluid-borne material to an analytic procedure during flow through an aperture.

Fluid-phase: Refers to particulate or soluble material suspended in a fluid medium.

Fluorescein isothiocyanate: The form of fluorescein, an orange-red material that fluoresces green in alkaline conditions, that can be coupled to antibodies and other proteins.

Fluorescence: Emission of light at a wave length slightly longer than that of the absorbed light source, hence emission of a color different from that of the original material or the light source applied.

Fluorescent treponemal antibody test: A test in which specific antitreponemal antibodies are demonstrated by indirect immunofluorescence, with fixed treponemal organisms used as target.

Fluorometric: Assay technique in which a fluorescent end point is subjected to quantitative analysis.

Follicle: A saclike mass; used to describe aggregates of lymphocytes in lymph nodes, spleen, or tissue undergoing immune-mediated inflammation.

Foreign: In immunology, pertaining to material of genetic constitution different from that of the host; of "non-self" origin.

Freund's adjuvant: A preparation widely used to enhance immunogenicity of injected antigens. Consists of a water-in-oil emulsion of mineral oil (called Freund's incomplete adjuvant) to which killed mycobacteria may be added (then called Freund's complete adjuvant).

Gamma globulin: Plasma proteins with the slowest (gamma) migration pattern on electrophoresis at pH 8.6. Because most immunoglobulins have gamma mobility, term is sometimes used to denote immunoglobulin concentration or antibody content.

Gammopathy: Any condition of abnormal immunoglobulin synthesis, including global and partial deficiencies, global and monoclonal excesses, and synthesis of abnormally constituted immunoglobulins.

Gene: The segment of DNA that directs synthesis of an individual protein.

Gene rearrangement: Modification of DNA sequence within a gene locus to select certain segments for expression and to delete material unnecessary for synthesis of the specific polypeptide.

Genome: The entire complement of genes possessed by an individual; all the information encoded in a complete set of chromosomes.

Genotype: Often used to denote the alleles present on both chromosomes at an individual locus or segment, but more general meaning is synonymous with genome.

Germ line: The deoxyribonucleic acid (DNA) sequence of genes in their unmodified state, before rearrangement for active synthesis of the relevant protein.

Gm markers: Allotypic differences in amino acid sequence in specific segments of the gamma heavy chain. Individual Gm sequences are associated with specific subclasses.

Graft-versus-host disease: The pathophysiologic consequences of cell-mediated immunity occurring when engrafted immunocompetent T cells recognize as foreign and react against antigens of an immunodeficient host.

Haploid: Characterized by a single set of chromosomes, as found in normal ova and sperm.

Haploidentical: Having in common one haplotype.

Haplotype: A sequence of closely linked alleles present in a defined segment of a single chromosome and characteristically transmitted as a genetic unit.

Hapten: A small epitope that cannot, by itself, elicit an immune response but that, when linked to a larger carrier molecule, is recognized by an antigen-specific receptor. Molecules of hapten can interact with antibody, once formed.

Heavy chain: The larger of the two paired polypeptide chains that constitute the immunoglobulin monomer. Heavy chains comprise approximately 440 amino acids, arranged in one variable domain and three or four constant domains.

Helper cells: The subpopulation of T lymphocytes that possess the CD4 antigen and cooperate with B lymphocytes or other T lymphocytes to generate immune reactivity.

Hemagglutination: Agglutination system in which the antigen-bearing particles are red blood cells.

Hemolysis: Damage to the membrane of red blood cells that results in escape of hemoglobin.

Heterodimer: A compound molecule consisting of two dissimilar units.

Heterogeneous assay: A receptor-ligand assay in which the bound material must be separated from the unbound material before the end point is measured.

Heterologous: Deriving from a species different from that of the host.

Heterozygous: Possessing different alleles at a given locus on the two members of a chromosome pair.

High endothelial venules: The postcapillary portion of venules, characterized by surface properties that allow lymphocytes to escape from the bloodstream into the tissue fluid.

Hinge region: The flexible portion of the immunoglobulin heavy chain lying between the first and second constant domains. Shape change necessary for binding with antigen occurs in this area, which is the site of the disulfide bonds that link the two heavy chains and may be the target for enzymatic cleavage.

Histamine: A small molecule present in many sites, including the granules of basophils, that causes short-lived increased vascular permeability, vasodilatation, smooth muscle contraction, and secretion by several types of epithelial cells.

Histocompatibility: The degree to which two individuals share antigens important for survival of tissue grafts.

HLA: The antigens, determined by numerous genes within the major histocompatibility complex, that most significantly affect survival of engrafted tissue. Initials are usually said to stand for "human leukocyte antigens" but occasionally are said to derive from "histocompatibility locus A."

Homogeneous assay: A receptor-ligand assay in which it is unnecessary to separate the bound and unbound materials before measuring the end point.

Homologous: In immunology, deriving from an individual of the same species as, but of different genetic composition from, the host.

Homozygous: Possessing the same alleles at a given locus on the two members of a chromosome pair.

Host: The individual exposed to immune stimulation.

Humoral: Referring to material in body fluids (the "humors" of the body); used especially to denote antibodies, the fluid-borne products of immune reactivity, in contrast to cell-mediated immune effects.

Hyperacute rejection: Rejection of a tissue graft occurring within minutes or hours of transplantation, owing to actions of preformed antibodies in the host against antigens on the donor tissue.

Hypersensitivity: A general term denoting harmful effects of immune actions. Often classified as "immediate," resulting from release of preformed substances following interaction of antigen with cell-bound antibody; and "delayed-type," resulting from effects of lymphokines released by T cells after contact with antigen.

Hypervariable regions: Short segments within the variable domains of immunoglobulin light and heavy chains, in which different immunoglobulin molecules exhibit pronounced differences in amino acid sequence. These sequences (three in light chains and four in heavy chains) determine the idiotypic specificity of the molecule.

I region: The segment of the major histocompatibility complex (MHC) at which the genes controlling immune reactivity are located.

Ia antigens: Antigens, on B cells and accessory cells of the mouse, that are determined by immune-response genes. Analogous to MHC class II products on human macrophages and B lymphocytes, and on cells manifesting immune activation; term is sometimes used for these human antigens.

Idiotope: The antigenic determinant that resides in the idiotypic configuration of an antigen-receptor molecule.

Idiotype: The structural configuration unique to that portion of an antigen receptor molecule that recognizes a specific antigen. The unique amino acid sequence can, itself, serve as an antigen. By extension, the term denotes the specificity of the antigen-recognition part of the receptor.

Immediate hypersensitivity: The form of immune-mediated pathophysiologic event that reflects actions of mediator substances released from the subjacent cells after cell-bound antibody unites with antigen.

Immune: Pertaining to the presence and actions of cells and proteins of the lymphoreticular system in its responses to antigenic stimulation.

Immune adherence: Attachment of a cell or particle coated with antibody or with C3 to cells that have receptors for the Fc portion of antibody or for C3 fragments.

Immune complex: The macromolecular complex formed when antibody unites with antigen.

Immune response genes (IR genes): Genes that determine degree of reactivity to antigens. These have been identified within the histocompatibility region (H-2) of the mouse and are thought to exist in the human major histocompatibility complex (MHC).

Immunity: The consequences of immune reactivity, in which the occurrence and nature of the response depend upon the specificity of the agent inducing the reaction.

Immunoblast: The enlarged form of a lymphocyte that is undergoing deoxyribonucleic acid (DNA) synthesis preparatory to cell division.

Immunodominant: The portion of an epitope that most significantly affects its specificity.

Immunoelectrophoresis: A semiquantitative technique in which proteins are first separated by electrophoresis and then participate in double diffusion with one or several antibodies against the individual proteins.

Immunofixation electrophoresis: A technique to identify proteins by inducing precipitin bands at the site where a specific antibody interacts with proteins that have first been separated by electrophoresis.

Immunogen: A material capable of eliciting an immune response.

Immunoglobulin: The category of glycoproteins composed of two identical light chains and two identical heavy chains, attached in a longitudinally symmetrical fashion to create two identical sites capable of combining with antigen.

Immunotherapy: Manipulation of immune actions or products to achieve therapeutic goals. Includes active and passive immunization; transplantation of immunologically active tissue; immunosuppression; immune enhancement with adjuvants or pharmacologic agents; and hyposensitization.

Inflammation: A cellular, vascular, and chemical reaction to injury in which the occurrence and nature of the response is not affected by the specificity of the agent inducing the injury.

Interferon: A group of small polypeptide cytokines produced either by non-specific cells after viral infection or other stimuli, or by antigen-stimulated T lymphocytes.

Interiorization: Incorporation into the cell cytoplasm of material that was on the external membrane surface.

Interleukins: A group of cytokines produced by macrophages or T lymphocytes that affect the activation, proliferation, and function of many different target cells but especially of lymphocytes and hematopoietic cells.

Interstitial fluid: The fluid, normally low in proteins and cells, that is outside of blood and lymphatic vessels and surrounds the cells and structural elements of all tissues.

Isoantibody: Antibody that reacts with antigens derived from individuals of the same species but of different genetic constitution as the host.

Isotype: Structural and potentially antigenic elements characteristic of all molecules of a given class or subclass.

Isotype switch: Attachment of the genetic material determining immunoglobulin idiotype from one segment that determines isotypic constant region to a segment determining a different isotype.

J chain: A 15 kD glycoprotein present in all polymeric immunoglobulins, hence present in IgM and secretory IgA but not in IgD, IgE, or IgG.

K cell: A killer cell, of lymphocyte origin, that has receptors for the Fc portion of IgG and exerts cytotoxic effects on cells to which antibody has attached. K cells, lacking receptors for specific antigens, can attack a wide variety of target cells.

Kappa chain: One of two light-chain isotypes. Synthesized under direction of a gene on chromosome 2 and present in approximately two thirds of human immunoglobulin molecules.

Kinin system: A system of precursor and activator proteins that eventuates in evolution of kinins—polypeptides that promote increased vascular permeability, contraction of smooth muscle, and activation of the coagulation and fibrinolytic systems.

Kuppfer cells: Cells of the monocyte/macrophage system located in the sinusoids of the liver and active in phagocytizing and processing material present in blood brought to the liver by the portal venous system.

Lambda chain: One of two light-chain isotypes, synthesized under control of a gene on chromosome 22; present in approximately one third of human immunoglobulin molecules.

Langerhans cells: Dendritic cells present in skin, lymph nodes, spleen, and thymus; derived from the monocyte/macrophage lineage, they express major histocompatibility complex (MHC) class II products and serve as antigen-presenting cells.

Large granular lymphocytes: Lymphocytes that lack receptors for specific antigen; they are characterized by numerous granules in abundant cytoplasm and are responsible for most killer (K) and natural killer (NK) cell activities.

Lectins: Proteins that can be extracted from plants and bind to various sugars and glycoproteins on cell membranes, inducing agglutination, mitosis, or activation of cells that express the appropriate receptor.

Ligand: A molecule that binds to a receptor molecule of complementary configuration.

Light chain: The smaller of the two paired polypeptide chains that constitute the immunoglobulin monomer. Containing approximately 220 amino acids, light chains have a variable domain that contributes to the antigen-combining site and a single constant domain.

Linkage disequilibrium: Simultaneous presence of alleles on the same chromosome at a frequency greater than that dictated by the distribution of those alleles in the population.

Locus: The position on a chromosome occupied by the gene for a specific characteristic.

Lymph fluid: The fluid present in lymphatic vessels, derived from interstitial fluid and reentering the bloodstream when the thoracic duct empties into the venous system.

Lymph nodes: Aggregates of lymphocytes and macrophages present in groups along the course of lymphatic vessels; the site of much antigen processing and presentation, antibody production, and lymphocyte proliferation.

Lymphocyte: A small mononuclear cell with dense nuclear chromatin and sparse cytoplasm, present in blood, lymphatic fluid, and tissues of the lymphoreticular system. Lymphocytes are the effector cells for immune reactivity and for certain types of chronic inflammation.

Lymphocyte-defined antigens: HLA antigens that cannot be identified with antibodies and can be detected only by appropriate reagent lymphocytes in cell-culture techniques.

Lymphocytotoxicity: An end point used in serologic examination for HLA antigens, in which complement-binding antibodies cause lethal damage to lymphocytes expressing the appropriate antigens.

Lymphoid: Pertaining to lymphocytes, lymphatic fluid, or the tissues of the lymphoreticular system.

Lymphokines: Soluble small polypeptides secreted by antigen-stimulated lymphocytes and capable of affecting functional events in other cells and tissues.

Lymphokine-activated killer cells (LAK cells): Large granular lymphocytes that have been exposed, *in vitro,* to the lymphokine interleukin 2 (IL-2) and are then reintroduced into the host, where their heightened state of activation exerts more effective natural killer (NK) cell actions.

Lymphoreticular system: A collective term for all the cells and tissues involved in the afferent and efferent aspects of immunity. Includes especially the lymph nodes, spleen, bone marrow, liver, thymus, and mucosa-associated lymphoid tissue.

M spike: The sharply defined peak on a densitometer tracing of protein electrophoresis that reflects the presence of monoclonal protein in the fluid examined.

Macrophage: A phagocytic cell derived from monocytes originating in bone marrow and exhibiting greater phagocytic, secretory, and chemotactic capacity than monocytes, which are less fully differentiated.

Major histocompatibility complex (MHC): Linked genes that determine cell-membrane antigens significant in survival of allogeneic tissue grafts. In humans, the major histocompatibility complex is on chromosome 6 and includes genes for at least six series of HLA antigens, for several proteins of the complement system, and for other activities associated with immunity.

Mast cells: Basophilic granulocytes present in tissues; characterized by receptors for the Fc portion of IgE antibodies and by cytoplasmic granules that contain histamine and other mediators of inflammation.

Mediator: A substance that exerts a characteristic effect on a target cell, usually through combination with a specific receptor.

Medulla: The inner portion of an organ or structure.

Meiosis: The process of cell division in which one diploid precursor cell generates four haploid gametes.

Membrane immunoglobulin: The immunoglobulin monomers, IgM and sometimes IgD, that are present on the exterior of the B-lymphocyte membrane and serve as antigen receptors.

Memory cells: Clonal progeny of an antigen-stimulated T or B lymphocyte, which exist in a state of potential activation and respond to antigen exposure with increased speed and intensity of immune response.

MHC restriction: The phenomenon in which T lymphocytes recognize their specific antigen only when it is presented on a cell expressing the same MHC class I or class II antigens as those of the host. CD4-positive T cells require class II antigens, and CD8-positive cells are restricted by class I antigens.

Micelle: A molecular aggregate that retains discrete existence suspended in plasma or other aqueous media.

Mitogen: Material that combines with specific non-antigen receptors on cell membranes to stimulate deoxyribonucleic acid (DNA) synthesis and cell division.

Mitosis: The process of cell division in which a diploid cell reproduces into two diploid daughter cells with the same genetic characteristics.

Mixed lymphocyte culture (or **reaction**)**:** A laboratory procedure in which lymphocytes of different genetic composition are cultured together and allowed to exert antigenic stimulation that promotes deoxyribonucleic acid (DNA) synthesis and immunoblast transformation.

Modulation: Disappearance of membrane receptors from a cell surface following interiorization of the receptor-ligand complex.

Monoclonal: Pertaining to or arising from daughter cells of a single clone, all of which have the same genetic composition and the capacity to synthesize the same products.

Monocyte: A large leukocyte with an ovoid or indented nucleus, derived from the same hematopoietic precursor as granulocytic leukocytes and capable of differentiation into macrophages characteristic of many different tissue locations.

Monokine: A soluble mediator secreted by monocytes or macrophages after stimulation by agents or events other than recognition of a specific antigen.

Monomer: A molecule consisting of a single, non-repeated structural unit.

Motility: Ability to move spontaneously. Macrophages and neutrophils exhibit motility, and lymphocytes do not.

Mucosa-associated lymphoid tissue: The stratified mass of lymphocytes present beneath the epithelial surface of respiratory, alimentary, excretory, and reproductive tracts.

Myeloid: Pertaining to the bone marrow, particularly to cells of the granulocytic series.

Myeloma (often, **multiple myeloma**)**:** A neoplasm of immunoglobulin-secreting plasma cells, usually characterized by aggregates of neoplastic cells in bones or other sites and by the presence in serum or urine of monoclonal protein produced by these cells.

Native: The unmodified or unprocessed form of a substance or activity.

Nephelometry: Measurement of the turbidity of a fluid, used to quantify precipitated immune complexes in a fluid medium.

NK cells: Natural killer cells. Large granular lymphocytes that exert cytotoxic effects on target cells without restriction by antigenic specificity.

Null cells: Lymphocytes that lack surface markers that allow assignment to T or B categories.

Oligo-: A combining form that means "few." Oligosaccharides, for example, have no more than 10 sugar residues.

Oncogene: A gene capable of producing neoplastic transformation, if suitably activated. The normal mammalian genome contains many oncogenes in unactivated form. Also present in many viruses.

Opsonins: Materials that, when present on the surface of a cell or particle, enhance phagocytosis. IgG antibodies and cleavage fragments of C3 are the major opsonins in humans.

Opsonization: Enhancement of phagocytosis by the presence, on the surface of a cell or particle, of molecules for which the phagocytic cell has receptors.

Papain: The proteolytic enzyme used to cleave the immunoglobulin monomer into two Fab and one Fc segment.

Passive agglutination: A laboratory technique in which soluble antigen is adsorbed to the surface of inert particles. Combination with antibody thus induces agglutination rather than precipitation.

Passive immunity: Immune protection achieved by transfer of effector material, usually antibody, from an immunized individual into an individual not previously exposed to the antigen.

Patching: Movement of molecules on a cell membrane, from a diffuse distribution into discrete clusters.

Pepsin: The proteolytic enzyme used to cleave the immunoglobulin monomer into a single F(ab)$'_2$ fragment plus immunologically inert fragments of heavy chain.

Peptide bond: The covalent bond that links amino acids into protein chains. Formed between the COOH group of one amino acid and the NH_2 group of the other.

Phagocytosis: Ingestion of particulate material by macrophages, neutrophils, and other leukocytes.

Phenotype: The aggregate of genetically determined characteristics expressed by an individual.

Phytohemagglutinin: A substance, derived from the kidney bean plant, that provokes lymphoblast transformation in T lymphocytes, independent of contact with specific antigen.

Pluripotential: Having the capacity to express any of several different developmental characteristics.

Poly-: Combining form meaning "many." Sometimes used to denote anything above one, but usually denotes a number greater than "several."

Polymer: In immunology, immunoglobulin molecules consisting of more than one immunoglobulin monomer joined covalently.

Polymorphism: The presence, in a population, of different forms of a characteristic determined by alleles at a single locus.

Postzone: An informal term used to describe failure of agglutination or precipitation occurring when there is pronounced antigen excess.

Precipitation: Formation of an insoluble immune complex after combination of soluble antigen with soluble antibody.

Precipitin line: The deposit of precipitated immune complex seen in the supporting medium when soluble antigen and soluble antibody meet in suitable proportions.

Presentation: In immunology, display of processed antigen on the surface of a cell capable of engaging in productive contact with effector cells that express the appropriate antigen receptor.

Primary immune response: The immune events, humoral or cell-mediated or both, that occur when an immunocompetent host encounters an antigen for the first time.

Processing: The modifications exerted upon native antigen to render it effectively immunogenic.

Progeny: Descendents or offspring. Used to describe cells that evolve from a single precursor.

Properdin: Factor P of the alternative pathway of complement activation. Present at serum concentration of approximately 25 µg/ml, it stabilizes the C3 convertase activity of C3b associated with activated factor B.

Proteolytic: Having the property to cleave proteins by dividing polypeptide bonds.

Prozone: The failure to achieve visible agglutination or precipitation that occurs when antibody is present in excess.

Radial immunodiffusion: A single diffusion technique in which antigen can be quantified by the size of the precipitin ring formed when antigen diffuses radially from a well cut into antibody-containing gel.

Radioimmunoassay: An analytic procedure in which a radioisotope is used to label antigen or antibody participating in an immune reaction.

Radioisotope: An unstable form of an element, which emits radiation in decaying to a stable state.

Reagin: A term used for two different antibodies: (1) the anticardiolipin antibody demonstrated in non-treponemal tests for syphilis;

(2) any antibody that binds to basophilic granulocytes and elicits immediate-type hypersensitivity.

Receptor: A molecular configuration that interacts with a molecule, usually smaller, that exhibits a complementary configuration. The combination of receptor with its ligand mediates subsequent biologically significant events.

Recombinatorial diversity: The variability in deoxyribonucleic acid (DNA) sequences that results from imprecise joining of segments selected from groups of alternative sequences (libraries) during the gene rearrangement that precedes synthesis of immunoglobulin chains.

Restriction endonuclease: An enzyme of bacterial origin that cleaves deoxyribonucleic acid (DNA) at specific sequences, generating fragments of reproducible properties that can be used to detect the presence of complementary sequences in unknown specimens being tested.

Reticulin: A protein found in fibrillar supporting elements in tissues of the immune system.

Reverse passive agglutination: A technique in which antibody is adsorbed to the surface of inert particles, so that combination with soluble antigen induces agglutination.

Rheumatoid factor: Antibody activity, present in the serum of patients with rheumatoid arthritis and other autoimmune conditions, that reacts with the Fc portion of IgG.

Rhodamine: A fluorescent dye that emits in the red spectrum after excitation by ultraviolet lightwaves.

Ribosomes: The spherical bodies in cytoplasm that are the site of ribonucleic acid (RNA)-directed protein synthesis.

Rocket electrophoresis: An analytic technique in which antigen moves in an electrical field through antibody-containing gel, leading to precipitation in tapered columns, the height of which is proportional to the concentration of antigen.

Secondary immune response: Immune events, either humoral or cell-mediated, that occur on second or subsequent exposure to an antigen and reflect the existence and activity of memory cells.

Secretory component: The glycoprotein chain that epithelial cells add to polymerized IgA as it traverses the cell to enter secreted fluid.

Self: In immunology, the cellular and soluble configurations characteristic of the host's genetic constitution.

Sensitization: 1. Induction of an immune response, especially one with deleterious consequences to the host. 2. Attachment of antibody to the surface of antigen-bearing particles, without formation of the lattice that constitutes agglutination.

Series: A group of protein products of essentially similar nature but differing in characteristics determined by different alleles at the locus that directs their synthesis.

Seroconversion: Development of positive results on a test for specific antibody after previous demonstration that antibody was absent.

Serodiagnosis: Diagnosis of infectious or other diseases from the results of tests for appropriate antibodies.

Serologically defined antigen: In the HLA system, an antigen that can be detected and identified through reactions with antibodies, without the need for tests of cell-mediated immunity.

Serology: The study of serum, especially tests for the presence of antibodies.

Single diffusion: A precipitation technique in which one reactant is uniformly dispersed in the suspending medium and one reactant diffuses through the immunologically active material.

Sinusoid: A vascular channel, carrying either blood or lymph fluid, that has a lumen wider and more irregular than that of capillaries and often allows prolonged or intimate contact between the moving fluid and the cells lining the channel.

Solid phase: The portion of a heterogenous system that consists of solid material, as opposed to fluid or gaseous constituents.

Specificity: In immunology, characterized by a unique, reproducible configuration that restricts steric interaction to a molecule of complementary configuration. The identifying term applied to individually characterized immune reactants.

Stem cell: An undifferentiated cell whose progeny can evolve along different lines of differentiation under suitable internal or external conditions.

Staphylococcal protein A: A cell-wall protein of *Staphylococcus aureus*, which interacts with the Fc portion of IgG through a receptor-ligand association.

Subclass: In immunology, the categories of immunoglobulin determined by isotypic variants within heavy-chain classes.

Suppressor cells: A subset of T lymphocytes that express the CD8 antigen and act to inhibit the effector actions of B cells or other T cells.

Terminal deoxynucleotidyl transferase: An enzyme that catalyzes rearrangement of deoxyribonucleic acid (DNA) in the nucleus of immature hematopoietic cells. Present in pre-pre-B cells, in stage I and stage II thymocytes, and in approximately 2 percent of cells in the normal bone marrow.

Thoracic duct: The collecting vessel that connects the central accumulation of lymphatic fluid with the bloodstream. It passes from the region of the lumbar vertebrae upward through the diaphragm to enter the venous system at the left internal jugular and/or subclavian vein.

Thymocytes: Cells of lymphoid origin present in the thymus, where they undergo progressive differentiation and maturation before exiting to become T lymphocytes.

Thymosins: A collective term for proteins intrinsic to the thymus that have the capacity to promote differentiation and maturation of lymphoid precursors into immunocompetent T lymphocytes.

Thymus-dependent antigen: Any antigen that elicits antibody only when there is concomitant stimulation of B lymphocytes by T lymphocytes and/or their secreted products.

Thymus-independent antigen: Any antigen capable of promoting antibody production in the absence of concomitant T-cell activity.

Titer: A figure that denotes the relative concentration of an antibody or other reactant; the titer is the reciprocal of the highest dilution that produces a reaction.

Titration: In serology, the process of testing serially diluted material to determine relative concentration. Each dilution is tested against a standard indicator to demonstrate the highest dilution at which reaction occurs. The reciprocal of this dilution is the titer of the test material.

Tolerance: In immunology, the state in which an otherwise immunocompetent host fails to react against a specific antigen.

Transformation: In immunology, the change that T or B lymphocytes exhibit after stimulation by specific antigen or by a suitable mitogen. The stimulated cell transforms into an immunoblast, characterized by increased nuclear size and synthesis of deoxyribonucleic acid (DNA).

Tuberculin test: An *in vivo* test for established cell-mediated immunity to proteins of the tubercle bacillus. Intradermal injection of the prepared antigen elicits a delayed hypersensitivity reaction in individuals who have had previous immunizing exposure to the organisms.

Turbidimetry: A technique for analyzing the concentration of precipitated material suspended in a fluid medium, by measuring the reduction of light transmitted through the material.

Vaccination: Now used as a general term describing introduction of microbial antigens with the intent of inducing immunity. Originally, introduction of cowpox (vaccinia) antigens to induce crossreactivity that protected against smallpox.

Van der Waals forces: Weak but universally present attractive forces exerted between molecules, arising from oscillation of electrical forces.

Variable region: The amino-terminal half of the light chain and approximately quarter of the heavy chain, in which pronounced variations in amino acid sequence confer idiotypic specificity.

Variolation: Introduction of material from a smallpox (variola) lesion, with the intent of inducing immunity to the disease and avoiding disabling or fatal native infection.

Virgin lymphocyte: Immunocompetent T or B lymphocyte that has not undergone activation or contact with its specific antigen.

Wasserman test: The first serologic test for syphilis; a complement fixation procedure that is now known to demonstrate presence of an anticardiolipin antibody strongly associated with syphilis, and not antibody to any specific antigen of *T. pallidum*.

Western blot: An immunoprecipitation procedure in which the test serum is reacted with a preparation of antigens separated by electrophoresis and then transferred ("blotted") to a supporting medium.

Xenogeneic: Originating from a source other than the species to which the host belongs.

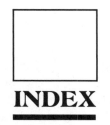

INDEX

A "*t*" following a page number indicates a table. A page number in *italics* indicates a figure.